ADVANCES IN

Pediatrics

Editor-in-Chief
Michael S. Kappy, MD, PhD

Professor of Pediatrics, University of Colorado
School of Medicine, Children's Hospital Colorado,
Aurora, Colorado

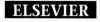

PHILADELPHIA   LONDON   TORONTO   MONTREAL   SYDNEY   TOKYO

ADVANCES IN
Pediatrics

VOLUMES 1 THROUGH 60 (OUT OF PRINT)

Vice President, Global Medical Reference: Mary Gatsch
Editor: Kerry Holland
Developmental Editor: Donald Mumford

Printed in the United States of America.

Editorial Office:
Elsevier
1600 John F. Kennedy Blvd,
Suite 1800
Philadelphia, PA 19103-2899

International Standard Serial Number: 0065-3101
International Standard Book Number: 13: 978-0-323-35542-1

ADVANCES IN
Pediatrics

Editor-in-Chief

MICHAEL S. KAPPY, MD, PhD, Professor of Pediatrics, University of Colorado School of Medicine, Children's Hospital Colorado, Aurora, Colorado

Associate Editors

LESLIE L. BARTON, MD, Professor Emerita, Department of Pediatrics, Steele Memorial Children's Research Center, University of Arizona, Tucson, Arizona

CAROL D. BERKOWITZ, MD, Executive Vice Chair, Department of Pediatrics, Harbor-UCLA Medical Center; Distinguished Professor of Pediatrics, David Geffen School of Medicine at UCLA, Torrance, California

JANE CARVER, PhD, MS, MPH, Professor, Department of Pediatrics and Molecular Medicine, University of South Florida College of Medicine, Tampa, Florida

MORITZ ZIEGLER, MD, Retired Surgeon-in-Chief, Pediatric Surgery, Children's Hospital Colorado, Retired, Professor of Surgery, University of Colorado School of Medicine, Denver, Colorado

CONTRIBUTORS

LALIT BAJAJ, MD, MPH, Associate Professor of Pediatrics and Emergency Medicine, Section of Emergency Medicine, Children's Hospital Colorado, University of Colorado School of Medicine, Aurora, Colorado

JENNIFER M. BARKER, MD, Associate Professor of Pediatrics, Section of Endocrinology, Children's Hospital Colorado, University of Colorado School of Medicine, Aurora, Colorado

CHRISTIE J. BRUNO, DO, Attending Neonatologist, The Children's Hospital at Montefiore; Assistant Professor, Department of Pediatrics, Albert Einstein College of Medicine, Bronx, New York

FERNANDO J. BULA-RUDAS, MD, Fellow, Pediatric Infectious Diseases and Immunology, University of Florida College of Medicine-Jacksonville, Jacksonville, Florida

LISA J. CHAMBERLAIN, MD, MPH, Associate Professor of Pediatrics, Stanford University School of Medicine, Stanford, California

ARLENE V. DRACK, MD, Ronald Keech Associate Professor of Pediatric Genetic Eye Disease, Department of Ophthalmology and Visual Science, Stephen A. Wynn Institute for Vision Research, University of Iowa, Iowa City, Iowa

ALINA V. DUMITRESCU, MD, Ophthalmology Resident, KU Eye Department, Kansas University Medical School, Kansas City, Kansas; Assistant Professor, Department of Ophthalmology and Visual Sciences, University of Iowa, Iowa City, Iowa

DIALA FADDOUL, MD, Pediatrician, Descanso Pediatrics, Huntington Medical Foundation, La Canada, California

NATALIA FESTA, BA, Division of General Pediatrics, Department of Pediatrics, Lucile Packard Children's Hospital, Stanford University School of Medicine, Stanford, California

ELLYNORE FLORENDO, MS, Division of General Pediatrics, Department of Pediatrics, Children's Hospital Los Angeles, University of Southern California Keck School of Medicine, Los Angeles, California

LISA S. FOLEY, MD, Surgical Resident, Division of Pediatric Surgery, Department of Surgery, Children's Hospital Colorado, University of Colorado School of Medicine, Aurora, Colorado

JAIME L. FRÍAS, MD, FAAP, FACMG, Emeritus Professor, Department of Pediatrics, University of South Florida, Tampa, Florida

REBECCA J. HAMBLIN, PhD, Postdoctoral Fellow, Department of Pediatrics, University of South Florida, St. Petersburg, Florida; Rogers Behavioral Health - Tampa Bay, Tampa, Florida

THOMAS HAVRANEK, MD, Attending Neonatologist, The Children's Hospital at Montefiore; Associate Professor, Department of Pediatrics, Albert Einstein College of Medicine, Bronx, New York

JANET S. HESS, DrPH, MPH, Assistant Professor, Department of Pediatrics, University of South Florida Morsani College of Medicine, Tampa, Florida

JOYCE R. JAVIER, MD, MPH, Assistant Professor, Clinical Pediatrics, Division of General Pediatrics, Department of Pediatrics, Children's Hospital Los Angeles, University of Southern California Keck School of Medicine, Los Angeles, California

MICHAEL S. KAPPY, MD, PhD, Department of Pediatrics, University of Colorado Denver School of Medicine, Children's Hospital Colorado, Aurora, Colorado

NANCY KELLY, MD, MPH, Associate Professor of Pediatrics, University of Texas Southwestern Medical Center, Dallas, Texas

SHERYL KENT, PhD, Clinical Director, Pain Consultation Service, Children's Hospital of Colorado; Assistant Professor, Department of Anesthesiology, University of Colorado, Anshutz Medical Center, Aurora, Colorado

ANN M. KULUNGOWSKI, MD, Assistant Professor, Division of Pediatric Surgery, Department of Surgery, Children's Hospital Colorado, University of Colorado School of Medicine, Aurora, Colorado

NIZAR F. MARAQA, MD, FPIDS, Assistant Professor, Pediatric Infectious Diseases and Immunology, University of Florida College of Medicine-Jacksonville, Jacksonville, Florida

JAZMINE S. MATEUS, MPH, Data Analyst, All Children's Hospital Johns Hopkins Medicine, St. Petersburg, Florida

FERNANDO S. MENDOZA, MD, MPH, Professor of Pediatrics, Division of General Pediatrics, Department of Pediatrics, Lucile Packard Children's Hospital, Associate Dean for Minority Advising and Programs, Stanford University School of Medicine, Stanford, California

AYESHA MIRZA, MD, FAAP, FPIDS, Department of Pediatrics, University of Florida Center for HIV/AIDS Research, Education and Service (UF CARES); Pediatric Infectious Diseases and Immunology, Wolfson Children's Hospital, Jacksonville, Florida

CRISTINA PELAEZ-VELEZ, MD, Assistant Professor, Department of Pediatrics, University of South Florida Morsani College of Medicine, Tampa, Florida

MOBEEN H. RATHORE, MD, CPE, FAAP, FPIDS, FSHEA, FIDSA, FACPE, Professor and Chief, Department of Pediatrics, University of Florida College of Medicine-Jacksonville; Pediatric Infectious Diseases and Immunology, Wolfson Children's Hospital, University of Florida Center for HIV/AIDS Research, Education and Service (UF CARES), Jacksonville, Florida

ROBIN SLOVER, MD, Medical Director, Pain Consultation Service, Children's Hospital of Colorado; Associate Professor, Department of Anesthesiology, University of Colorado, Anshutz Medical Campus, Aurora, Colorado

ERIC A. STORCH, PhD, All Children's Hospital Guild Endowed Chair and Professor, Department of Pediatrics, University of South Florida, St. Petersburg, Florida; Departments of Psychology, Psychiatry and Behavioral Neurosciences' Health Policy and Management, University of South Florida, Tampa, Florida; Clinical Director, Rogers Behavioral Health – Tampa Bay, Tampa, Florida; Director of Research for Developmental Pediatrics, Mind-Body Branch, All Children's Hospital, Johns Hopkins Medicine, St. Petersburg, Florida

DIANE M. STRAUB, MD, MPH, Professor and Chief, Division of Adolescent Medicine, Department of Pediatrics, University of South Florida Morsani College of Medicine, Tampa, Florida

MONICA S. WU, MA, Graduate Research Assistant, Department of Pediatrics, University of South Florida, St. Petersburg, Florida; Department of Psychology, University of South Florida, Tampa, Florida

ADVANCES IN
Pediatrics

CONTENTS   VOLUME 62 • 2015

Childhood Tuberculosis: An Overview
Diala Faddoul

Child Advocacy in the Twenty-first Century
Lisa J. Chamberlain and Nancy Kelly

Children in Immigrant Families: The Foundation for America's Future

Joyce R. Javier, Natalia Festa, Ellynore Florendo, and Fernando S. Mendoza

Preparing for Transition from Pediatric to Adult Care: Evaluation of a Physician Training Program

Janet S. Hess, Diane M. Straub, Jazmine S. Mateus, and Cristina Pelaez-Velez

Evidence-Based Psychological Treatments of Pediatric Mental Disorders

Monica S. Wu, Rebecca J. Hamblin, and Eric A. Storch

Gene Therapy for Blinding Pediatric Eye Disorders

Alina V. Dumitrescu and Arlene V. Drack

▶ Videos of subretinal injection for gene replacement therapy accompany this article

Screening for Critical Congenital Heart Disease in Newborns
Thomas Havranek and Christie J. Bruno

Vascular Anomalies in Pediatrics
Lisa S. Foley and Ann M. Kulungowski

Hypo and Hyper: Common Pediatric Endocrine and Metabolic Emergencies
Jennifer M. Barker and Lalit Bajaj

Pediatric Headaches
Robin Slover and Sheryl Kent

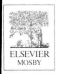

ELSEVIER
MOSBY

ADVANCES IN PEDIATRICS

Introduction

Michael S. Kappy, MD, PhD

The Editorial Board is pleased to present volume 62 of *Advances in Pediatrics*, an over 60-year publication dedicated to publishing updates in a wide variety of pediatric topics, medical, surgical, and others.

Several years ago, we instituted a feature entitled "Foundations of Pediatrics," which honored men and women in our field whose contributions enabled us to stand "on the shoulders of giants." Our current honoree is David Smith, whose contributions to the field of genetics and general pediatrics were exemplary. Dr Frias' tribute is a moving testimony to Dr Smith's career.

We continue to offer articles that offer advances in pediatric infectious diseases (Rathore et al, Faddoul), general pediatrics (Chamberlain et al, Mendoza et al, Straub et al, Storch), surgery (Drach et al, Kulongowski), cardiovascular disorders (Bruno et al), endocrinology (Bajaj and Barker), and the evaluation and treatment of headache in children (Slover).

Our hope is that these articles will better enrich the primary care and sub-specialty care pediatric practice. Any comments regarding this volume as well as suggestions for future articles can be directed to:

Michael S. Kappy, MD, PhD
Department of Pediatrics
University of Colorado School of Medicine
Children's Hospital Colorado
13123 East 16th Avenue
B-265, Aurora, CO 80045, USA

E-mail address: michael.kappy@childrenscolorado.org

0065-3101/15/$ – see front matter
http://dx.doi.org/10.1016/j.yapd.2015.05.001

Advances in Pediatrics 62 (2015) 1–10

ADVANCES IN PEDIATRICS

ELSEVIER
MOSBY

David Weyhe Smith, MD (1926–1981)—The Father of Dysmorphology

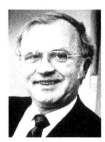

David Weyhe Smith, MD

Jaime L. Frías, MD

Department of Pediatrics, University of South Florida, Tampa, FL, USA

Keywords
* • Dysmorphology • Endocrinology • Congenital anomalies • Teratology
* • Fetal alcohol syndrome

" A leader in the field of dysmorphology, Dr Smith contributed to the understanding of embryologic derangement leading to congenital defects." Thus starts the record of David W. Smith's induction to the Johns Hopkins Society of Scholars in 1979 [1]. Indeed, he was an unquestionable leader in the field, one who brought new vision to the study of congenital anomalies by stressing the importance of defining the nature of the problem, its time of origin during development, and the likely pathogenetic mechanisms leading to the anomaly.

David W. Smith was born September 24, 1926, in Oakland, California. He received his bachelor's degree in 1946 from the University of California, Berkeley, where, according to Dave Smith lore, he played for the Golden Bears football team. However, I have been unable to corroborate this story and a

E-mail address: jlfrias@comcast.net

0065-3101/15/$ – see front matter
http://dx.doi.org/10.1016/j.yapd.2015.04.011

careful search of University of California, Berkeley football team rosters from 1942 to 1946 failed to show his name [2]. Perhaps it is in Dave's favor to debunk this legend, because during the years he was at Berkeley the Golden Bears' performance was at a historic low: record low scoring, fewest rushing yards, and fewest total yards.

Following graduation from Berkeley, he went to medical school at Johns Hopkins University and obtained his MD degree in 1950. His residency in pe-diatrics at the Johns Hopkins Hospital was interrupted by 2 years of military service as a Captain in the US Army, which he spent mostly in Germany. Once relieved of military duties, he returned to Johns Hopkins to complete his residency. Subsequently, he did a 1-year fellowship in pediatric endocri-nology with Lawson Wilkins. During that year he published his first scientific paper ("The mental prognosis in hypothyroidism in infancy and childhood: A review of 128 cases" [3]) with Robert Blizzard and Lawson Wilkins as coau-thors. It is quite possible that it was this study that kindled Dave's interest in abnormal prenatal development, which would soon become the focus of his academic endeavors.

After a year in pediatric practice in Los Gatos, California, he received an offer to join a pediatric practice in Madison, Wisconsin. While considering this opportunity, he called Nathan Smith (no relation), who at the time chaired the Department of Pediatrics at the University of Wisconsin School of Medi-cine, to find out about the feasibility of doing some teaching in his department if he joined the pediatrics group in Madison. Instead, Nathan offered him a full-time position as the endocrinologist in his young department. Dave, in a typical show of modesty, demurred and suggested a fellow trainee in Lawson Wilkins' program because he regarded him as a better scientist and, therefore, a more appropriate person for the job. Nathan refused to take "no" for an answer and rapidly convinced Dave, who accepted the challenge and joined the Uni-versity of Wisconsin faculty in 1957 as an Instructor in Pediatrics.

Dave set himself to work and, with his characteristic enthusiasm and power-ful drive, promptly established a strong and productive clinical and training program in pediatric endocrinology. Soon, however, because of his long-term interest in human development he veered his attention toward the study of congenital anomalies. The period from 1960 to 1965 represents Dave's transi-tional years from pediatric endocrinology to clinical genetics. In fact, as of 1962 he simultaneously had fellows in both subspecialties: Luc Lemli (1963–1964) and Arlan Rosenbloom (1964–1966) in endocrinology, and John Opitz (1962–1964), Donna Daentl (1965–1966), and this author (1965–1967) in clin-ical genetics.

The same overlap was evident in his publications, which provided important contributions to both fields. Noteworthy are a phenomenal series of ground-breaking papers in the then-nascent area of clinical cytogenetics that started ap-pearing in 1960, a short year after the report of the first chromosomal anomaly in humans, trisomy 21, by Jerome Lejeune in France [4]. This series of papers included the first description of trisomy 13, together with Patau and associates

[5], and the description of trisomy 18 [6] that closely followed the initial report by Edwards and colleagues [7]. It is of interest to recall that Edwards, whose name is commonly used as an eponym for trisomy 18 syndrome, and his coauthors identified the extra chromosome in the patient they reported as chromosome 17. Smith and colleagues [6], however, identified the extra chromosome in their two patients as an E group chromosome (numbers 16–18), but in the addendum to that publication they reported four more patients and the definitive identification of the extra chromosome as number 18.

Within that period, Dave also published the first report on the Cornelia de Lange syndrome in the English language medical literature [8]. In that paper, he and his coauthors described nine patients and postulated a dominant mutation as the most likely cause of the syndrome. Forty-one years later, in 2004, their suggestion was confirmed when two different groups simultaneously reported the identification of dominant mutations in the *NIPBL* gene, the human homolog of *Drosophila melanogaster* nipped-B gene, as the cause of the Cornelia de Lange syndrome [9,10]. Two other seminal papers on congenital anomalies were published in that period. One was a study of minor congenital anomalies in the newborn [11], and the other a description of the syndrome that is now recognized by the eponymous designation of Smith-Lemli-Opitz syndrome [12].

At the same time, Dave's productivity as an endocrinologist continued, as evidenced by a series of papers that were important contributions to the pediatric endocrinology literature of the time. This series included the use of zinc glucagon in the management of idiopathic hypoglycemia [13,14], urinary excretion of dopa in children with short stature and malnutrition [15], the importance of the route and site of insulin administration in the management of diabetes mellitus [16], the effects of medroxyprogesterone (Depo-Provera) in girls with idiopathic isosexual precocity [17], the lack of concordance of idiopathic anterior hypopituitarism in two identical twins [18], the scholastic performance of children with hypopituitarism [19], and the variability of salt losing in related patients with congenital adrenal hyperplasia [20]. An additional group of publications from that period, including two studies on sex chromatin in newborn females [21,22], and reports on Klinefelter syndrome [23], Turner syndrome [24], and the natural history of metaphyseal dysostosis [25], may be considered as bridging the two fields.

Perhaps Dave's pivotal moment was when he decided to spend a sabbatical year (1964–1965) studying embryology with Gian Töndury, Professor of Anatomy and Histology at the University of Zürich. Dave later recognized him as the teacher "from whom I gained knowledge of embryology and the interpretation of errors of morphogenesis" [26].

I had my first contact with Dave when he was in Switzerland. I was in Chile, my native country, and after completion of my pediatric training, I was awarded an American College of Physicians/Kellogg Foundation fellowship for subspecialty training in the United States. I had the good fortune of meeting Nathan Smith, who had stepped down as chair of Pediatrics at the University of Wisconsin and was doing a sabbatical year at the University of Chile. When

I mentioned to Nathan my interest in pursuing training in clinical genetics, he put me in contact with Dave, who accepted my application for a fellowship starting September 1965.

When I arrived in Wisconsin, Dave received me with his distinctive spontaneous warmth, and as the days and weeks went on, I realized how lucky I was to have him as my mentor. It is uncommon to find such an enthusiastic and motivating teacher, one whose intellectual inquisitiveness stimulates curiosity while at the same time nurtures independent thinking. During the year I was in Madison (1965–1966) I was also lucky to have worked closely with John Opitz who, even in those early days, was a fountain of encyclopedic knowledge. It was also a pleasure to share responsibilities with the other fellows on Dave's team, Arlan Rosenbloom and Donna Daentl, and with the graduate students who participated in some of our clinical activities, such as Jules Leroy and Frank Walker.

At that time, Dave was working on an article that might be considered his manifesto which was published in 1966 [27]. This paper, aimed at general pediatricians and subspecialists, summarized Dave's basic concepts on altered human morphogenesis and proposed the use of the term "dysmorphology," which he coined "to identify the general category of disease which encompasses abnormalities in development of structural tissue regardless of etiology, timing of origin, or severity" [27,28]. He further suggested the use of this term as a substitute for "teratology," rightly considering that the term "teratology" was inappropriate for clinical use for the following reasons: first, its literal meaning from the Greek, "study of monsters," is incongruous because most common human malformations tend to be minor; second, by implying abnormal formation at an early stage, up to the end of the fetal period, it excludes developmental abnormalities of postnatal origin; and, third, because by common usage the term "teratology" implies an environmental cause for developmental abnormalities, it seems to ignore the important role of genetic factors in their causation.

Early in 1966, Dave accepted a position as Professor and Head of the Dysmorphology Unit at the University of Washington (UW) Department of Pediatrics, and invited me to move with him. Although I had some regret when leaving Madison and the exciting academic environment of both the Pediatrics and the Genetics departments, my strong desire to continue training with Dave made the decision easier and in the summer of 1966 my family and I moved to Seattle.

Initially, Dave's office, and by extension mine, was in the building across the street from Harborview Medical Center, then King County Hospital. But because most of our clinical activities were at University Hospital, he persuaded the department administrators to give him a new location in the main campus. And that is how a couple of months later we ended up in the Coach House, an old motel (some said of ill repute) near campus purchased by the UW and used to temporarily house different programs while the construction of new medical center buildings was being completed. The suite had two bedrooms that we used as our offices, a tiny kitchen that doubled as a cytogenetics laboratory, a small dining room with a drawing table and graphics materials, and a good-sized living room that served as a library and office for a part-time secretary.

Before leaving Madison, Dave had been diligently preparing a manuscript that summarized the characteristics of several syndromes with short stature. He completed this task while in Seattle and the paper was published in 1967 with the title "Compendium on Shortness of Stature" as a supplement to the *Journal of Pediatrics* [29]. This compendium was the basis for the book that would become his magnum opus [26], which he started writing a few months after our move to Seattle. Under his direction, we prepared poster-sized tables to summarize the findings reported in the literature on each of the disorders that would be included in the book. Out of these, he assigned me the responsibility of writing up 15 syndromes and, in addition, I helped identify references needed for the description of many others.

This work was greatly facilitated by having a permanently reserved carrel at the UW Medical School Library and a wonderful, most efficient research librarian, Mrs Lyle Harrah, who would find for us any and all references we requested. Dave and I would formally review the progress of this and other projects at least once a week. Sometimes, weather-permitting, we would rent a canoe from the UW boat house and paddle to a nice spot near the arboretum where we would eat our lunch, get our work done, and have relaxed conversations. These were precious moments during which we would fix the world's maladies and talk about our plans for the future. One of the first times we did this, Dave suggested we explore Lake Union to enjoy its scenic views of Seattle. Evidently, we had not recalled that the lake was part of the ship canal that joins Lake Washington to Puget Sound until we saw what looked like a huge tug boat beelining in our direction, no matter how hard we tried to correct our course. Lots of sweat and paddling like hell finally took us out of its way.

Recognizable Patterns of Human Malformation [26], published by WB Saunders in 1970, was an instant success and became the obligatory consultation text in dysmorphology. In its introduction, Dave stated what I recognized as his mantra, "Every malformation represents an inborn error in morphogenesis. Just as the study of inborn metabolic errors has extended our understanding of normal biochemistry, so the accumulation of knowledge concerning defects in morphogenesis may assist us in further unraveling the story of structural development." Now in its seventh edition, under the able direction of Ken Jones, the book continues to be considered the leading work in the field.

Dave's bibliography lists 174 papers, seven books, and five book chapters, which denotes unusual productivity, especially if we consider that his academic career spanned only 24 years. In addition to *Recognizable Patterns of Human Malformation* [26], three of his books merit special mention either because they reflect Dave's compassionate and thoughtful way to deal with his patients and their families or because they cover some of his other areas of keen academic interest. The first, *The Child with Down Syndrome* [30], was written "for parents, physicians and persons concerned with his education and care" in collaboration with Ann A. Wilson, a research associate. The book contains a review of chromosome behavior and the faulty distribution that results in trisomy 21, and is written in clear and concise language suited for parents and the nonspecialist. It continues with an appraisal of the physical, mental, and social characteristics of persons with Down syndrome that is especially well done, aiming at helping the family understand the child's potential beyond his or her physical or intellectual limitations. Two other chapters in the book, the first a photo album of children with Down syndrome, and the second on family adaptation to the child with Down syndrome, have been an excellent resource for parents to understand the range of their child's capabilities and potential.

Growth and its Disorders [31], published in 1977, brought together Dave's background as a pediatric endocrinologist and a morphologist as it reviewed the basic principles of human growth and its alterations caused by endocrine, genetic, or environmental causes. In a recent note to me, Arlan Rosenbloom pondered, "Noteworthy, that the six people Dave credits for the studies and knowledge greatly influencing the content of the book are Nancy Bayley, Stan Garn, Andrea Prader, Jim Tanner, Reginald Whitehouse, and, of course, Lawson Wilkins."

The third book, *Recognizable Patterns of Human Deformations* [32], published posthumously in 1981 and now in its third edition under the leadership of John Graham, reviews the effect of mechanical forces in normal and abnormal morphogenesis and describes the response of different body parts to unusual mechanical forces. In its introduction, Dave credits Dr Peter Dunn of Bristol, England for sparking his interest in human deformations when he heard Dunn's talk about the subject at one of a series of international meetings held to define the classification and nomenclature of defects in morphogenesis in which Dave was an active participant [33–36].

Among Dave's many legacies are his dysmorphology fellows. We constitute a rather small group, because he only took one fellow at a time, each for a period of 2 years. After I completed my fellowship and returned to Chile in 1967, I was followed, in succession, by John Aase, Bryan Hall, Ken Jones, Jim Hanson, John Graham, and Margot van Allen. All of them have had successful and productive academic careers, developed strong programs in dysmorphology, and trained many of the dysmorphologists that now serve as leaders in the field. In 1980, the group started a summer meeting that includes about 125 participants chosen by the quality of their submitted abstracts on new research in selected areas of dysmorphology. The meeting strives to be a colloquium that allows for plenty of discussion, dialogue, and debate among participants. The David Smith Workshop on Malformations and Morphogenesis is now in its 35th year.

Dave is also universally recognized for the first description of the fetal alcohol syndrome (FAS). In a 1981 letter to the editor of *Nutrition Today* [37], Dr Sterling Clarren, former faculty member at the UW Department of

Pediatrics, narrated how the first recognition of FAS occurred. In a nutshell, he relates that Dr Christy Ulleland was doing a study on small-for-gestational age infants and realized that several of them were the offspring of alcoholic mothers. She brought this information to Dave's attention. He examined these children with Ken Jones, his fellow at that time, and recognized a specific pattern of anomalies that subsequently became known as FAS. Together with Dr Ulleland and Dr Streissguth, a clinical psychologist who also evaluated the children, they published an article in *Lancet* [38] that attracted worldwide attention. Further studies have demonstrated that FAS is the most common cause of intellectual disability due to an environmental factor [39].

Despite the fame Dave achieved as the father of dysmorphology and as one of the true giants of pediatrics, a model teacher, a scholar, and a superb clinician, his curriculum vitae is sparse, brief, and to the point, reflecting his humble personality and his dislike for hyperbole and the limelight. In it, he briefly lists his editorial responsibilities, his society memberships (former Vice-President of the Society for Pediatric Research, council member of the American Pediatric Society, former council member of the Teratology Society, and former President of the Western Society for Pediatric Research), and the recognitions and awards he received (Josiah Macy Faculty Scholar Award in 1975, and induction in the Johns Hopkins Society of Scholars in 1979).

Any reminiscence about Dave would be incomplete if it did not mention his love for and dedication to his family (his wife, Ann and his four sons) or if it did not make reference to his outgoing personality, and his honesty, integrity, and loyalty. Beverly Morgan, chair of the Department of Pediatrics during part of Dave's tenure at UW, reflected on some of these attributes at the Festschrift in his honor held September 1981: "David Smith was a faculty member who always put the good of others – his patients, students, fellows, laboratory associates, and other faculty members as well as the Departments of Pediatrics in which he served – above his personal goals and gains. He had little use for bureaucratic detail and suffered poorly issues of turf and power. In controversial meetings he would stand up, hands in his pockets, and make comments such as, 'Why don't we stop all this arguing and just get together and chop wood?' [40].

And, how can one forget his spontaneous, stentorian laughter? Or his singing, whether it was an aria of Carmen, or the Ein Prosit song, or that one about Uncle George and Auntie Mabel? Or his yodeling? Or his harmonica? This brings to memory the day he was chairing a session at a Birth Defects meeting in Vancouver, BC. Cedric Carter from England gave the last talk of the session and Dave went to the podium to congratulate him for his excellent talk. He then whipped out his always-ready little harmonica from the front pocket of his jacket and in honor of Dr Carter proceeded to play… the "Deutschlandlied" ("Song of Germany")"!!! During the break I told him about his faux pas, and when everyone had congregated back in the auditorium, he simply stood up at front and said, "Dr Carter, I understand I made a lapsus harmonicae," and proceeded to play "Britannia Rules the Waves."

Although it happened in 1979, I remember the call as if it was today. One of his associates in the dysmorphology unit called to say that Dave was hospitalized with the diagnosis of retroperitoneal lymphoma. As I learned afterward, he was going to Saudi Arabia with his wife, invited as a Visiting Professor by Dr Nadia Sakati, and on the flight to Riyadh, he developed severe edema of a lower extremity. On arrival, he was taken to King Faisal Hospital, where they discovered a retroperitoneal mass and strongly suspected the diagnosis of lymphoma. Rather than returning immediately to the United States, as most of us would have done, in a demonstration of his incredible stamina and sense of responsibility, Dave insisted on giving his planned lectures while sitting in a wheelchair.

I talked with Dave several times throughout the following months, but did not see him until March, 1980 in Orlando when both of us were there to testify at the first Bendectin trial. He was in great shape and good spirits, and the lymphoma was in remission. We met again in September of that year in Washington, DC to participate in a Food and Drug Administration hearing on Bendectin. He again looked fine, but on the second day there he started having problems that forced him to go back to Seattle. That was the last time I talked with him. In mid-January 1981, I received a call from Ken Jones telling me that Dave was in his last days. I flew to Seattle to say good-bye, but I do not know if he realized I was there. Two days later, on January 23, 1981, he was gone at the age of 54 years. The world had lost a wonderful man, a consummate physician, a giant of pediatrics, and a brilliant teacher. I had lost a dear friend and the most influential person in my professional life.

Acknowledgments

The author expresses his deep appreciations to Arlan L. Rosenbloom, MD, Distinguished Service Professor Emeritus of Pediatrics at the University of Florida College of Medicine, and John M. Opitz, MD, Professor of Pediatrics, Human Genetics, Pathology, and Obstetrics & Gynecology, University of Utah School of Medicine, for the invaluable help they provided by confirming several aspects of this biography; and to Sonja A. Rasmussen, MD, MS, Editor-in-Chief, *Morbidity and Mortality Report*, Centers for Disease Control and Prevention, for her critical review of the article.

References

[1] Available at: https://archive.org/stream/commencement1979/commencement1979_djvu.txt. Accessed October 29, 2014.
[2] Available at: http://www.lostlettermen.com/football/california/players/alpha/s. Accessed November 7, 2014.
[3] Smith DW, Blizzard RM, Wilkins L. The mental prognosis in hypothyroidism in infancy and childhood: a review of 128 cases. Pediatrics 1957;19:1011–22.
[4] Lejeune J, Turpin R, Gautier M. Le Mongolisme: premier exemple d'aberration autosomique humaine. Ann Génét 1959;1:41–9.
[5] Patau K, Smith DW, Therman E, et al. Multiple congenital anomaly caused by an extra autosome. Lancet 1960;1:790–3.

[6] Smith DW, Patau K, Therman E, et al. A new autosomal trisomy syndrome: two cases of multiple congenital anomaly caused by an extra chromosome. J Pediatr 1960;57: 338–45.

[7] Edwards JH, Harnden DG, Cameron AH, et al. A new trisomic syndrome. Lancet 1960;1: 787–90.

[8] Ptacek L, Opitz JM, Smith DW, et al. The Cornelia De Lange syndrome. J Pediatr 1963;63: 1000–20.

[9] Krantz ID, McCallum J, DeScipio C, et al. Cornelia de Lange syndrome is caused by mutations in NIPBL, the human homolog of Drosophila melanogaster nipped-B. Nat Genet 2004;36:631–5.

[10] Tonkin ET, Wang TJ, Lisgo S, et al. NIPBL, encoding a homolog of fungal Scc2-type sister chromatid cohesion proteins and fly nipped-B, is mutated in Cornelia de Lange syndrome. Nat Genet 2004;3(6):636–41.

[11] Marden PM, Smith DW, McDonald MJ. Congenital anomalies in the newborn, including minor variations: a study of 4412 babies by surface examination and buccal smear for sex chromatin. J Pediatr 1964;64:357–71.

[12] Smith DW, Lemli L, Opitz JM. A newly recognized syndrome of multiple congenital anomalies. J Pediatr 1964;64:210–7.

[13] Kushner RS, Lemli L, Smith DW. Zinc glucagon in the management of idiopathic hypoglycemia. J Pediatr 1963;63:1111–5.

[14] Rosenbloom AL, Smith DW, Cohan RC. Zinc glucagon in idiopathic hypoglycemia of infancy. Efficacy of long term control. Am J Dis Child 1966;112:107–11.

[15] Copps SG, Gerritsen T, Smith DW, et al. Urinary excretion of 3,4-dihydroxyphenylalnine (DOPA) in two children of short stature with malnutrition. J Pediatr 1963;62:208–16.

[16] Nora J, Smith DW, Cameron JR. The route of insulin administration in the management of diabetes mellitus. J Pediatr 1964;64:547–51.

[17] Lemli L, Aron M, Smith DW. The action of Depo-Provera in three girls with idiopathic isosexual precocity. J Pediatr 1964;65:888–94.

[18] Rosenbloom AL, Smith DW. Idiopathic anterior hypopituitarism in one of identical twins. J Pediatr 1965;67:84–8.

[19] Rosenbloom AL, Smith DW, Loeb DG. Scholastic performance of short-statured children with hypopituitarism. J Pediatr 1966;69:1131–3.

[20] Rosenbloom AL, Smith DW. Varying expression for salt losing in related patients with congenital adrenal hyperplasia. Pediatrics 1966;38:215–9.

[21] Smith DW, Marden P, McDonald MJ, et al. Lower incidence of sex chromatin in buccal smears of newborn females. Pediatrics 1962;30:707–10.

[22] Wegmann T, Smith DW. Lower incidence of sex chromatin in newborn females delivered by cesarean section. Pediatrics 1964;34:419–21.

[23] Wegmann TG, Smith DW. Incidence of Klinefelter's syndrome among juvenile delinquents and felons. Lancet 1963;1:274.

[24] Lemli L, Smith DW. The XO syndrome: a study of the differentiated phenotype in 25 patients. J Pediatr 1963;63:577–88.

[25] Rosenbloom AL, Smith DW. The natural history of metaphyseal dysostosis. J Pediatr 1965;66:857–68.

[26] Smith DW. Recognizable patterns of human malformation. 1st edition. Philadelphia: WB Saunders Company; 1970.

[27] Smith DW. Dysmorphology (teratology). J Pediatr 1966;69:1150–69.

[28] Jones KL, Carey JC. The importance of dysmorphology in the identification of new human teratogens. Am J Med Genet C Semin Med Genet 2011;157:188–94.

[29] Smith DW. Compendium on shortness of stature. J Pediatr 1967;70:463–519.

[30] Smith DW, Wilson AA. The child with Down syndrome. Philadelphia: WB Saunders Company; 1973.

[31] Smith DW. Growth and its disorders. Philadelphia: WB Saunders Company; 1977.

[32] Smit DW. Recognizable patterns of human deformation. Philadelphia: WB Saunders Company; 1981.

[33] Classification and nomenclature of malformation. Lancet 1974;1:798.

[34] Classification and nomenclature of morphological defects. Lancet 1975;1:513.

[35] Benirschke K, Lowry RB, Opitz JM, et al. Developmental terms: some proposals: first report of an international working group. Am J Med Genet 1979;3:297–302.

[36] Spranger J, Benirschke K, Hall JG, et al. Errors of morphogenesis: concepts and terms. Recommendations of an international working group. J Pediatr 1982;100:160–5.

[37] Clarren SK. Fetal alcohol syndrome. Letter to the editor. Nutr Today 1981;16:31.

[38] Jones KL, Smith DW, Ulleland CN, et al. Pattern of malformation in offspring of chronic alcoholic mothers. Lancet 1973;1:1267–71.

[39] May PA, Baete A, Russo J, et al. Prevalence and characteristics of fetal alcohol spectrum disorders. Pediatrics 2014;134:855–66.

[40] Morgan B. Reminiscences. J Pediatr 1982;101:799–800.

Advances in Pediatrics 62 (2015) 11–27

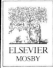

Immunization Update V

Ayesha Mirza, MD[a,b],
Mobeen H. Rathore, MD, CPE[a,b],*

[a]Department of Pediatrics, University of Florida Center for HIV/AIDS Research, Education and Service (UF CARES), 653-1 West 8th Street, Jacksonville, FL 32209, USA; [b]Pediatric Infectious Diseases and Immunology, Wolfson Children's Hospital, 800 Prudential Drive, Jacksonville, FL 32207, USA

Keywords

- Immunizations • Seasonal influenza vaccines • Adolescent vaccines
- Pediatric vaccines • Pertussis • Measles • Human papillomavirus • Poliovirus

Key points

- With all the new vaccines and strategies for prevention, the most important challenge that we must continue to talk about globally and at home is the one presented by ongoing transmission of diseases for which excellent vaccines already exist.
- As pediatricians this presents a constant reminder that we must keep the conversation about the importance of vaccine-preventable diseases with patients and their families going at every possible opportunity possible.
- We also need to constantly remind ourselves that every case of a vaccine-preventable disease is a missed opportunity for prevention.
- Keeping a broader perspective for global eradication of vaccine preventable diseases in mind and advocating for availability of vaccines at an affordable cost as well as encouraging local vaccine development should be part of our mission as advocates for children globally.

INTRODUCTION

News of Ebola Virus Disease (EVD) overshadowed the news for the mid to latter parts of the year 2014. While the epidemic raged primarily in West Africa, this time it succeeded in grabbing the attention of the rest of the world as imported cases were seen in other parts of the world including the United States (US) and Europe. Even though it seems such a cliché, it has never been true now more so than ever before, that the world is an ever shrinking place and an infectious agent is only an airplane ride away. So whether it is

*Corresponding author. 653-1 West 8th Street, Jacksonville, FL 32209. E-mail address: mobeen.rathore@jax.ufl.edu

0065-3101/15/$ – see front matter
http://dx.doi.org/10.1016/j.yapd.2015.04.004

EVD in West Africa or polio in Pakistan or measles in the Philippines, one cannot become complacent in the United States that children are protected until it is ensured that every child and every adolescent globally is adequately immunized. Although there is no available vaccine for EVD, there are effective vaccines available for measles. Yet, there is ongoing transmission not only of measles but also of pertussis, another vaccine-preventable disease, in the United States year after year. The reasons for ongoing transmission of these vaccine-preventable diseases, as discussed in previous updates, are multifactorial: importation of measles virus from areas of the world where disease transmission is ongoing, issues related to declining immunogenicity with the currently available pertussis vaccines, and last but not least the vaccine naysayers all contribute to the ongoing transmission of these diseases in the United States and other developed countries around the world.

This article discusses the current state of influenza vaccines including the quadrivalent vaccine, ongoing measles and pertussis transmission in the United States, human papillomavirus virus (HPV) vaccine uptake, the updated recommendations for meningococcal vaccines, updates on the pneumococcal vaccines, and finally other updates from around the globe.

INFLUENZA VACCINES

The American Academy of Pediatrics (AAP) and the Centers for Diseases Control and Prevention (CDC) continue to recommend annual influenza vaccines for all infants older than 6 months, children, and adolescents, with special emphasis on immunization of children with chronic medical conditions (CMCs). These recommendations also include annual immunization of all health care personnel, pregnant women and women who are considering pregnancy or breast feeding during the current influenza season, and all child care providers and staff [1].

Overall, the percentage of outpatient visits for influenza-like illness (ILI) during the 2013–14 season decreased when compared with the previous 2012–13 season. Severe cases of influenza were reported predominantly among people 18 to 64 years of age who accounted for nearly 60% of influenza-associated hospitalizations. Individuals aged 50 to 64 years had the second highest hospitalization rate (rates remained highest for those 65 years and older) [2]. The cumulative hospitalization rate (per 100,000 population) by age group for the period between October 1, 2013, to April 30, 2014, was as follows: 46.9 (0–4 years), 9.5 (5–17 years), 22.0 (18–49 years), 54.3 (50–64 years), and 88.1 (>65 years) [3].

As in previous years, 43% of hospitalized influenza cases in children were reported in those with no underlying CMC. Asthma and reactive airway disease continued to top the list of CMCs that predisposed children with influenza most frequently to hospitalization. About 91% of individuals (both adults and children) admitted to the intensive care unit had not received their influenza immunization [1].

A total of 109 influenza-related pediatric deaths were reported to the CDC as of August 24, 2014 [4]. Of 107 deaths, 87 were attributable to influenza A viruses, 16 were associated with influenza B viruses, 2 deaths were associated with dual infection with both viruses, and 2 deaths were associated with an undetermined type of influenza virus. More than 50% of these deaths were in children with CMCs of which neurologic disorders and pulmonary diseases accounted for the majority. About 47% of these children, however, had no underlying CMC [1]. A total of 133 influenza related pediatric deaths were reported for the 2014–15 influenza season through the week of April 25, 2015 [5].

The predominant circulating virus during the 2013–14 influenza season was the 2009 H1N1 virus, with influenza B also becoming predominant during the latter part of the season and mainly affecting the northeastern part of the United States. Cases of ILI were first observed in November with the numbers reaching a peak by the last week of November and declining by early January [3].

For the 2014–15 influenza season, both trivalent (TIV) and quadrivalent vaccines are available. Both vaccines contain 2 strains of influenza virus (A/California/2009 [H1N1] and A/Texas/50/2012 [H3N2] viruses), as well as a B strain (B/Massachusetts/2/2012-like virus). The quadrivalent vaccine also contains an additional B virus (B/Brisbane/60/2008-like virus). The influenza vaccine strains for the 2014–15 are the same as those used during the previous 2013–14 season [6]. Available vaccines are detailed in Table 1.

The presence of identical strains from the 2013–14 influenza vaccine to the 2014–15 vaccines raises the question of whether it is necessary to immunize

Table 1
Vaccines available for the 2014–15 influenza season in the United States

Trade name	Age indication	Route
Inactivated influenza vaccines quadrivalent		
Fluarix	≥3 y	im
Flulaval	≥3 y	im
Fluzone	≥3 y	im
Inactivated influenza vaccines trivalent		
Afluria	≥9 y	im
Fluarix	≥9 y via syringe/18–64 y via jet injector	im
FluLaval	≥3 y	im
Fluvirin	≥4 y	im
Fluzone	≥36 mo & ≥6 mo	im
Fluzone Intradermal	18–64 y	im
Inactivated influenza vaccine trivalent cell culture based		
Flucelvax	≥18 y	im
Inactivated influenza vaccine trivalent high dose		
Fluzone High Dose	≥65 y	im
Recombinant influenza vaccines trivalent		
FluBlok	18–49 y	im
Live attenuated influenza vaccine quadrivalent		
Flumist Quadrivalent	2–49 y	Intranasal

Abbreviation: im, intramuscular.
Adapted from CDC. Weekly U.S. influenza surveillance report. Available at: http://www.cdc.gov/flu/weekly/#S3. Accessed December 12, 2014; and Available at: http://www.cdc.gov/flu/pdf/protect/vaccine/influenza-vaccines-table-2014-15.pdf. Accessed May 8, 2015.

those individuals who received the vaccine during the previous season. The simple answer is yes, these individuals do need to be immunized again. Although the 2014–15 influenza virus vaccine is the same as that of the previous year, repeat immunization is recommended for all individuals because immunity does tend to wane, with antibody titers decreasing to 50% of their original levels approximately 6 to 12 months after vaccination.

For the 2014–15 influenza season, the CDC Advisory Committee on Immunization Practices (ACIP) recommended preferential administration of live attenuated influenza vaccine (LAIV) in children 2 to 8 years of age based on data that demonstrated increased efficacy in this age group as compared with the inactivated influenza vaccine (IIV). The AAP did not make a preferential recommendation for LAIV in the 2- to 8-year-olds. Regardless of which recommendation is being followed by clinicians, the important point is to give the available vaccine without waiting for LAIV if it is not available for administration.

Observational data from the US Flu Vaccine Effectiveness Network and 2 additional studies conducted during the 2013–14 influenza season showed that LAIV was not as effective against pandemic influenza A (H1N1) virus as compared with the IIV in children 2 to 8 years of age and that children in this age group were not protected against the pandemic influenza A strain if they were immunized with LAIV. However, the CDC did not make any changes to their vaccine recommendations based on these findings. Guidance from the AAP did not express any preference for LAIV versus IIV. The number of vaccines recommended for each child would depend on receipt of influenza vaccine in the previous year (Fig. 1). Guidance has also been provided for individuals with egg allergy and administration of influenza vaccine (Fig. 2).

The question of vaccine uptake remains another issue. Multiple studies have shown that provider recommendation remains the single most important factor when it comes to influenza vaccine administration [7,8]. In many communities, influenza vaccine is also being offered to children in their schools. School-associated influenza vaccine administration is likely to become more commonplace and help increase vaccine uptake.

Many institutions across the country have instituted different policies requiring influenza vaccine administration for health care workers (HCWs) [9]. Data available support institutional requirements for influenza vaccination for all HCWs [10]. Universal administration of influenza vaccine to school children has also been shown to have many benefits, including improved immunization rates, decreased absenteeism in schools, and benefits to the community by decreasing health care use and improving influenza-related hospitalizations [11–13]. The question of whether to mandate universal influenza immunization of all HCWs despite all the scientific literature supporting this has sparked a debate on the ethics of such a move and generated much controversy. The main objection of those who opposed was the infringement on autonomy of individuals, whereas those in favor of mandatory vaccination argue that patient safety, enhancement of public trust, and strengthening of the health care workforce are all at stake [14].

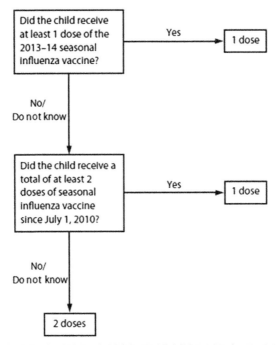

Fig. 1. Influenza vaccine dosing algorithm for children aged 6 months through 8 years—Advisory Committee on Immunization Practices, United States, 2014–15 influenza season. Two approaches are recommended for determination of the necessary doses for the 2014–15 season; both are acceptable. The first approach considers only doses of seasonal influenza vaccine received since July 1, 2010. In cases in which adequate vaccination history from before the 2010–11 season is available, the second approach may be used. (*From* CDC. Weekly U.S. influenza surveillance report. Available at: http://www.cdc.gov/mmwr/preview/mmwrhtml/mm6332a3.htm. Accessed May 8, 2015.)

Because influenza vaccine recommendations are updated before every influenza season, pediatricians are advised to check both the CDC and the AAP Web sites for updates as they become available. Appropriate resources include the AAP at Red Book Online Influenza Resource Page http://redbook.solutions.aap.org/self serve/ssPage.aspx?SelfServeContentId=influenza-resources and CDC at http://www.cdc.gov/flu/.

MENINGOCOCCAL VACCINES

Since 2005, 800 to 1200 cases of meningococcal cases have been reported annually in the United States, representing an annual incidence of 0.3 cases per 100,000 population [15]. Despite the low incidence, the case fatality ratio remains high at 10% to 15% and 11% to 19% of survivors have significant long-term sequelae such as neurologic disability, loss of a limb, and hearing loss.

In 2005, routine use of meningococcal vaccines was recommended for adolescents starting at age 11 years. Groups at high risk for meningococcal disease

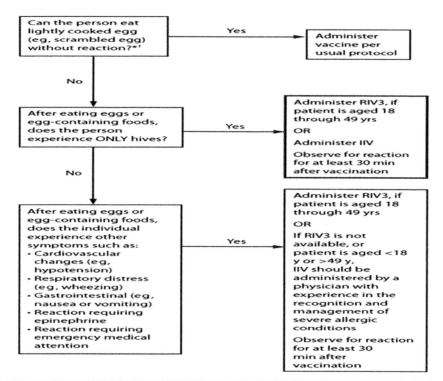

Fig. 2. Recommendations regarding influenza vaccination of persons who report allergy to eggs—Advisory Committee on Immunization Practices, United States, 2014–15 influenza season. Persons with a history of egg allergy who have experienced only hives after exposure to egg should receive influenza vaccine. Because few data are available for use of live attenuated influenza vaccine in this setting, inactivated influenza vaccines (IIV) or trivalent recombinant influenza vaccine (RIV3) should be used. RIV3 may be used for persons aged 18 through 49 years who have no other contraindications. However, IIV (egg or cell culture based) may also be used, with certain additional safety measures. * Persons with egg allergy might tolerate egg in baked products (e.g., bread or cake). Tolerance to egg-containing foods does not exclude the possibility of egg allergy (Erlewyn-Lajeunesse M, Brathwaite N, Lucas JS, Warner JO. Recommendations for the administration of influenza vaccine in children allergic to egg. BMJ 2009;339:b3680). † For persons who have no known history of exposure to egg, but who are suspected of being egg-allergic on the basis of previously performed allergy testing, consultation with a physician with expertise in the management of allergic conditions should be obtained before vaccination. Alternatively, RIV3 may be administered if the recipient is aged 18 through 49 years. (*From* CDC. Weekly U.S. influenza surveillance report. Available at: http://www.cdc.gov/mmwr/preview/mmwrhtml/mm6332a3.htm. Accessed May 8, 2015.)

for whom the vaccination is recommended include college students living in residential facilities, those with certain medical conditions such as anatomic or functional asplenia and complement deficiencies, travelers to endemic areas of the world, and microbiologists. All should be routinely immunized against meningococcal disease using age-appropriate vaccines. Meningococcal vaccines available at present are listed in Table 2.

Although serogroups B, C, and Y are the major causes of outbreaks in the United States, it was only in October of 2014 that the US Food and Drug Administration (FDA) approved the first vaccine against serogroup B [16]. This new vaccine licensed under the trade name of Trumenba (Wyeth Pharmaceuticals Inc, Philadelphia, PA, USA), can be used in individuals aged 10 to 25 years [17]. Another meningococcal serogroup B vaccine is under review by the FDA at this time [18]. The challenges associated with the development of vaccines against serogroup B have been discussed in detail in previous updates [19].

Two recent college outbreaks of *Neisseria meningitides* serogroup B disease in 2013 on 2 large college campuses on the east and west coast of the United States (total 13 cases and 1 death) highlighted the critical need for a vaccine that provided protection against serogroup B. During these particular outbreaks, in the absence of an FDA-approved vaccine in the United States, an interim guidance for control of meningococcal disease due to serogroup B in organizational settings was published by the CDC. The serogroup B meningococcal vaccine used to immunize more than 15,000 individuals during the outbreaks on these campuses was originally approved under the FDA's expanded access program and sponsored by the CDC. However, since then the vaccine was approved for use in the US on January 23, 2015. It is manufactured and supplied by Novartis Vaccines (Cambridge, MA) and marketed under the trade name of Bexsero™. It was already licensed for use in Europe, Australia and Canada [18].

MEASLES AND PERTUSSIS

With 22 states reporting 603 cases of measles between January 1 and October 31, 2014, the numbers of measles cases in 2014 are the highest seen since measles was eliminated from the United States in 2000 (Fig. 3) [20]. This occurrence is a direct result of the ongoing measles outbreak in the Philippines because most of the US cases were secondary to cases imported from there. It is no surprise that most of these secondary cases of measles were unvaccinated because it is well-known that measles is a highly contagious disease with a high basic reproduction number close to 12 to 18, which is equivalent to the number of secondary cases resulting from 1 case introduced into a fully susceptible population [21].

Similarly, cases of pertussis continue to be reported to the CDC (Fig. 4). The total number of cases reported to the CDC in 2012 was 48, 277 [22]. In 2013, the total number of cases reported was 28,639 and the incidence in those younger than 6 months was 160 per 100,000. Twelve deaths were reported in infants younger than 3 months.

Emphasis on adolescent and adult immunization with Tdap, as well as the immunization of pregnant women with each pregnancy, needs to continue to prevent ongoing transmission in infants and young children who remain the most susceptible to pertussis. Reasons for declining immunity as well as

Table 2
Commercially available meningococcal vaccines in the United States

Vaccine	Manufacturer & year of licensure	Type	Age range	Meningococcal antigens
MPSV4	Sanofi Pasteur, Inc, Swiftwater, PA, USA, 1981 (Menomune)	Polysaccharide	≥2 y	A, C, Y, W,
MenACWY-D	Sanofi Pasteur, Inc, Swiftwater, PA, USA, 2005 (Menactra)	Protein conjugate (with diphtheria toxoid)	Single dose 2–55 y 2 doses 9–23 mo	A, C, Y, W
Men ACYW-CRM	Novartis Vaccines, Cambridge, MA, USA, 2010 (Menveo)	Protein conjugate (with diphtheria toxoid)	Single dose 2–55 y	A, C, Y, W
Hib-MenCY-TT	GlaxoSmithKline, Middlesex, UK, 2012 (MenHibRix)	Protein conjugate (with tetanus toxoid)	4-dose series 6 wk through 18 mo	C, Y
4CMenB	Wyeth Pharmaceuticals Inc, Philadelphia, PA, USA, 2014 (Trumenba)	Recombinant protein conjugate	3-dose series, 0, 2, 6 mo	B

January 1 to May 1, 2015[a]

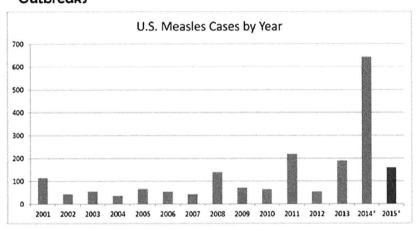

169
Cases

reported in 20 states and the District of Columbia: Arizonia, California, Colorado, Delaware, Florida, Georgia, Illinois, Massachusetts, Michigan, Minnesota, Nebraska, New Jersey, New York, Nevada, Oklahoma, Pennsylvania, South Dakota, Texas, Utah, Washington

5
Outbreaks

representing 89% of reported cases this year

U.S. Measles Cases by Year

Fig. 3. Measles cases and outbreaks. [a] Provisional data reported to CDC's National Center for Immunization and Respiratory Diseases. [b] Updated once a month. (*From* CDC. Available at: http://www.cdc.gov/measles/cases-outbreaks.html. Accessed May 8, 2015.)

strategies for effective immunization were detailed in a previous update [23]. As with influenza, immunization of HCWs should also be an important consideration here.

HUMAN PAPILLOMAVIRUS

The CDC published 2 reports on sexually transmitted infections (STIs) in 2013 in the United States that estimated the human and economic burden of STIs in the United States [24,25]. The estimates showed that there are 20 million new STIs, with an estimated direct medical cost of 16 billion dollars annually [26]. HPV infection accounts for approximately two-thirds of these new STIs, 90% of which would resolve spontaneously; however, approximately 10% may lead to potentially serious diseases such as cervical cancer.

Unfortunately, the uptake of HPV vaccine in children and adolescents remains abysmal. Multiple studies addressing the barriers to HPV vaccination that detail the attitudes and concerns among health care providers as well as among parents and patients have been published. Some of them are founded in fact, such as those related to costs, whereas others such as the vaccine's effect

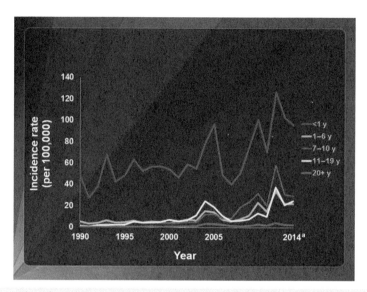

Fig. 4. Reported pertussis incidence (per 100,000 persons) by age group in the United States from 1990 to 2014. Infants younger than 1 year, who are at greatest risk for severe disease and death, continue to have the highest reported rate of pertussis. School-aged children 7 to 10 years continue to contribute a significant proportion of reported pertussis cases. [a] 2014 Data are provisional. (*From* CDC. National notifiable diseases surveillance system and supplemental pertussis surveillance system. Available at: http://www.cdc.gov/pertussis/surv-reporting.html. Accessed May 8, 2015.)

on sexual behavior are misplaced. However, these misperceptions continue to exert a pervasive negative effect on vaccine uptake and immunization rates [27–29]. Physician recommendation also remains less than optimal. Concerns about vaccine costs as well as lack of time to educate parents about the vaccine continue to top the list of physician concerns when surveyed about factors related to low vaccine recommendation rates particularly among low- and middle-income patient populations [30]. There also seems to be a geographic variation in HPV vaccine uptake in the United States, with 13- to 17-year-old girls in the southern states less likely to initiate and complete the 3-part vaccine series [31]. In addition to race, ethnicity and income also affect vaccine uptake, and although low-income and minority populations are as likely to initiate HPV vaccination, they are less likely to complete the vaccine series and also less likely to receive provider vaccine recommendation [32,33]. To further complicate matters, vaccine coverage in populations with Medicaid is also less than optimal, suggesting that at least in this population factors other than cost may play an important role in suboptimal immunization rates [34].

Immunization of male patients is another challenging issue. Data show that the vaccine is immunogenic against the vaccine strains and affords good protection [35]. The vaccine also showed reduced rates of anal intraepithelial neoplasia in men who have sex with men with no safety concerns [36]. There is a need for ongoing public and provider education and reinforcement as to the importance of vaccination against HPV. Parental questions about need for vaccination are best addressed by explaining the different modalities by which HPV can be acquired and by ongoing education [37].

Discussions are ongoing to consider possibly changing the current recommended HPV vaccine schedule from a 3-dose to 2-dose schedule in the United States. There is immunologic basis for this recommendation. The bivalent HPV vaccine is already approved in Europe for a 2-dose schedule. The quadrivalent HPV vaccine, although not approved in Europe for a 2-dose schedule, was favorably reviewed by the European drug approval agency for a 2-dose schedule. Some provinces in Canada are also using a 2-dose schedule, and a 2-dose schedule is also under consideration in Mexico. Strategic Advisory Group of Experts (SAGE) of the World Health Organization (WHO) has already made the recommendation for a 2-dose schedule for HPV vaccine for girls if the vaccination is initiated before age 15 years.

A new 9-valent HPV vaccine (Gardasil 9; Merck & Co, Inc, Whitehouse Station, NJ, USA) approved by the FDA includes the 4 HPV types 6, 11, 16, and 18 contained in Gardasil and an additional 5 HPV types 31, 33, 45, 52, and 58. These additional HPV types protect against an additional 20% of cervical cancers that the previous vaccines did not cover. Gardasil 9 has been approved for females aged 9 through 26 years and males aged 9 through 15 years. It is to be administered in 3 doses, with the same schedule as the quadrivalent HPV vaccine. ACIP recommendations should be forthcoming [38].

PNEUMOCOCCAL VACCINES

Two pneumococcal conjugate vaccines (PCVs) have been introduced during the last 2 decades. The 7-valent PCV (PCV7) was introduced in 2000, and subsequently, the 13-valent PCV (PCV13) was introduced in 2010. As expected, rates of invasive pneumococcal disease (IPD) decreased after the introduction of the PCV7; however, there were sharp relative increases in nonvaccine serotypes, specifically 19A and 6C [39]. PCV13 contains 6 additional serotypes (1, 3, 5, 6A, 7F, and 19A) accounting for 67% of IPD in US children younger than 5 years in 2007 [40]. Some early trends have shown decreases in PCV13 serotype–associated disease [41]. Initial data also suggest that nonvaccine serotypes are more common in children with CMCs who continue to be at greater risk of hospitalization and morbidity from IPD than healthy children [42]. Further, a Poisson model used to assess progress in the prevention of IPD in the United States after introduction of PCV13 also suggests that the amount of serotype replacement as a result of PCV13 is unlikely to greatly affect the overall number of cases prevented by the vaccine [43].

In addition to being used for vaccination of normal healthy children, PCV13 is also recommended for vaccination of adults 65 years and older as well as for individuals 19 years or older with underlying CMC that predispose them to IPD such as human immunodeficiency virus infection, leukemia, lymphoma, severe kidney disease, and organ transplantation [44].

Given that PCV13 has been used only in clinical practice since 2010, ongoing active surveillance will further reveal the long-term effects on IPD both in adults and children, as well as the effects on pneumococcal carriage.

A recently published article studied models for changing the current dosing schedule of 4 doses of the conjugated pneumococcal vaccine to a 3-dose schedule [45]. Some experts have serious reservations about changing the current conjugated pneumococcal vaccine schedule in the United States. A 3-dose PCV schedule is already standard in 21 high-income and 13 upper middle-income countries, with decrease in IPD in those countries. Some Canadian provinces and some countries had switched from a 4-dose to a 3-dose PCV with a no negative impact on IPD. There are, however, no direct comparisons of a 3-dose with a 4-dose PCV schedule. The article determined that changing the schedule from 4 doses to 3 doses in the United States may only slightly increase IPD from its current level and may cause a very slight increase in IPD-related mortality.

GLOBAL IMMUNIZATION ACHIEVEMENTS AND CHALLENGES

Globally, many challenges remain as far as vaccine-preventable diseases are concerned, and new ones are constantly emerging such as mentioned earlier, namely, EVD. However, there have also been some achievements to celebrate. Many malaria vaccine candidates remain in development, with one from GlaxoSmithKline (Middlesex, UK) the RTS,S currently in phase 3 studies, making it the first such vaccine candidate to advance this far [46]. In addition, India was certified polio-free by the WHO in March 2014. Given the considerable challenges and population of more than 1 billion in India, eradication of polio in that country was considered a near-insurmountable task by many. Now polio is endemic only in Pakistan, Afghanistan, and Nigeria [47]. Nigeria seems to be on the verge of being polio-free. However, major challenges remain in Afghanistan and Pakistan. The other good news about polio eradication is that wild poliovirus type 2 has been eradicated from circulation, allowing for the change in the oral polio vaccine from a trivalent to a bivalent vaccine. WHO has developed a comprehensive, long term strategy, the polio Eradication and Endgame Strategic Plan 2013–18 with the goal to deliver a polio free world by 2018. This is a multi-pronged approach which includes the transition from OPV to IPV as well as the transition from trivalent OPV to bivalent OPV [48].

At present, India is preparing to introduce the pentavalent vaccine (DTP, Hib, and hepatitis B vaccines) to further conquer other vaccine-preventable diseases in that country.

There is also a new vaccine against Japanese encephalitis virus manufactured in China, which would be more readily available to children in developing countries and can be given as a single dose [49].

Ongoing challenges include the eradication of polio from the 3 previously mentioned polio-endemic countries and the long-standing WHO goal of eradication of measles. Given the lack of an animal reservoir, it was expected that measles eradication was achievable.

The outbreak of EVD in Africa has presented yet another opportunity for vaccine development. Other emerging but not entirely new viruses, such as Chikungunya, Enterovirus D-68, although not vaccine preventable at this point, give scientists and vaccine developers much food for thought.

TYPHOID VACCINE

Typhoid vaccines have been available for decades. Although immunization with the typhoid vaccine may not prevent infection, it does enhance resistance to developing typhoid fever disease. Two typhoid vaccines are available; however, there is no vaccine against *Salmonella* Paratyphi A, B, and C (another major agent that causes enteric fever) available currently. The previously available typhoid and paratyphoid A and B (TAB) vaccine is no longer available because the components were ineffective. Although the FDA has approved both available typhoid vaccines for use in children, the lower ages of cutoffs are different for the 2 vaccines. The Vi capsular polysaccharide (ViCPS) vaccine is approved starting at age 2 years or older and the live oral TY21a vaccine for use in children 6 years or older. Typhoid vaccine is recommended for individuals in the United States traveling to areas of the world where they may be at risk of exposure to *Salmonella* Typhi, people with intimate exposure to a documented typhoid fever carrier, laboratory workers with frequent contact with *Salmonella* Typhi, and people living in areas outside the United States with endemic typhoid infection [50].

The efficacy of the oral Ty21a vaccine is estimated to be 35% in the first year and 58% in the second year postimmunization. The cumulative efficacy of the vaccine for the first 3 years postvaccination is approximately 55%. On the other hand, the efficacy of the ViCPS vaccine is estimated to be 69% for the first year and 59% for the second year after immunization. For ViCPS vaccine, there was no benefit in the third year after receiving the vaccine [51]. (For more details, please see the *Salmonella* article by Bula-Rudas and colleagues elsewhere in this issue.)

The WHO recommends use of typhoid vaccine to control typhoid disease and outbreaks. In the 48 countries of the WHO's Southeast Asian and Western Pacific regions where typhoid is common, between 2009 and 2013, only 23 countries collected data on typhoid cases and 9 countries implemented some sort of a typhoid vaccination program or recommended vaccine use. Most of these countries targeted high-risk groups and/or food handlers. In addition, 11 countries reported that the typhoid vaccine was used in the private sector. Three countries initiated public sector typhoid vaccination programs before 2008, targeting preschool or school-aged children in selected geographic areas. One country implemented a narrow school-based vaccine program in 2011, with plans to expand the program to school-aged children and food handlers. In addition, in one country a mass typhoid vaccination campaign was conducted [52].

YELLOW FEVER VACCINE

For travelers, there is some good news; the long-standing recommendation that booster doses were required after 10 years for yellow fever vaccine no longer holds true.

Yellow fever is a mosquito-borne disease responsible for 200,000 cases annually with 30,000 deaths. The case fatality rate for severe yellow fever disease is 20% to 50%. Only 1 yellow fever vaccine is approved and available in the United States (YF-Vax, Sanofi Pasteur, Inc, Swiftwater, PA, USA). This vaccine is approved for 1 subcutaneous dose followed by a booster every 10 years for individuals traveling to or living in an area where there is a risk for yellow fever infection and for laboratory workers who may be at risk for exposure to yellow fever virus. This vaccine is recommended for the first dose at age 9 months or older. There are no human studies to determine the efficacy of yellow fever vaccine, and no correlate of protection from yellow fever infection has been determined.

Since 1965, International Health Regulations (IHR) of the WHO has allowed countries to require yellow fever vaccine for permission to entry. More than 540 million doses of yellow fever vaccine have been distributed worldwide, with only 18 documented vaccine failures in vaccine recipients. SAGE has reviewed existing evidence and concluded that a single dose of yellow fever vaccine confers lifelong immunity against yellow fever disease [53]. In April 2013, SAGE recommended that only 1 dose of yellow fever vaccine is sufficient and no booster dose is necessary. The World Health Assembly of the WHO adopted the recommendations of IHR to remove the booster dose requirements starting June 2016. At this time, ACIP still recommends a booster dose of yellow fever vaccine every 10 years. ACIP is also considering changing the decennial yellow fever vaccine requirements. In addition, ACIP has asked the Committee on Infectious Diseases of the AAP for their recommendations for booster doses in children.

EBOLA VIRUS VACCINE

The outbreak of EVD in Africa has brought renewed attention to the development of Ebola virus vaccine and doubling up on the efforts to get a human vaccine approved for use in humans [54]. Several Ebola virus vaccines have been studied in rodents and nonhuman primates with encouraging results [55]. Several investigational vaccines are potential candidates for human trials, and a few of them are advanced enough in their development that they will be evaluated in humans. The most promising vaccines are recombinant Adenovirus vector (rAd3; GlaxoSmithKline, Middlesex, UK, and the US National Institute of Health), recombinant vesicular stomatitis virus (rVSV; NewLink Genetic, Ames, IA, USA, and Public Health Administration of Canada), and MVA-BN (Bavarian Nordic, Kvistgaard, Denmark, and Johnson & Johnson, New Brunswick, NJ, USA) and are being fast tracked for clinical trials.

SUMMARY

With all the new vaccines and strategies for prevention, the most important challenge that one continues to talk about globally and at home is the one presented by ongoing transmission of diseases for which excellent vaccines already exist. As pediatricians, this presents a constant reminder to keep the conversation about the importance of vaccine-preventable diseases with the patients and their families going at every possible opportunity possible. One needs to constantly remind oneself that every case of a vaccine-preventable disease is a missed opportunity for prevention. One must also have a broader perspective for global eradication of vaccine-preventable disease and advocate for availability of vaccines globally at affordable cost and encourage local vaccine development.

References

[1] American Academy of Pediatrics, Committee on Infectious Diseases. Recommendations for prevention and control of influenza in children, 2014–2015. Pediatrics 2014;134: 1–17.

[2] CDC. 2013–2014 Influenza season. Questions and answers. Available at: http://www.cdc.gov/flu/pastseasons/1314season.htm. Accessed October 25, 2014.

[3] Epperson S, Blanton L, Kniss K, et al, Influenza Division, National Center for Immunization and Respiratory Diseases, CDC. Influenza activity - United States, 2013–2014 season and composition of the 2014–2015 influenza vaccines. MMWR Morb Mortal Wkly Rep 2014;63:483–90.

[4] Centers for Disease Control and Prevention. Influenza associated pediatric mortality. Fluview. Available at: http://gis.cdc.gov/GRASP/Fluview/PedFluDeath.html. Accessed October 26, 2014.

[5] CDC Weekly US Influenza Surveillance Report. 2014–2015 Influenza Season Week 16 ending April 25, 2015. Available at: http://www.cdc.gov/flu/weekly/index.htm. Accessed May 7, 2015.

[6] Centers for Disease Control and Prevention. Prevention and control of seasonal influenza with vaccines: recommendations of the Advisory Committee on Immunization Practices (ACIP) - United States, 2014–15 influenza season. MMWR Morb Mortal Wkly Rep 2014;63:691–7.

[7] Mirza A, Subedar A, Fowler SL, et al. Influenza vaccine: awareness and barriers to immunization in families of children with chronic medical conditions other than asthma. South Med J 2008;101:1101–5.

[8] Pandolfi E, Marino MG, Carloni E, et al. The effect of physician's recommendation on seasonal influenza immunization in children with chronic diseases. BMC Public Health 2012;12:984–9.

[9] Stewart AM, Cox MA. State law and influenza vaccination of health care personnel. Vaccine 2013;31:827–32.

[10] Miller BL, Ahmed F, Lindley MC, et al. Increases in vaccination coverage of healthcare personnel following institutional requirements for influenza vaccination: a national survey of U.S. hospitals. Vaccine 2011;29:9398–403.

[11] Reichert TA, Sugaya N, Fedson DS, et al. The Japanese experience with vaccinating school children against influenza. N Engl J Med 2001;344:889–96.

[12] Kwong JC, Ge H, Rosella LC, et al. School-based influenza vaccine delivery, vaccination rates, and healthcare use in the context of a universal influenza immunization program: an ecological study. Vaccine 2010;28:2722–9.

[13] Kwong JC, Stukel TA, Lim J, et al. The effect of universal influenza immunization on mortality and health care use. PLoS Med 2008;5:e211–23.

[14] Ottenberg AL, Wu JT, Poland GA, et al. Vaccinating healthcare workers against influenza: the ethical and legal rationale for a mandate. Am J Public Health 2011;101:212–6.

[15] Centers for Disease Control and Prevention. Prevention and control of meningococcal disease: recommendations of the advisory committee on immunization practices (ACIP). MMWR Recomm Rep 2013;62:1–22.

[16] Mirza A, Rathore MH. Immunization update III. Adv Pediatr 2011;58:41–64.

[17] FDA News Release. First vaccine approved by FDA to prevent serogroup B meningococcal disease. Available at: http://www.fda.gov/NewsEvents/Newsroom/PressAnnouncements/ucm420998.htm. Accessed November 11, 2014.

[18] FDA News Release: FDA approves a second vaccine to prevent serogroup B meningococcal disease. Available at: http://www.fda.gov/NewsEvents/Newsroom/PressAnnouncements/ucm431370.htm. Accessed May 8, 2015.

[19] Trumenba® - meningococcal group B vaccine. Full prescribing information. Available at: http://labeling.pfizer.com/ShowLabeling.aspx?id=1796. Accessed November 12, 2014.

[20] Centers for Disease Control and Prevention. Measles. Available at: http://www.cdc.gov/measles/. Accessed November 9, 2014.

[21] Centers for Disease Control and Prevention. Herd immunity thresholds for selected vaccine preventable diseases. Available at: http://www.bt.cdc.gov/agent/smallpox/overview/intro-to-smallpox.pdf. Accessed November 10, 2014.

[22] Centers for Disease Control and Prevention. 2013 Final pertussis surveillance report. Available at: http://www.cdc.gov/pertussis/downloads/pertuss-surv-report-2013.pdf. Accessed November 12, 2014.

[23] Mirza A, Rathore MH. Immunization update IV. Adv Pediatr 2013;60:11–31.

[24] Satterwhite CL, Torrone E, Meites E, et al. Sexually transmitted infections among U.S. women and men: Prevalence and incidence estimates, 2008. Sex Transm Dis 2013;40:187–93.

[25] Owusu-Edusei K, Chesson HW, Gift TL, et al. The estimated direct medical cost of selected sexually transmitted infections in the United States, 2008. Sex Transm Dis 2013;40:197–201.

[26] Centers for Disease Control and Prevention. Incidence, prevalence and cost of sexually transmitted infections in the United States. Available at: http://www.cdc.gov/std/stats/STI-Estimates-Fact-Sheet-Feb-2013.pdf. Accessed November 2014.

[27] Holman DM, Benard V, Roland KB, et al. Barriers to human papillomavirus vaccination among US adolescents: a systematic review of the literature. JAMA Pediatr 2014;168:76–82.

[28] Hendry M, Lewis R, Clements A, et al. "HPV? Never heard of it!": a systemic review of girls' information needs, views and preferences about human papillomavirus vaccination. Vaccine 2013;31:5152–67.

[29] Perkins RB, Clark JA, Apte G, et al. Missed opportunities for HPV vaccination in adolescent girls: a qualitative study. Pediatrics 2014;134:e666–74.

[30] Bruno DM, Wilson TE, Gany F, et al. Identifying human papillomavirus vaccination practices among primary care providers of minority, low-income and immigrant patient populations. Vaccine 2014;32:4149–54.

[31] Rahman M, McGrath CJ, Berenson AB. Geographic variation in human papillomavirus vaccination uptake among 13–17 year old adolescent girls in the United States. Vaccine 2014;32:2394–8.

[32] Heudin P, Liveright E, Del Carmen MG, et al. Race, ethnicity, and income factors impacting human papillomavirus vaccination rates. Clin Ther 2014;36:24–37.

[33] Niccolai LM, Mehta NR, Hadler JL. Racial/ethnic and poverty disparities in human papillomavirus vaccination completion. Am J Prev Med 2011;41:428–33.

[34] Vadaparampil ST, Staras SA, Malo TL, et al. Provider factors associated with disparities in human papillomavirus vaccination among low income 9 to 17 year old girls. Cancer 2013;119:621–8.

[35] Goldstone SE, Jessen H, Palefsky JM, et al. Quadrivalent HPV vaccine efficacy against disease related to vaccine and non-vaccine types in males. Vaccine 2013;31:3849–55.

[36] Palefsky JM, Giuliano AR, Goldstone S, et al. HPV vaccine against anal HPV infection and anal intraepithelial neoplasia. N Engl J Med 2011;365:1576–85.

[37] Grimes RM, Benjamins LI, Williams KL. Counseling about the HPV vaccine: desexualize, educate and advocate. J Pediatr Adolesc Gynecol 2013;26:243–8.

[38] FDA. Approval of Gardasil 9. Available at: http://www.fda.gov/NewsEvents/
     Newsroom/PressAnnouncements/ucm426485.htm. Accessed December 12, 2014.
[39] Centers for Disease Control and Prevention. Invasive pneumococcal disease in children five
     years after conjugate vaccine introduction – eight states, 1998–2005. MMWR Morb Mor-
     tal Wkly Rep 2008;57:144–8.
[40] Pilishvili T, Laxau C, Farley MM, et al. Sustained reductions in invasive pneumococcal dis-
     ease in the era of conjugate vaccine. J Infect Dis 2010;201:31–41.
[41] Kaplan SL, Barson WJ, Lin PL, et al. Early trends in invasive pneumococcal infections in
     children after the introduction of the 13-valent pneumococcal conjugate vaccine. Pediatr
     Infect Dis J 2013;32:203–7.
[42] Iron Tam PY, Madoff LC, Coombes B, et al. Invasive pneumococcal disease after implemen-
     tation of 13-valent conjugate vaccine. Pediatrics 2014;134:210–7.
[43] Link-Gelles R, Taylor T, Moore MR, et al. Forecasting invasive pneumococcal disease trends
     after the introduction of the 13-valent pneumococcal conjugate vaccine in the United States,
     2010–2010. Vaccine 2013;31:2572–7.
[44] Centers for Disease Control and Prevention. Pneumococcal vaccination. Available at:
     http://www.cdc.gov/pneumococcal/vaccination.html. Accessed November 11,
     2014.
[45] Stoecker C, Hampton LM, Link-Gelles R, et al. Cost-effectiveness of using 2 vs 3 primary
     doses of 13-valent pneumococcal conjugate vaccine. Pediatrics 2013;132:e324.
[46] World Health Organization. Questions and answers on malaria vaccines. Available at:
     http://www.who.int/immunization/research/development/malaria_vaccine_qa/en/.
     Accessed November 12, 2014.
[47] World Health Organization. Poliomyelitis. Available at: http://www.who.int/media
     centre/factsheets/fs114/en/. Accessed November 12, 2014.
[48] Polio Global Eradication Initiative: Polio Eradication and Endgame Strategic Plan 2013–
     2018. Available at: http://www.polioeradication.org/resourcelibrary/strategyandwor-
     k.aspx. Accessed May 8, 2015.
[49] World Health Organization. Japanese encephalitis virus. Available at: http://www.who.int/
     mediacentre/news/releases/2013/japanese_encephalitis_20131009/en/. Accessed
     November 12, 2014.
[50] Committee on Infectious Diseases. Salmonella infections. In: Kimberlin DW, Brady MT,
     Jackson MA, et al, editors. Red Book: 2015 Report of the Committee on Infectious Diseases.
     Elk Grove Village (IL): American Academy of Pediatrics; 2015. p. 695–702.
[51] Anwar E, Goldberg E, Fraser A, et al. Vaccines for preventing typhoid fever. Cochrane Data-
     base Syst Rev 2014;(1):CD001261.
[52] Centers for Disease Control and Prevention. Typhoid fever surveillance and vaccine use—
     South-East Asia and Western Pacific Regions, 2009–2013. MMWR Morb Mortal Wkly Rep
     2014;63(39):855–60.
[53] World Health Organization. Yellow fever. Available at: http://www.who.int/media
     centre/news/releases/2013/yellow_fever_20130517/en/. Accessed November 12,
     2014.
[54] Levine MM, Tapia M, Hill AV, et al. How the current West African Ebola virus disease
     epidemic is altering views on the need for vaccines and is galvanizing a global effort to
     field-test leading candidate vaccines. J Infect Dis 2015;211:504–7.
[55] Marzi A, Feldmann H. Ebola virus vaccines: an overview of current approaches. Expert Rev
     Vaccines 2014;13(4):521–31.

Advances in Pediatrics 62 (2015) 29–58

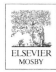

ADVANCES IN PEDIATRICS

Salmonella Infections in Childhood

Fernando J. Bula-Rudas, MD[a],
Mobeen H. Rathore, MD, CPE, FPIDS[a,b,c,*],
Nizar F. Maraqa, MD, FPIDS[a]

[a]Pediatric Infectious Diseases and Immunology, University of Florida College of Medicine-Jacksonville, 653-1 West 8th Street, LRC-3, Pediatrics, L-13, Jacksonville, FL 32209, USA; [b]Infectious Diseases and Immunology, University of Florida Center for HIV/AIDS Research, Education and Service (UF CARES), 653-1 West 8th Street/LRC-3, Pediatrics, L-13, Jacksonville, FL 32209, USA; [c]Pediatric Infectious Diseases, Wolfson Children's Hospital, 800 Prudential Drive, Jacksonville, FL 32207, USA

Keywords

- Salmonellosis • Nontyphoidal *Salmonella* • Typhoid • Enteric fever

Key points

- *Salmonella* are gram-negative bacilli within the family Enterobacteriaceae. They are the cause of significant morbidity and mortality worldwide.
- Animals (pets) are an important reservoir for nontyphoidal *Salmonella*, while humans are the only natural host and reservoir for *Salmonella* Typhi.
- *Salmonella* infections are a major cause of gastroenteritis worldwide. They account for an estimated 2.8 billion cases of diarrheal disease each year.
- The transmission of *Salmonella* is frequently associated with the consumption of contaminated water and food of animal origin, and it is facilitated by conditions of poor hygiene.
- The most important measures to prevent the spread and outbreaks of *Salmonella* infections and typhoid fever are adequate sanitation protocols for food processing and handling as well as hand hygiene.
- In the United States, 2 vaccines are commercially available against *Salmonella* Typhi. The World Health Organization recommends the use of these vaccines in endemic areas and for outbreak control.

*Corresponding author. 653-1 West 8th Street/LRC-3, Pediatrics, L-13, Jacksonville, FL 32209. *E-mail address:* mobeen.rathore@jax.ufl.edu

0065-3101/15/$ – see front matter
http://dx.doi.org/10.1016/j.yapd.2015.04.005

INTRODUCTION

Salmonella species were discovered more than a century ago by the American scientist Salmon, after whom they are named. They are recognized worldwide as a common cause of childhood infections, particularly gastroenteritis, bacteremia, and typhoid (enteric) fever. *Salmonella* serotype Typhi and *Salmonella* serotype Paratyphi A, B, and C (ie, typhoidal *Salmonella*) are responsible for causing typhoid fever in humans, an illness that is most burdensome in the developing world. The World Health Organization (WHO) estimates 16 to 33 million cases of typhoid fever causing 500,000 to 600,000 deaths worldwide annually. In the United States, it is estimated that approximately 200 to 300 cases occur annually. In a surveillance report from 1999 to 2006 in the United States, a total of 1902 cases of typhoid fever and 3 deaths were recorded [1]. The majority (about 80%) of cases in the United States are acquired while traveling internationally, especially to countries in south-central Asia.

Nontyphoidal *Salmonella* (NTS) species, which are found widely in animals, are estimated to cause more than 90 million illnesses worldwide and to account for approximately 155,000 deaths each year. In the United States, more than 40,000 NTS infections are reported annually to the Centers for Disease Control and Prevention (CDC); however, many milder illnesses go unreported, thus underestimating the true burden of these infections. Despite the mild and self-limiting nature of most NTS infections in healthy hosts, they are responsible for more than 450 US deaths annually [2]. The transmission of these organisms is frequently associated with the consumption of contaminated water and food of animal origin (eg, eggs, meat, dairy products), and to be facilitated by conditions characterized by poor hygiene. Young children are at risk for acquiring *Salmonella* infections, and young infants as well as children with certain underlying conditions (such as hemoglobin disorders, infection with human immunodeficiency virus [HIV], malignancy, or other causes of immune suppression) have an increased risk of severe disease and death from complications.

MICROBIOLOGY AND NOMENCLATURE

The organisms that belong to the genus *Salmonella* are motile, gram-negative, facultative anaerobic bacilli and are classified within the family Enterobacteriaceae. *Salmonella* organisms are not difficult to identify in the laboratory. These bacteria grow under both aerobic and anaerobic conditions. They ferment glucose but not lactose, are oxidase-negative, are indole-negative, and reduce nitrate to nitrite. Most *Salmonella* species produce hydrogen sulfide, a property commonly used for easy identification using selective media (eg, Salmonella-Shigella agar) [3].

The genus *Salmonella* consists of 2 species: *enterica* and *bongori*. Recently, DNA hybridization studies have suggested that most clinically important *Salmonella* organisms may be included into a single species: *Salmonella enterica* subspecies *enterica*. More than 2500 serotypes can be identified by serologic studies, which can be performed at reference laboratories, but serotyping is rarely of any clinical utility.

Microbiology laboratories use a combination of antigenic and biochemical reactions to further classify *Salmonellae*. Identification of serogroups is made by agglutination using antisera directed against specific O (somatic) antigens, which determine (but are not limited to) serogroups A, B, C_1, C_2, D, and E. Unique serotypes are then further characterized by reactions to other O (lipopolysaccharide), H (flagellar), and Vi (capsular) antigens.

Because the nomenclature of *Salmonella* may be very complex, and for better clarification, the CDC published guidelines for consistent terminology that provide easy interpretation for clinical and epidemiologic use, as shown in Table 1 [4]. For named serotypes, to emphasize that they are not separate species, the serotype name is not italicized and the first letter is capitalized. At the first citation of a serotype, the genus name "*Salmonella*" is given followed by the word "serotype" and then the serotype name (eg, *Salmonella* serotype Enteritidis). The word serotype may then be omitted from subsequent citations.

Salmonella organisms that cause typhoid fever belong to *S enterica* subspecies *enterica* serotype Typhi (*Salmonella* Typhi) and serotype Paratyphi (*Salmonella* Paratyphi) A–C. On the other hand, most (~ 80%) nontyphoidal *Salmonella* organisms responsible for human illness belong to *S enterica* subspecies *enterica* serotypes Typhimurium (ie, *Salmonella* serotype Typhimurium) and Enteritidis (ie, *Salmonella* serotype Enteritidis).

EPIDEMIOLOGY

Salmonella infections are a major cause of acute gastroenteritis worldwide, accounting for an estimated incidence of 2.8 billion cases of diarrheal disease each year. Because of the self-limited nature of most intestinal *Salmonella* infections, the data collected by public health authorities usually represent a fraction of the total cases. The WHO established the Foodborne Disease Burden Epidemiology Reference Group for the purpose of obtaining more accurate and representative data for these illnesses. However, estimating the global burden of *Salmonella* infections is hampered by the lack of sufficient health systems infrastructure in many countries, to support creating programs for the surveillance of food-borne illnesses. The epidemiology of NTS infections is quite different from that of typhoid fever. NTS infections have a worldwide distribution, whereas most typhoidal *Salmonella* infections in the United States are acquired abroad.

Table 1
Salmonella nomenclature

Complete name	CDC designation
Salmonella enterica subsp *enterica* ser Typhi	*Salmonella* ser Typhi
Salmonella enterica subsp *enterica* ser Paratyphi A	*Salmonella* ser Paratyphi A
Salmonella enterica subsp *enterica* ser Typhimurium	*Salmonella* ser Typhimurium
Salmonella enterica subsp *enterica* ser Enteritidis	*Salmonella* ser Enteritidis
Salmonella enterica subsp *enterica* ser Dublin	*Salmonella* ser Dublin

Abbreviations: subsp, subspecies; ser, serotype.

Nontyphoidal *Salmonella* in the United States

Nontyphoidal *Salmonella* infections in the United States increased steadily from World War II through the 1980s. There was a substantial decline seen in the mid-1990s; however, cases have increased again since the mid-2000s and more than 45,000 cases of nontyphoidal salmonellosis were reported annually by the CDC. Forty percent of these culture-proven infections occurred in children less than 15 years of age [5]. These figures continue to be an underestimate of the true incidence of NTS infections. In 2004, the Foodborne Diseases Active Surveillance Network (FoodNet), established in 1996 as a collaborative active surveillance program that involves 10 state public health departments, the CDC, US Food and Drug Administration (FDA), and the US Department of Agriculture, estimated that there are 39 cases of undocumented salmonellosis for every culture-confirmed case [6]. Since FoodNet started surveillance, from 1996 through 1999, about 1.4 million diarrheal illnesses annually are estimated to be attributed to *Salmonella* infections in the United States that account for approximately 15,000 hospitalizations and 400 deaths per year [7].

Salmonella infection was the most common food-borne–associated infection in 2010. Its incidence rate was 17.6 illnesses per 100,000 persons. Children aged less than 5 years had the highest incidence rate (69.5 infections per 100,000 children). *Salmonella* Enteritidis was the most common serotype isolated (22% of cases), followed by *Salmonella* Newport (14%) and *Salmonella* Typhimurium (13%) [8].

Among the food-borne disease outbreaks with confirmed or suspected cause reported to the CDC between 1998 and 2008, *Salmonella* species were the most common identified cause. NTS outbreaks were most commonly associated with poultry and eggs. Food products that contain raw or undercooked eggs can also be contaminated. The eggs may be contaminated in 2 ways: organisms on the shell surface penetrate the egg, or there may be a direct transovarian inoculation of the organism into the egg yolk. However, the egg-related *Salmonella* outbreaks have decreased over time due to extensive use of antimicrobials in the poultry industry and more strict preventive measures. In the United States, the current estimated frequency of egg contamination with *Salmonella* is 1 in 20,000 eggs.

In Great Britain, it is required by law that all hens be immunized against *Salmonella*. This protection measure, enacted in the late 1990s, has seen *Salmonella* cases in Britain drop from 14,771 in 1997 to just 581 cases in 2009. In the United States, the FDA provided guidance (nonbinding recommendations) for the industry regarding egg production, storage, and transportation. Various preventive measures are recommended and *Salmonella* vaccines are considered a very effective component of any *Salmonella* prevention program. However, the efficacy of a vaccination program depends on various parameters, some of which include the vaccination program used, effectiveness of administration by the vaccination crew, age of the birds when the vaccine is administered, and the local environmental load of *Salmonella*. If individual producers identified a vaccination program that is effective for their particular farms, the FDA would encourage the use of the program as an additional *Salmonella* prevention measure and not as a substitute to a more comprehensive prevention program (US Department of Health and Human Services Food and Drug Administration: Center for Food Safety and Applied Nutrition. August, 2012. Available at: http://www.fda.gov/downloads/Food/GuidanceRegulation/UCM313781.pdf).

Nontyphoidal *Salmonella* outbreaks have also been associated with fresh produce, meat, milk, peanut butter, spices, and other foods. Contamination has occurred at all points along the food-processing pathway. For example, one outbreak by *Salmonella* Enteritidis causing more than 200,000 cases nationwide was attributed to ice cream made in one state and then distributed nationally. The source of contamination was tankers used for transporting the ice cream base that were used previously to transport liquid eggs [9].

Most NTS infections are food-borne infections whose transmission is associated with agricultural products. However, transmission can also occur from contact with pet reptiles and amphibians (most commonly turtles, iguanas, frogs, lizards, snakes), live poultry, pet rodents (eg, hamsters, hedgehogs, mice, rats), cats and dogs, and even from handling pet foods. In Michigan, between January 2001 and June 2003, reptile-associated salmonellosis, mostly associated with turtles, was estimated to cause 12% of cases of salmonellosis in children 5 years of age or younger [10]. More recent outbreaks associated with small turtles have been reported. In October 2013, the CDC reported a multistate outbreak in which a total of 473 cases from 41 states occurred from May 23, 2011 to September 9, 2013. Most of the reported cases occurred in California (n = 106), New York (n = 55), and Texas (n = 45). The median age of the affected persons was 4 years. Seventy percent of ill persons were children 10 years of age or younger and 31% were infants 1 year of age or younger [11]. The sale of small turtles still occurs despite a federal law prohibiting it. Recommendations for people who have turtles as pets are available on the CDC Web site: http://www.cdc.gov/healthypets/pets/reptiles/turtles.html [12].

Live poultry has also been reported as a source of NTS infection. Between 2004 and 2011, 316 cases caused by *Salmonella* Montevideo were reported from multiple states mostly in children younger than 5 years of age who reported having purchased the live young poultry as pets. In early 2013, the national molecular subtyping network for food-borne bacteria, PulseNet, identified 4 clusters of human *Salmonella* infection. Many of these ill people reported contact with live poultry from a single mail-order hatchery of chicks and ducklings in Ohio. A total of 158 people from 30 states, 42% of whom were 10 years of age or younger, were reported to have been infected with these *Salmonella* serotypes: Infantis, Lille, Newport, and Mbandaka [13]. More recently, in May 2014, a new *Salmonella* outbreak was detected in the United States. At the time of writing this article, the outbreak seemed to have ended (last reported case was on September 27, 2014) after causing illness in 363 persons from 43 states and Puerto Rico. The outbreak was linked to live poultry from Mt. Healthy Hatcheries in Ohio. *Salmonella* Infantis, *Salmonella* Newport, and *Salmonella* Hadar were the serotypes identified. Children 10 years of age or younger accounted for 37% of the cases. Among 233 ill persons with available information, 76 (33%) were hospitalized and no deaths were reported [14].

A major reservoir of NTS is the gastrointestinal tract of asymptomatic animals that may contribute significantly to the public health burden attributed to NTS infections.

Symptoms of infection with NTS depend on the number of ingested bacteria. In general, the amount of bacteria that must be ingested for a healthy human host to have a symptomatic disease ranges from 10^6 to 10^8 organisms. In infants and immunocompromised children, disease can be caused by ingestion of a smaller bacterial inoculum. Direct, person-to-person transmission has also been documented, but is more likely to occur in hosts with compromised immunity [15]. Transplacental and perinatal infections following vaginal delivery have been reported to occur. Nosocomial infections may be associated with the use of contaminated medical equipment and therapeutic or diagnostic preparations, mainly those of animal origin.

Several risk factors have been associated with NTS infections in children. These risk factors include riding in a shopping cart with meat or poultry placed next to the child, exposure to reptiles, travel abroad, attending a childcare center with an infected infant, and ingestion of contaminated infant formula. Ingestion of contaminated infant formula is most likely related to the inappropriate storage and handling of opened cans of concentrated formula. Case control studies suggest that breast-feeding is a strong protective factor against acquiring *Salmonella* infection in infancy [16].

After infection with NTS and without antimicrobial treatment, the organism is excreted in feces for approximately 4 to 6 weeks. Although older children and adults excrete *Salmonella* in their stool for no more than 8 weeks following the infection, children younger than 5 years of age may have a more prolonged excretion for as long as 20 weeks after the illness. Extremes of age, immunosuppression, and antimicrobial therapy are well-established reasons for prolonged fecal excretion.

Nontyphoidal *Salmonella* outside the United States

The global burden of NTS gastroenteritis has been difficult to establish. In general, gastroenteritis is a major cause of morbidity and mortality around the world in both children and adults. Obtaining epidemiologic data from developing countries has been challenging because of insufficient surveillance systems in many of these countries. Also, the definitive diagnosis of NTS is made based on laboratory analysis and determination of serotypes; therefore, it mostly goes undiagnosed in persons who present with uncomplicated diarrheal illness. In fact, testing is performed only when the severity of the case requires more extensive evaluation and possibly hospital management. Laboratory-based surveillance systems, for adequate data collecting, require that an infected person must seek medical attention in a health care facility, submit a stool specimen, and have this laboratory-confirmed infection notified to public health authorities. Many countries lack such a system or the public health resources to support it.

In 2000, the global burden of typhoid fever was estimated by extrapolating available data to countries and regions where epidemiologic data were lacking. The WHO recommended a similar model for estimating the global burden of food-borne diseases, including NTS. In 2010, Crump and Mintz [17] estimated that 93.8 million illnesses worldwide were caused by NTS, of which more than 80 million were food-borne–associated. The total annual number of diarrheal illnesses was estimated to be around 2.8 billion with *Salmonella* infections representing approximately 3% of these illnesses [17,18]. Prospective studies that evaluate real incidence would be the gold standard to determine more accurate data regarding the burden of *Salmonella* infections. However, high cost precludes conducting such studies in many countries.

It is necessary to obtain more data about the burden of *Salmonella* infections worldwide because of the growth in mass production and distribution of food products. *Salmonella* infections in developing countries seem to be associated more with water contamination than being a food-borne–related illness. This fact is thought to be determined by more frequent contamination at the source of the produce as well as lack of disinfection during transport and during household storage. However, to determine more accurate data, there is a need for improvement in public health surveillance for food-borne illnesses, especially in Asia, Africa, and Latin America [18].

Typhoidal *Salmonella* (*Salmonella* Typhi and *Salmonella* Paratyphi)

In 2000, typhoid fever was estimated to have caused 21.6 million illnesses and 216,500 deaths globally. In 2010, a systematic review included data from 47 countries and estimated that 13.5 million episodes of typhoid fever occurred globally, which is comparable to a crude estimate of 10.8 million episodes. Such estimates are recognized to have important limitations, such as limited surveillance data from some regions of the world, particularly sub-Saharan Africa. Paratyphoid fever is estimated to have caused an additional 5.4 million illnesses in 2000 [19].

Typhoidal *Salmonella* is known to have a significant impact on impoverished children in developing countries despite the limitations of currently available epidemiologic data. According to worldwide surveillance, countries within south-central and southeast Asia (eg, Bangladesh, India, Indonesia, Nepal, Pakistan, and Vietnam) and southern Africa have the highest incidence of typhoid fever, estimated to be more than 100 cases per 100,000 population per year. Poor sanitation and lack of access to clean water in urban areas are the main reasons behind such high incidence. In rural areas, contaminated water is also the main risk factor for transmission. The incidence of typhoid fever is lower (10–100 cases per 100,000) in the rest of Asia, Africa, Latin America, and Oceania (excluding Australia and New Zealand) [19,20]. In Europe and North America, the incidence is lowest and its decline is attributed to the provision of clean water and development of more sophisticated sewage systems.

About 200 to 300 cases of *Salmonella* Typhi are reported each year in the United States, and most of these cases (around 80%) occur among travelers to regions where typhoid fever is endemic, mainly south-central Asia. Children account for about 40% of these cases [1]. Between 1997 and 2007, the GeoSentinel Surveillance Network reported 580 cases of vaccine-preventable diseases among international travelers from resource-rich countries. Typhoid fever was the most commonly reported disease among these travelers and only 38% of them had a pretravel clinical encounter [21].

Humans are the only natural host and reservoir for *Salmonella* Typhi. It can survive in any type of water for days and in contaminated eggs and frozen oysters for months. The amount of bacteria needed to cause infection ranges from a thousand to one million organisms, and most infections occur through the ingestion of food or water contaminated with human feces. Risk factors associated with the transmission of *Salmonella* Typhi include a history of contact with people infected with the organism, not using soap for hand washing, and poor personal hygiene. Other factors include consuming flavored iced drinks or food from street vendors, and eating raw fruits and vegetables either grown on fields fertilized with sewage or irrigated with contaminated water.

Paratyphoid fever requires higher infective doses of ingested organisms, and it is more likely to be acquired by consuming food from street vendors as opposed to household factors (eg, poor personal hygiene). In the United States, approximately 30% of *Salmonella* Paratyphi infections are related to exposure to chronic carriers. *Salmonella* Paratyphi is responsible for a growing proportion of enteric fever in many developing countries, especially in Asia [20].

There also seems to be a genetic predisposition to infection with *Salmonella* Typhi. A report from Vietnam in 2001 suggested that human leukocyte antigen (HLA)-linked genes play a role in determining susceptibility or resistance to this infection. No similar data have since been obtained from other ethnic groups, and future studies may help define common HLA genes and their role in susceptibility [20].

The National Typhoid Fever Surveillance conducted in the United States identified 1902 cases of typhoid fever between 1999 and 2006. More than half of the cases were reported from California, New York, and New Jersey. The age was known for 1685 of the cases reported. Among these, 64 cases (4%) were younger than 2 years, 205 (12%) were 2 to 5 years old, and 423 (25%) were 6 to 17 years old. The overall rate of travel-associated typhoid fever during this reporting period was 1.6 per 1,000,000 travelers arriving in the United States. Approximately 78% of the total cases reported visiting a single country. India, Pakistan, and Bangladesh (countries whose combined populations constitute approximately one-third of the world's population) were the countries visited by 67% of the patients with travel-associated typhoid infection. The surveillance also reported 391 domestically acquired cases. Approximately 17% of these cases were traced to a typhoid carrier, and 75 (22%) cases were part of typhoid outbreaks. Three such outbreaks were reported to the CDC Foodborne Outbreak Reporting System during this period: one outbreak in Texas with 6 confirmed cases from contaminated oysters harvested in the US Gulf Coast; one outbreak in Florida with 3 confirmed cases from beverages prepared from frozen imported fruit; and one outbreak in Maryland with 4 confirmed cases associated with a restaurant [1].

The most recent outbreak of *Salmonella* Typhi in the United States occurred in 2010: 12 cases were reported from 3 states (California, Nevada, and Oregon). This outbreak was associated with frozen mamey fruit pulp that is used to prepare smoothies. Nine of these cases required hospitalization, and no fatalities were reported [22].

PATHOGENESIS

Multiple risk factors present in a host may predispose to *Salmonella* infections, and in addition to the dose of organisms ingested, may determine the incubation period, symptoms, and severity of an acute *Salmonella* infection. Gastric acidity is the first defensive barrier to the ingested organism, and any situation that decreases the degree of acidity facilitates the survival of *Salmonella*. Neonates are particularly vulnerable to symptomatic salmonellosis because of their hypochlorhydria and rapid gastric emptying time. Immunocompromised hosts with altered cellular and humoral immune defenses are also vulnerable to severe *Salmonella* infections. Persons with sickle cell disease are particularly susceptible to developing septicemia and osteomyelitis with NTS because of impaired phagocytic and opsonizing capacity. Table 2 lists some of the principal predisposing factors to *Salmonella* infection or dissemination.

Table 2
Predisposing factors to *Salmonella* infection or dissemination

Impaired system	Condition
Gastrointestinal system	Achlorhydria
	Conditions with rapid gastric emptying
	Anatomic alterations of the stomach (eg, gastrectomy)
	Inflammatory bowel disease
	Alteration in normal gut flora from antimicrobial therapy
Immune system	Impaired cell-mediated immunity
	• HIV/AIDS
	• Malnutrition
	• Therapeutic agents (corticosteroids or other immunosuppressants)
	Impaired complement opsonization
	• Sickle cell anemia
	Defects of neutrophils
	• Chronic granulomatous disease
Reticuloendothelial system	Hemoglobinopathies
	• Hemolytic anemias (sickle cell anemia, thalassemia)
	• Malaria
	Malignancies
	• Leukemia
	• Lymphoma
Other	Schistosomiasis
	Solid tumors
	Gallbladder disease

Pathogenesis of nontyphoidal *Salmonella*

Salmonella are facultative intracellular pathogens that can survive within host macrophages. Most isolates of NTS cause inflammatory enterocolitis and diarrhea. They are rarely invasive beyond the lamina propria or the intestinal lymphatic system in immunocompetent hosts. However, serotypes like *Salmonella* Choleraesuis and *Salmonella* Dublin may cause bacteremia rapidly, with little or no intestinal involvement. In most instances, the acidic environment of the stomach easily eradicates *Salmonella* and other enteric pathogens. However, when exposed to a moderately acidic gastric environment, *Salmonella* organisms may become tolerant to acidity, an ability termed the acid tolerance response.

The organisms that survive the gastric acidity must then compete with the normal intestinal microbial flora for survival. The use of oral antimicrobials is associated with a reduction of the intestinal microbiota, which allows the *Salmonella* organisms to out-compete the normal gut microbiota and enhance their virulence in an inflammatory environment.

Adherence and invasion

Attachment to epithelial cells in the intestinal lumen is an important factor for survival of the pathogen and its subsequent invasion of the gastrointestinal tract. Multiple genes mediate adherence. Fimbriae and fimbrial operons facilitate adherence to the cell surface. The role of biofilm formation has been described as well. *Salmonella* attaches to the epithelial cells, called M (microfold) cells, which overlie the Peyer patches in the colon. The M cells have endocytic activity and they transfer the pathogen from the lumen to the basal area, triggering a rapid immune response. In vivo studies have also suggested that nonphagocytic cells, such as enterocytes, may also play a role internalizing *Salmonella*.

The invasion by *Salmonella* can also occur through the dendritic cells that extend between epithelial cells or through foci of solitary intestinal lymphoid tissues (SILTs) in the setting of a strong inflammatory response. A study performed on small intestines of a murine model suggested that foci of SILTs may act as portals of entry of *Salmonella* at early stages of infection [23]. After invading the cell, the pathogen is contained within a modified phagosome known as the *Salmonella*-containing vacuole, where it can survive and replicate, contributing to the microorganisms' ability to disseminate to the circulation and the reticuloendothelial system. The intracellular bacterial growth is limited by innate macrophage mechanisms. Thus, persons with impaired phagocytic activity, such as those with chronic granulomatous disease, are at risk for developing more severe, invasive NTS infections.

Inflammatory response and virulence

The interaction of the organism with host cells in the intestine usually triggers the activation of pro-inflammatory cytokines that attract neutrophils to the site and cause the symptoms of gastroenteritis. NTS induces migration of neutrophils to the gastrointestinal tract to facilitate its own uptake. The migration of neutrophils also causes the paracellular flux of fluids and electrolytes. This theory is supported by the fact that strains that usually do not cause enteritis, such as *Salmonella* Typhi, do not induce neutrophil migration. *Salmonella* also induces other proinflammatory cytokines, such as granulocyte macrophage-colony stimulating factor, monocyte chemotactic protein-1, and tumor necrosis factor-α. Certain features of the lipid A, present in *Salmonella*, may correlate with virulence or with activation of the immune response, the details of which are not yet fully elucidated.

Several genes related to virulence are also responsible for the severity of the disease. For example, most *Salmonella* carry an *iro* gene cluster (*iroN, iroBCDE*). These gene clusters can provide resistance to the peptide lipocalin 2 by encoding a lipocalin-resistant siderophore that supplies iron to the inflamed gut [24].

In addition, 2 *Salmonella* pathogenicity islands (SPI) have been identified and termed SPI-1 and -2. These SPIs are compounds of 40 kilobases of DNA that encode multiple virulence factors. One of these, called type III secretions systems, is responsible for injecting proteins into the targeted cells, facilitating the uptake of the bacteria into those cells. SPI-1 encodes for genes that trigger intestinal secretory and inflammatory responses. SPI-2 is only induced once *Salmonella* is within the cell, and its encoded products account for survival and replication within macrophages [25].

In addition, some strains of NTS carry plasmids that induce bacteremia and persistence within the reticuloendothelial system. *Salmonella* Typhimurium has a plasmid that increases the growth rate within the macrophages and also stimulates interleukin (IL)-12 production, which may lead to attenuated T-cell proliferation, as identified in mouse models [26].

Pathogenesis in immunocompromised hosts
Other host factors that predispose to severe NTS infection include impaired cell-mediated and humoral immunity as well as impaired phagocytic function. T-cell impaired immunity is a major factor in the predisposition to invasive NTS. This impairment is very well evidenced by the increased susceptibility to invasive NTS in HIV-infected individuals. In this population, there are 3 immunologic factors that contribute to the invasive presentation of NTS. First, the gastrointestinal tract is an important site where profound CD4 T-cell depletion occurs during HIV infection. With this depletion, several mechanisms of defense associated with cytokine production are altered, especially IL-17, -21, -22, and -26. These cytokines are important in maintaining the integrity of the epithelial mucosal barrier and in inducing epithelial cell expression of peptides, such as β-defensins and lipocalin, which play an antimicrobial role. Moreover, IL-17-producing T cells (Th17 cells) mediate neutrophil chemoattraction and therefore stimulate the immune response. Absence of these cells during HIV infection may explain the mechanism by which *Salmonella* disseminate from the gut and the lack of symptoms of enteritis and diarrheal disease during HIV-associated invasive NTS.

Second, persistence and recurrence of invasive NTS seem to be caused by altered cytokine production during intracellular infection. Quantitative blood and bone-marrow cultures revealed similar quantities of bacteria in both compartments in HIV-infected adults with invasive NTS at first presentation, but a 6 times greater concentration of *Salmonella* in bone marrow compared with blood during relapse. The latter suggests persistence and replication. More-over, bacterial load negatively correlates with cytokine concentrations and CD4 cell count. Therefore, failure of immunologic control allows *Salmonella* to escape from the intracellular compartment and then causes symptomatic relapse [24].

Third, humoral immunity is important for both serum and intracellular killing of *Salmonella*. However, the impairment seems to be associated more with the presence rather than the absence of immunoglobulin G antibodies directed against *Salmonella*. A study performed in Malawian adults infected with HIV showed that antibodies directed against *Salmonella* lipopolysaccharide impaired immunity by blocking or competing with coexisting effective bacteri-cidal antibodies directed against *Salmonella* outer membrane proteins [27].

Impaired phagocytic function increases the risk for NTS invasive infection. Children with chronic granulomatous disease, hemoglobinopathies, and ma-laria are the principal examples of this group. Phagocytic activity using lyso-somal enzymes and defensins limit the growth of *Salmonella* intracellularly. When impaired, phagocytic activity cannot limit this growth, which facilitates the dissemination of the microorganism from the submucosa to the circulation.

Pathogenesis of typhoidal *Salmonella*

Typhoid fever is a syndrome characterized by severe systemic illness with fever and abdominal pain that is classically associated with *Salmonella* Typhi. Never-theless, other *Salmonellae* may cause a similar syndrome (eg, *Salmonella* Paraty-phi A, *Salmonella* Schottmuelleri, *Salmonella* Choleraesuis). The term enteric fever refers mainly to both typhoid and paratyphoid fever. The pathogenesis of *Salmonella* Typhi shares similar aspects and predisposing factors with NTS infection. The mechanism for attachment to the intestinal epithelium is similar, and the severity of the infection depends on the amount of ingested organisms. Similar to NTS, individuals with predisposing conditions and immunosuppres-sion are at greater risk for typhoid fever and may present with more severe illness with smaller amounts of ingested organisms.

Unlike NTS, *Salmonella* Typhi does not trigger an early inflammatory response in the gut of the human host. *Salmonella* Typhi eludes this inflamma-tory response and uses a more subtle approach to invade and colonize different tissues of the body. The ingested organisms adhere to the intestinal epithelium of the small bowel and penetrate the mucosa through the lymphatic tissue of the Peyer patches. Subsequently, the organisms disseminate through the lymphatic system or via the bloodstream.

Salmonella Typhi uses 2 mechanisms for entering the submucosa; they can pass through the specialized antigen-sampling epithelial M cells or directly penetrate around the epithelial tissue [28,29]. The organism interacts with the cystic fibrosis transmembrane conductance regulator (CFTR) that partici-pates in the entry of *Salmonella* Typhi into the epithelial cell. A study in Indonesia performed genetic analysis of a case control cohort and showed that a specific polymorphism that affects CFTR seemed to confer modest protection against *Salmonella* Typhi [30].

Salmonella Typhi then recruits monocytes and lymphocytes, causing hypertrophy of the Peyer patches. This along with necrosis of the intestinal tissue may be the mechanisms responsible for the abdominal cramping and intestinal perforation seen in typhoid fever. The organisms engulfed by monocytes or macrophages reach the liver, spleen, and bone marrow via the bloodstream. Replication of the organism occurs within the reticuloendothelial system and manifests with the classic symptoms of severe malaise, hepatosplenomegaly, and generalized sepsis. This intestinal invasion and primary bacteremia occur within 24 hours of ingesting the organisms [31]. Dissemination of the *Salmonella* organisms through the bloodstream occurs mainly during the first week of illness and is characterized by frequent episodes of high-grade bacteremia [32]. As the clinical illness progresses, the organisms continue to be shed back into the bloodstream at lower levels of bacteremia throughout the course. In addition, the bone marrow is an important site for *Salmonella* Typhi replication, hence its importance as a diagnostic source for culture in the setting of a patient who has had a prolonged illness or who has already received antibiotic therapy [33].

The chronic carriage state is defined as excretion of the organism in stool or urine for more than 1 year after the acute infection. The mechanism for the persistence of *Salmonella* in the host seems to be associated with a particular allele present in the *Nramp1* and expressed on the macrophages of mice models [20,34]. In these models, mice that expressed the allele *Nramp1* did not die after oral inoculation with *Salmonella* Typhimurium but presented with persistent infection. The organism remained in small quantities mainly inside the macrophages of the reticuloendothelial system, and its reactivation was triggered by the administration of antibodies that neutralize interferon γ. The latter suggests a role for interferon γ in suppressing the replication of *Salmonella* [20,35].

CLINICAL MANIFESTATIONS
Nontyphoidal *Salmonella*
Nontyphoidal *Salmonella* generally causes a self-limited gastroenteritis in immunocompetent hosts in industrialized countries. However, a small percentage of individuals may present with invasive disease and extra-intestinal infections, such as meningitis and osteomyelitis, depending on special characteristics of the host and serotypes of the pathogen. Immunocompromised individuals are more susceptible to severe illness, and individuals with pre-existing anatomic abnormalities are prone to metastatic infection. In developing countries, NTS presents more commonly with a systemic disease that cannot be distinguished clinically from enteric fever. In these countries, children are more prone to develop serious complications from NTS infections. Herein, the focus is mainly on the clinical presentation of NTS in children residing within industrialized nations. The clinical features of NTS can be arranged into 4 main categories: acute gastroenteritis, bloodstream infection, extraintestinal focal infections, and asymptomatic carriage.

Acute gastroenteritis

Acute self-limiting gastroenteritis is the most common clinical presentation of NTS infection. Clinically, it presents with the similar features of any acute gastroenteritis caused by other pathogens. Symptoms include fever, abrupt onset of nausea and vomiting, abdominal cramping in the periumbilical and right lower quadrant area, followed by watery diarrhea. Stools are usually non-bloody, but dysentery can be present. The incubation period ranges from 6 to 72 hours after the ingestion of contaminated food or water. A higher dose of ingested bacteria correlates with more severe disease and prolonged duration of illness as discussed in previous sections. Clinical symptoms may be mild or the person may be asymptomatic; for this reason, the data about true incidence of infection are underestimated. A definitive diagnosis can be confirmed by stool culture. Dehydration and electrolyte imbalance are the most common complications of NTS gastroenteritis.

All symptoms usually resolve within 1 week in healthy hosts. Fever is likely to resolve within 48 to 72 hours, and diarrhea is expected to last no more than 10 days. If diarrhea persists, other diagnoses should be considered. In neonates, infants, and immunocompromised children, symptoms may persist for several weeks with an increased risk for complications. Bacteremia can occur in infants with NTS gastroenteritis and most require hospitalization. Bacteremia can lead to extra-intestinal manifestations, such as endocarditis, meningitis, and osteomyelitis [36]. Persons with ulcerative colitis infected with NTS may present with invasion of the bowel wall, toxic megacolon, systemic involvement, and death. Reactive arthritis, without clinical joint infection, following NTS gastroenteritis has been reported to occur in 2% of the cases. This complication is usually seen in individuals who possess the HLA-B27.

Bloodstream infection

Overall, transient bloodstream infection (BSI) occurs as a complication in 1% to 5% of patients with NTS gastroenteritis. *Salmonella* Choleraesuis, Heidelberg, and Dublin seem to be more invasive and are more frequently associated with bacteremia [37,38]. Antibiotic-resistant strains of *Salmonella* Typhimurium have been associated with a 2- to 3-fold increased risk of developing bacteremia [39]. The incidence and associated morbidity and mortality of NTS BSI depend on the age and presence of predisposing underlying conditions of the host. BSI occurs more frequently in infants as well as immunocompromised and malnourished children [40–42]. In the United States, the incidence of invasive NTS was estimated to be 7.8 cases per 100,000 infants less than 1 year of age [43]. These infants are also prone to developing metastatic foci of infection and death.

There is no reliable laboratory marker to predict which children with NTS infection will develop BSI. *Salmonella* bacteremia usually presents with fever or signs of sepsis, but it also has been reported in infants without such presentation. For this reason, there is an emphasis on obtaining a blood culture in infants with suspected or confirmed NTS gastroenteritis.

Immunocompromised children are at risk for developing serious focal infections during NTS BSI, such as meningitis, brain abscess, osteomyelitis, pyogenic arthritis, or pneumonia. Previously healthy children have a significantly lower risk (3%) of developing such focal infections compared with the immunocompromised (35%) [44,45]. In children with acquired immunodeficiency syndrome (AIDS), septicemia without an obvious focus may occur as a severe complication of NTS infection, despite antibiotic therapy. Patients who have underlying conditions associated with hemolytic anemia (eg, sickle cell disease or malaria) are at a higher risk for BSI. In Africa, the high prevalence of malaria has been established as an important predisposing factor for invasive NTS. Surveillance studies have identified *Salmonella* Typhimurium and *Salmonella* Enteritidis as the most common invasive serotypes. Invasive NTS infection can occur during pregnancy. The prognosis is good in otherwise healthy women, but transplacental transmission of the organism may lead to infection of the fetus and, possibly, to fetal death.

Focal nontyphoidal Salmonella *infections*

NTS is able to spread via the bloodstream to any organ during infection. Underlying anatomic abnormalities in the host potentiate the risk for metastatic infections. Moreover, children with underlying conditions such as sickle cell disease have an increased risk for focal infections. Infarcted bone in patients with sickle cell disease predisposes to the development of *Salmonella* osteomyelitis. *Salmonella* suppurative arthritis may also occur in individuals with preceding bone and joint trauma.

Infants with *Salmonella* BSI are at a particularly higher risk of developing *Salmonella* focal infection. Meningitis can occur in neonates and infants younger than 3 months of age and is associated with a high rate of mortality or neurologic sequelae in survivors [46]. Other focal infections include cholangitis and pneumonia, alone or as a co-infection with tuberculosis or *Streptococcus pneumoniae*.

Asymptomatic carriage

Asymptomatic fecal excretion of the *Salmonella* bacilli is very common after symptomatic or asymptomatic NTS infection. The duration of excretion seems to be longer after symptomatic infection, and it is common to have intermittent shedding. The average duration of excretion in patients less than 5 years of age is approximately 7 weeks. Eighteen percent of these children may have a positive stool culture 6 months after the initial infection. Therefore, routine follow-up stool cultures are not recommended after an uncomplicated NTS gastroenteritis in immunocompetent patients [47]. Younger age, symptomatic infection, treatment with antibiotics, and infection with a strain of *Salmonella* different than *Salmonella* Typhimurium were identified as factors associated with prolonged excretion [48]. Stool cultures that yield *Salmonella* should not suggest the need for treating NTS gastroenteritis with antibiotics. Although prolonged duration of *Salmonella* excretion has been demonstrated in some patients, this state of carriage does not seem to correlate with the development of antimicrobial resistance by the pathogen [49].

Chronic carriage of NTS is defined as the shedding of a *Salmonella* species for more than 1 year, confirmed by an initial positive stool culture from a sample obtained at least 1 month after resolution of acute gastroenteritis and then subsequent repeat positive cultures. Chronic carriage of NTS is uncommon in children; it has been reported to occur in 2.6% of children less than 5 years of age [47]. If chronic carriage is detected, eradication should only be attempted in special circumstances such as the presence of an immunosuppressed family member living in the same household.

Typhoid fever

The clinical manifestations of typhoid fever vary from an isolated fever to severe toxemia and involvement of multiorgan systems. Typhoid fever, also referred to as enteric fever, is classically associated with *Salmonella* Typhi and Paratyphi, but other *Salmonellae* can cause disease manifestations similar to this syndrome. The onset of symptoms usually develops between 5 to 21 days after ingestion of the pathogen. During the first week of illness, there is a stepwise occurrence of symptoms starting with low-grade fever that increases insidiously and eventually becomes unremitting. Febrile seizures may occur, especially in children. The fever is then followed by the appearance of other manifestations of systemic disease, such as headache, malaise, myalgia, and lethargy. Constipation may be an early feature of typhoid fever, and other gastrointestinal symptoms, which include abdominal pain, nausea, vomiting, or diarrhea, may soon follow. At this stage, typhoid fever is indistinguishable from other nonspecific systemic illnesses caused by bacterial or viral pathogens.

High fever with chills continues during the second week of illness and may last for up to 4 weeks if left untreated. Relative bradycardia at the peak of high fever is a more common sign of typhoid in adults than in children [50]. Diarrhea with blood and fecal leukocytes is more frequently seen in children, and hepatosplenomegaly may occur during the first weeks of the illness. In this stage, lethargy and headache are replaced by stupor. Skin manifestations, although uncommon, are characterized by the appearance of rose spots, mainly seen on the chest and abdomen but have been described on the extremities as well [51]. These small erythematous maculopapular lesions are particularly seen in people with fair skin and are present in a quarter of typhoid fever cases [20].

Intestinal manifestations are common during the third and fourth week of illness. In fact, some patients may not develop diarrhea until the third week. The diarrhea may not resolve until 6 weeks after the onset of symptoms. Malaise and lethargy may also continue for a couple of months. Complications of typhoid fever are likely to develop at this stage of the illness. Patients may present with intestinal bleeding and perforation (which may be heralded by a sudden rapid drop in body temperature), along with bacteremia and peritonitis. Septic shock and death may result as a consequence of such complications. Extra-intestinal complications have also been described. These complications may involve the central nervous system (eg, encephalomyelitis, meningitis,

Guillain-Barré syndrome, or cranial or peripheral neuritis), cardiovascular system (eg, endocarditis or myocarditis), respiratory system (eg, pneumonia or empyema), bones and joints (eg, osteomyelitis, arthritis, or dactylitis), hepatobiliary system (eg, cholecystitis or splenic and liver abscesses), and the genitourinary system (glomerulonephritis or pyelonephritis) [20,51].

In children, a viral infection can easily be confused with *Salmonella* Typhi infection [15]. Clinical manifestations may vary in severity from region to region and among children of different ages. In a review of 552 culture-confirmed cases of typhoid fever in Bangladesh, intestinal perforation was not seen in patients less than 5 years of age [52]. Children with typhoid fever in Chile [53] were described to have a mild illness that usually did not require hospitalization; cases of typhoid fever had a fatality rate of 11%, and in Pakistan [54], children younger than 5 years of age with typhoid fever seemed to have more severe disease.

Usually, after 4 weeks of the illness, fever begins to decline gradually. Asymptomatic fecal excretion of *Salmonella* continues after resolution of the illness and may last for several months. A few patients may become chronic carriers with prolonged fecal excretion. It is important to differentiate between convalescing excretors and chronic carriers because of the varying risk for transmission. Fecal excretion during convalescence is more likely to be a source for contamination of food or water and transmission to others than during chronic carriage. Chronic carriers have high serum antibody titers against the Vi antigen, which facilitates the rapid identification of these patients and differentiation from individuals convalescing from an acute infection [55].

DIAGNOSIS

Because *Salmonella* infections are clinically indistinguishable from similar illnesses caused by other pathogens, confirmatory cultures are required for a definitive diagnosis. Clinical manifestations and type of exposure may suggest the diagnosis, but the inflammatory diarrhea with fever caused by *Salmonella* can also be associated with enteric pathogens, such as *Shigella,* enteroinvasive or enterohemorrhagic *Escherichia coli, Campylobacter jejuni, Yersinia enterocolitica,* and *Clostridium difficile.* Moreover, systemic manifestations present in typhoid fever are similar to other infections that can present with insidious prolonged fever like malaria, tuberculosis, Epstein-Barr virus infection, tularemia, ehrlichiosis, histoplasmosis, amebic liver abscess, and plague, among others [15]. Epidemiologic and travel history are important to determine the risk of having typhoid fever.

Gastroenteritis caused by NTS is best diagnosed with stool specimens cultured in selective media that inhibit growth of normal flora. Stool specimens are preferred over rectal swabs. Enrichment broths can be used to enhance isolation of *Salmonella,* especially when the number of bacteria is low.

Typhoid fever and NTS BSIs are confirmed with positive blood cultures. The volume of blood obtained for the sample correlates directly with the sensitivity of the test. A minimum of 1 to 15 mL of blood should be obtained for culture depending on the child's weight and age [56]. Bone marrow culture is more sensitive (80%–95% sensitivity) than blood culture for the diagnosis of typhoid fever, especially in those patients who have had prolonged fever or have received antibiotics for several days. Despite its invasive nature, culture of the bone marrow is recommended by some experts for diagnosis of typhoid fever in patients with a prolonged fever without an identified source of infection [32].

Stool cultures have a low sensitivity for the diagnosis of typhoid fever (30%) and rely on the volume of feces cultured. To identify asymptomatic and chronic carriers, several stool samples should be obtained because shedding of the bacteria occurs irregularly. Use of the agglutination reaction to Vi capsular antigen has been described as a screening tool for chronic carriers of *Salmonella* Typhi. This test has a sensitivity of 70% to 80% and a specificity of 80% to 95% when used for this purpose. However, the test would have limitations in settings where Vi-based typhoid vaccine use is widespread [55].

The Widal test is a serologic test with limited value for the diagnosis of typhoid fever. It detects antibodies against the somatic (O) and flagellar (H) antigens of *Salmonella* Typhi. The use of this test is discouraged because of the varying sensitivity, specificity, and predictive values obtained from different geographic areas. Nevertheless, the Widal test has been found to be helpful when used with locally determined cutoff points [56].

DNA probes and polymerase-chain-reaction assays are newer methods for the diagnosis of typhoid fever and are available in research laboratories. In developing countries where typhoid fever is endemic, access to molecular tests is usually not available because of cost. Some algorithms based on clinical criteria have been developed but have not been validated [56].

Clinical Laboratory Standards Institute methods and interpretative criteria should be followed when testing *Salmonella* antimicrobial susceptibility, especially when multidrug-resistant (MDR) isolates are a concern. Ampicillin, trimethoprim/sulfamethoxazole, and a fluoroquinolone should be tested for *Salmonella* isolated from stool. Extra-intestinal isolates should also be tested for extended-spectrum cephalosporins. Traditionally, resistance to nalidixic acid has been used as a surrogate for reduced *Salmonella* susceptibility to fluoroquinolones; however, nalidixic acid–susceptible *Salmonella* Typhi with reduced susceptibility to ciprofloxacin has been described [20].

MANAGEMENT
Nontyphoidal *Salmonella*
General supportive care is the mainstay in managing uncomplicated gastroenteritis in healthy adults and children with NTS infection. Antimicrobials are not recommended for treatment of immunocompetent adults or children more than 1 year of age who present with mild to moderate gastroenteritis caused by *Salmonella*. This recommendation is supported by a meta-analysis of 12 trials that found no significant benefit from antibiotic therapy on the duration of illness, diarrhea, or fever [57]. Antibiotic therapy has not been shown to

shorten the duration of symptoms and in fact may prolong colonization and carrier stage. In infants less than 3 months of age, antimicrobial treatment is recommended because these patients are at higher risk for bacteremia and extra-intestinal complications such as meningitis and osteomyelitis [40–42,58]. Use of antimicrobials should also be considered in children with underlying medical conditions, such as HIV infection, primary immunodeficiency disorders, sickle cell anemia, chronic gastrointestinal disease, and cancer; nevertheless, the efficacy of this measure is unproven [57].

Antimicrobial therapy should be targeted according to local epidemiology and pattern of antimicrobial resistance of *Salmonella*. Agents that have shown in vitro and in vivo activity against *Salmonellae* include ampicillin, amoxicillin, tetracycline, macrolides, trimethoprim-sulfamethoxazole, chloramphenicol, and fluoroquinolones. Fluoroquinolones may be considered more effective in the treatment of immunocompromised patients because of their potent intracellular activity. However, fluoroquinolones are not approved by the FDA for this indication in people younger than 18 years of age and are not recommended unless the benefits of therapy outweigh the potential risks with use of the drug [58]. The 2012 meta-analysis for treating NTS infection did not find studies that evaluated the effect of fluoroquinolones in infants and young children [57]. Resistance to ampicillin, amoxicillin, and trimethoprim-sulfamethoxazole is more common in developing countries. In this scenario, ceftriaxone, cefotaxime, azithromycin, and fluoroquinolones are recommended.

Infants less than 3 months of age require a blood culture when there is a confirmed stool culture with *Salmonella* species, even if they are afebrile and their appearance is nontoxic (Fig. 1). A blood culture is recommended in the initial evaluation of nontoxic, afebrile infants with diarrhea of duration less than 5 days, if there are epidemiologic data that raises suspicion for infection with *Salmonella*. If the infant is febrile, hospital admission and parenteral antibiotics are recommended initially pending blood culture results because clinical severity and fever are not reliable predictors of bacteremia [36,42,59]. If the blood culture remains negative, it is recommended to treat these infants with parenteral antibiotics for 5 to 7 days. If the infant is ill-appearing or the blood culture is grows *Salmonella*, a lumbar puncture should be performed [60]. Duration of antibiotic therapy should be at least 10 to 14 days for bacteremia alone, 4 weeks for meningitis, and 4 to 6 weeks for osteomyelitis or other focal metastatic infections [15].

In infants between 3 and 12 months of age (Fig. 2), a stool culture should be obtained if there is diarrhea for 5 days' duration or more. If the stool culture is positive for NTS but the infant is afebrile, no antibiotic treatment is recommended. In a febrile but non-toxic-appearing infant, a blood culture is recommended if stool culture is positive, but antibiotics may be held until result of the blood culture is reported. If the child has a positive stool culture for *Salmonella* and is an immunocompromised host or is ill-appearing, hospital admission is recommended and a more extensive evaluation that includes blood culture,

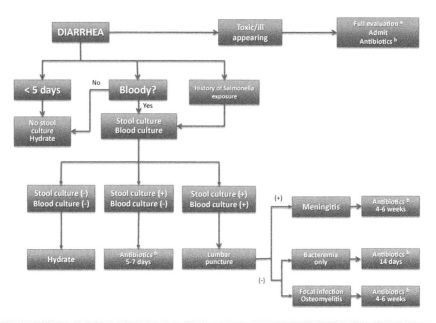

Fig. 1. Recommended management of nontyphoidal *Salmonella* infections in infants 0 to 3 months of age. [a]Evaluation for focal infection of meninges, bone, urinary tract, or other sites. [b]Cefotaxime or ceftriaxone.

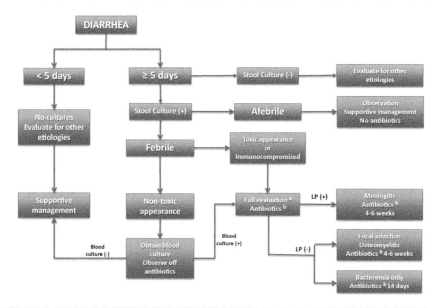

Fig. 2. Recommended management of nontyphoidal *Salmonella* infection in infants 3 to 12 months of age. [a]Evaluation for focal infection of meninges, bone, urinary tract, or other sites. [b]Cefotaxime or ceftriaxone.

lumbar puncture, and initiation of parenteral antibiotics should be undertaken. Duration of antibiotic treatment is similar to that recommended in infants less than 3 months of age and according to the results of cultures.

When osteomyelitis is a consideration, adequate bone imaging should be obtained for diagnosis. Osteomyelitis should be highly suspected in children with sickle cell disease. The usual length of treatment of *Salmonella* osteomyelitis is 4 to 6 weeks.

A third-generation cephalosporin (ceftriaxone or cefotaxime) is the treatment of choice and should be included for empiric treatment in persons with localized invasive disease (eg, osteomyelitis, abscess, meningitis, or bacteremia in HIV-infected patients). Antibiotic treatment should be extended beyond the minimum recommended length of therapy for the specific infection treated to reduce the chance of relapse (eg, at least 4 weeks of antibiotic therapy for *Salmonella* meningitis) [58].

Typhoid fever

Typhoid fever is not endemic in the United States, and a high index of suspicion for enteric fever should be based on a comprehensive history that includes travel to endemic areas or contact with possible chronic carriers of *Salmonella*. Prompt empiric antibiotic therapy is recommended in children to decrease fatality rates and likelihood of complications. Parenteral therapy should be reserved for those who are severely ill or who present with complications [61].

Antibiotic treatment of typhoid fever has become challenging because of the emergence of strains of *Salmonella* that are resistant to the classically used first-line agents: ampicillin, trimethoprim-sulfamethoxazole, and chloramphenicol. However, these remain the agents of choice for a fully susceptible strain of *Salmonella* Typhi. The choice of antibiotics for the empiric management of typhoid fever depends on the variable resistance patterns of *Salmonella* Typhi according to geographic location. More recent recommendations include an extended spectrum cephalosporin, azithromycin, or a fluoroquinolone as drugs of choice for empiric treatment pending susceptibility test results. Selecting which class of antibiotic to use should depend on local resistance patterns, age of the patient, and severity of illness. A single antibiotic agent is sufficient, as combination therapy has not been demonstrated to have superior efficacy [62]. It is appropriate to use oral antibiotic agents following parenteral administration when symptoms improve.

The appropriate duration of treatment with a third-generation cephalosporin in children with typhoid fever has not been conclusively determined, but a course of treatment for 10 to 14 days is usually recommended. A shorter, 7-day course has been suggested by some authors, but randomized trials in Pakistan and Egypt reported relapse in approximately 15% of children within 1 month of completing therapy with ceftriaxone [63].

In the United States, the Report of the Committee on Infectious Diseases of the American Academy of Pediatrics recommends the use of a third-generation cephalosporin (ceftriaxone, cefotaxime, or cefixime), azithromycin, or a fluoroquinolone (ciprofloxacin or ofloxacin) depending on the geographic area and the likelihood of being infected by an MDR *Salmonella* Typhi strain. The dosage, route, and duration of recommended antibiotics for the treatment of typhoid fever are shown in Table 3. Fluoroquinolones in the United States are not approved by the FDA for this indication in patients younger than 18 years of age, and their use is not recommended unless benefits of therapy outweighs the risks of using these drugs [58]. The concerns from use of fluoroquinolones in children are based on the cartilage toxicity attributed to these drugs in studies with beagles. Nevertheless, large series studies of children for whom fluoroquinolones have been used for treatment of typhoid fever report no evidence of adverse effects on growth, bone, or joints. A prospective cohort study in more than 300 Vietnamese children between 1 and 14 years of age, who were followed up for 2 years after receiving a short course of treatment with either ciprofloxacin for 7 days or ofloxacin for 3 to 5 days, found no evidence of acute joint toxicity nor joint symptoms attributable to fluoroquinolones. Moreover, in the same study, there was no difference found in height velocity when the groups who received fluoroquinolones were compared with children who were not known to become infected nor received treatment with these agents [64]. Based on these data, most experts agree that in areas where MDR *Salmonella* Typhi strains are common, fluoroquinolones are safe and efficacious (when susceptible) for treatment of enteric fever in children [65].

Salmonella Typhi isolates should be tested for resistance to nalidixic acid, ciprofloxacin, or ofloxacin because of emerging resistance to fluoroquinolones. Nalidixic acid–resistant *Salmonella* Typhi (NARST) strains have decreased ciprofloxacin susceptibility and seem to be treated less efficiently with a short course of fluoroquinolones. A single chromosomal mutation in the quinolone resistance region of the *gyr*A gene may be sufficient to reduce the susceptibility to ciprofloxacin. Ciprofloxacin susceptibility may also be reduced without exhibiting resistance to nalidixic acid [17,66]. Because of limited resources in

Table 3
Antibiotic regimens used for typhoid fever treatment in children in the United States

Drug[a]	Dose (mg/kg/d)	Route	Duration (d)
Ceftriaxone	100	IV	10–14
Cefotaxime	150–200	IV	10–14
Cefixime	20	IV	10–14
Ciprofloxacin	30	PO or IV	7–10
Ofloxacin	30	PO or IV	7–10
Azithromycin	10–20	PO or IV	5–7
Amoxicillin	100	PO	14
TMP-SMX	8–12 (TMP)/40–60 (SMX)	PO or IV	14
Chloramphenicol	75	IV	14–21

Abbreviations: IV, intravenous; PO, oral; TMP-SMX, trimethoprim-sulfamethoxazole.
[a]When *Salmonella* Typhi is susceptible.

the developing countries, susceptibility testing may not be easily available and NARST treatment should be considered with drugs other than fluoroquinolones.

The use of corticosteroids might be beneficial in patients with symptoms of severe enteric fever (delirium, obtundation, stupor, coma, or shock). This indication is based on a randomized, double-blind, prospective study in the 1980s that compared the use of chloramphenicol alone versus in combination with dexamethasone. The use of dexamethasone was associated with a significantly lower mortality (10% vs 55%) [67]. The dose of intravenous dexamethasone is the same for adults and children: an initial dose of 3 mg/kg, followed by 1 mg/kg every 6 hours for a total of 48 hours [58,68,69]. Relapses of typhoid fever can occur, even in immunocompetent patients, typically 2 to 3 weeks after resolution of the fever. A decrease in the rates of relapse has been observed because chloramphenicol is no longer considered the standard treatment of choice and is used less frequently or not at all. Studies performed with newer antibiotics and including for treatment of MDR *Salmonella* Typhi infections have shown a relapse rate of 1% to 6% compared with rates of 10% to 25% in the chloramphenicol era [70]. For treatment of relapses, an additional course of antibiotics using an agent with confirmed susceptibility is recommended.

Chronic carriage

Chronic carriage is not common in children. Most (80%–90%) chronic carriers can be successfully cured with a prolonged course of an antibiotic. Presence of gall-bladder stones may reduce the chance of success. The recommended therapy for chronic carriage of *Salmonella* in adult patients is ciprofloxacin. However, the chronic carriage state in children may be treated with high-dose (up to 100 mg/kg per day) oral ampicillin or amoxicillin in combination with probenecid for a total duration of 3 months. Other alternatives used include trimethoprim-sulfamethoxazole twice daily for 3 months or ciprofloxacin twice daily for 28 days [56].

PREVENTION
Nontyphoidal *Salmonella*

In general, the most important measures to prevent spread and outbreaks of *Salmonella* infections are adequate sanitation protocols for food transport and preparation, sanitation of water supplies and sewage disposal, appropriate hand hygiene, isolation of infected patients, and restriction of exposure of children younger than 5 years of age and immunocompromised hosts to reptile pets and rodents. Breast-feeding in young infants remains an important measure for protection from *Salmonella* infections [71]. There is no available vaccine against NTS. *Salmonella* infection is a notifiable disease and health care facilities must report cases to local public health authorities.

Strict industry protocols for food handling and transportation should be established because contaminated food products play a critical role in *Salmonella* infection outbreaks. Hand washing before handling food is a key factor. Eggs should be refrigerated for storing and cooked thoroughly before consumption. It is not recommended to ingest raw eggs or food containing raw eggs. Persons should not drink or consume unpasteurized milk or dairy products. Washing utensils and kitchen surfaces with soap and water after they have been in contact with raw meat or meat products is also important. It is recommended to cook thoroughly any food of animal origin, such as beef, pork, and poultry. Patients with salmonellosis should not prepare food, and many health departments in the United States require stool testing for restaurant workers with *Salmonella* infection to determine their carrier status before returning to work.

Reptile pets (turtles, iguanas, lizards, and snakes), ducklings, and mail-ordered chicks from hatcheries have caused important *Salmonella* outbreaks in the United States as noted in previous sections. For this reason, avoidance of these pets is recommended by the CDC. The sale of small turtles was banned in 1975 because they were identified as a common source of salmonellosis; nevertheless, they are still being sold, and cases associated with pet turtles are still being reported. Schools that keep pets in the classroom should avoid small turtles and other reptiles and must encourage hand-washing measures when children have contact with animals. Parents are advised to wash children's hands after handling pets.

Children who attend childcare centers and present with NTS infection need to be excluded until diarrhea resolves. There is no set requirement for negative stool cultures after NTS infection to be allowed to return to childcare. Similar recommendations apply for workers in childcare settings [58].

In the hospital setting, standard and contact precautions are recommended for symptomatic patients. Nonrandomized studies suggest the use of prophylactic antibiotics may control nosocomial *Salmonella* epidemics when used in addition to isolation measures. However, further validation of these results is needed before the routine use of prophylactic antibiotics can be recommended [47].

Typhoid fever

Enteric fever is acquired through the ingestion of food or water contaminated with *Salmonella*; therefore, handling food appropriately and having clean water and adequate sewage systems help prevent the transmission of the disease. For travelers to endemic areas, it is important to avoid consumption of food or water where sanitation measures and personal hygiene are poor. Typhoid immunization enhances resistance to developing typhoid fever but does not provide complete protection. Two vaccines are available against *Salmonella* Typhi, but there is no vaccine against *Salmonella* Paratyphi (another major agent that causes enteric fever). The Vi capsular polysaccharide (ViCPS) vaccine is approved by the FDA for use in children 2 years of age or older, and the live oral TY21a vaccine is approved for use in children 6 years of age or older (Table 4). In the United States, immunization is only recommended for travelers to areas where risk of exposure to *Salmonella* Typhi is recognized, people with intimate exposure to a documented typhoid fever carrier, laboratory

Table 4
Commercially available typhoid vaccines in the United States

Vaccine	Minimum age indicated (y)	Dose	Route	Booster dose	Adverse effects
Live-attenuated Ty21a (Vivotif)	6	1 capsule every 2 d for 4 doses	Oral	Every 5 y	Fever or headache (0%–5%)
ViCPS vaccine (Typhim Vi)	2	1 dose (25 μg)	Intramuscular	Every 2 y	Fever (0%–1%) Headache (1.5%–3%) Local reaction at site of injection (7%)

workers with frequent contact with *Salmonella* Typhi, and people living in areas outside the United States with endemic typhoid infection [58].

A systematic review in 2014 reported efficacy of the oral Ty21a vaccine between 35% and 58% at years 1 and 2 after one dose. The 3-year cumulative efficacy of the vaccine is approximately 55%. The efficacy or the ViCPS vaccine was 69% and 59% at year 1 and 2 after vaccination; however, no benefit was detected in the third year after vaccination [72]. Antimicrobials should be avoided for 7 days before or after vaccination with Ty21a. Both vaccines have caused mild adverse events that include fever, abdominal pain, nausea, vomiting, headache, rash, or urticaria. Local reaction, pain, and induration at the injection site are reported more commonly with the ViCPS vaccine. No serious adverse events have been attributed to either vaccine.

The WHO recommends the use of the ViCPS and Ty21a vaccines in endemic areas and for outbreak control. The recommendation for routine immunization of school-age children against *Salmonella* Typhi was released in a WHO statement in 2003. The statement supports the implementation of immunization for young children in areas where typhoid fever is a public health problem and where MDR strains of *Salmonella* Typhi have a significant prevalence [73]. The WHO also strongly recommends vaccination against typhoid fever during an outbreak as an effective tool for prevention. In addition, vaccination should be considered for those who already suffered from the disease if re-exposure is likely to occur, because natural infection does not provide lifelong immunity against *Salmonella* Typhi.

As a matter of practical concern, the available vaccines (ViCPS and Ty21a) are not ideal for use in wide-scale vaccination programs [74]. They require reimmunization every 2 to 3 years and are only indicated for persons 2 years of age or older. The urgent need for better control of typhoid fever leads to the development of a new agent by conjugation of the ViCPS vaccine with a nontoxic recombinant *Pseudomonas aeruginosa* exotoxin A. This vaccine has shown an efficacy of 91.5% in a double-blind, randomized trial in approximately 11,000 children between the ages of 2 and 5 years, from an area in Vietnam known to be endemic for typhoid fever. Further research is ongoing for evaluation and development of novel typhoid vaccines that are cheap, safe, and efficacious, especially among infants.

In a childcare setting, if a child or a staff member is identified with symptomatic *Salmonella* Typhi infection, the recommendation is to collect stool samples from all attendees and staff members and exclude all those who are infected. The length of exclusion depends on the age of the infected person. Generally, children younger than 5 years of age require 3 negative stool specimens before obtaining clearance to return to the site, whereas those 5 years of age and older should have 24 hours without a diarrheal stool before they are allowed to return. Local and state health departments should be consulted regarding regulations for testing and length of exclusion, because these may vary by jurisdiction [58].

SUMMARY

- *Salmonella* are gram-negative bacilli within the family Enterobacteriaceae. They are the cause of significant morbidity and mortality worldwide.
- Animals (pets) are an important reservoir for nontyphoidal *Salmonella*, whereas humans are the only natural host and reservoir for *Salmonella* Typhi.
- *Salmonella* infections are a major cause of gastroenteritis worldwide. They account for an estimated 2.8 billion cases of diarrheal disease each year.
- The transmission of *Salmonella* is frequently associated with the consumption of contaminated water and food of animal origin, and it is facilitated by conditions of poor hygiene.
- Nontyphoidal *Salmonella* infections have a worldwide distribution, whereas most typhoidal *Salmonella* infections in the United States are acquired abroad.
- In the United States, *Salmonella* is a common agent for food-borne–associated infections. Several outbreaks have been identified and are most commonly associated with agricultural products.
- Nontyphoidal *Salmonella* infection is usually characterized by a self-limited gastroenteritis in immunocompetent hosts in industrialized countries, but it may also cause invasive disease in vulnerable individuals (eg, children less than 1 year of age, immunocompromised).
- Antibiotic treatment is not recommended for treatment of mild to moderate gastroenteritis by nontyphoidal *Salmonella* in immunocompetent adults or children more than 1 year of age.
- Antibiotic treatment is recommended for nontyphoidal *Salmonella* infections in infants less than 3 months of age, because they are at higher risk for bacteremia and extraintestinal complications.
- Typhoid (enteric) fever and its potential complications have a significant impact on children, especially those who live in developing countries.
- Antibiotic treatment of typhoid fever has become challenging because of the emergence of *Salmonella* Typhi strains that are resistant to classically used first-line agents: ampicillin, trimethoprim-sulfamethoxazole, and chloramphenicol.
- The choice of antibiotics for the management of typhoid fever should be guided by the local resistance pattern. Recommendations include using an extended spectrum cephalosporin, azithromycin, or a fluoroquinolone.

- Fecal carriage of Salmonella is an important factor in the spread of the organism to healthy individuals.
- The most important measures to prevent the spread and outbreaks of *Salmonella* infections and typhoid fever are adequate sanitation protocols for food processing and handling as well as hand hygiene.
- In the United States, 2 vaccines are commercially available against *Salmonella* Typhi. The WHO recommends the use of these vaccines in endemic areas and for outbreak control.

References

[1] Lynch MF, Blanton EM, Bulens S, et al. Typhoid fever in the United States, 1999-2006. JAMA 2009;302(8):859–65.
[2] Scallan E, Hoekstra RM, Angulo FJ, et al. Foodborne illness acquired in the United States—major pathogens. Emerg Infect Dis 2011;17(1):7–15.
[3] Framer J. Enterobacteriaceae: introduction and identification. In: Murray P, Baron E, Pfaller M, et al, editors. Manual of clinical microbiology. Washington, DC: ASM Press; 1995. p. 438.
[4] Brenner FW, Villar RG, Angulo FJ, et al. Salmonella nomenclature. J Clin Microbiol 2000;38(7):2465–7.
[5] Hopkins RS, Jajosky RA, Hall PA, et al. Summary of notifiable diseases–United StateS, 2003. MMWR Morb Mortal Wkly Rep 2005;52(54):1–85.
[6] Centers for Disease Control and Prevention. Preliminary FoodNet data on the incidence of infection with pathogens transmitted commonly through food—10 states, 2009. MMWR Morb Mortal Wkly Rep 2010;59(14):418–22.
[7] Voetsch AC, Van Gilder TJ, Angulo FJ, et al. FoodNet estimate of the burden of illness caused by nontyphoidal Salmonella infections in the United States. Clin Infect Dis 2004;38(Suppl 3):S127–34.
[8] Centers for Disease Control and Prevention. Vital signs: incidence and trends of infection with pathogens transmitted commonly through food—foodborne diseases active surveillance network, 10 U.S. sites, 1996–2010. MMWR Morb Mortal Wkly Rep 2011;60(22):749–55.
[9] Hennessy TW, Hedberg CW, Slutsker L, et al. A national outbreak of Salmonella enteritidis infections from ice cream. The Investigation Team. N Engl J Med 1996;334(20):1281–6.
[10] Wells EV, Boulton M, Hall W, et al. Reptile-associated salmonellosis in preschool-aged children in Michigan, January 2001-June 2003. Clin Infect Dis 2004;39(5):687–91.
[11] CDC - Eight multistate outbreaks of human salmonella linked to small turtles - salmonella. Available at: http://www.cdc.gov/salmonella/small-turtles-03-12/index.html. Accessed November 23, 2014.
[12] Turtles kept as pets | healthy pets healthy people | CDC. Available at: http://www.cdc.gov/healthypets/pets/reptiles/turtles.html. Accessed November 23, 2014.
[13] Notes from the field: Multistate outbreak of human salmonella infections linked to live poultry from a mail-order hatchery in Ohio — March–September 2013. Available at: http://www.cdc.gov/mmwr/preview/mmwrhtml/mm6310a4.htm?s_cid=mm6310a4_w. Accessed November 23, 2014.
[14] Salmonella infections linked to live poultry | May 2014 | salmonella | CDC. Available at: http://www.cdc.gov/salmonella/live-poultry-05-14/index.html. Accessed November 23, 2014.
[15] Reller M. Salmonella species. In: Long S, Pickering L, Prober C, editors. Principles and practices of pediatric infectious diseases. 4th edition. Philadelphia: Elsevier; 2012. p. 814–9.
[16] Jones TF, Ingram LA, Fullerton KE, et al. A case-control study of the epidemiology of sporadic Salmonella infection in infants. Pediatrics 2006;118(6):2380–7.
[17] Crump JA, Mintz ED. Global trends in typhoid and paratyphoid fever. Clin Infect Dis 2010;50(2):241–6.

[18] Majowicz SE, Musto J, Scallan E, et al. The global burden of nontyphoidal Salmonella gastroenteritis. Clin Infect Dis 2010;50(6):882–9.

[19] Crump JA, Luby SP, Mintz ED. The global burden of typhoid fever. Bull World Health Organ 2004;82(5):346–53.

[20] Bhan M, Bahl R, Bhatnagar S. Typhoid and paratyphoid fever. Lancet 2005;366(9487): 749–62.

[21] Boggild AK, Castelli F, Gautret P, et al. Vaccine preventable diseases in returned international travelers: results from the GeoSentinel surveillance network. Vaccine 2010;28(46): 7389–95.

[22] Loharikar A, Newton A, Rowley P, et al. Typhoid fever outbreak associated with frozen mamey pulp imported from guatemala to the western United States, 2010. Clin Infect Dis 2012;55(1):61–6.

[23] Halle S, Bumann D, Herbrand H, et al. Solitary intestinal lymphoid tissue provides a productive port of entry for Salmonella enterica serovar typhimurium. Infect Immun 2007;75(4): 1577–85.

[24] Feasey NA, Dougan G, Kingsley RA, et al. Invasive non-typhoidal salmonella disease: an emerging and neglected tropical disease in Africa. Lancet 2012;379(9835): 2489–99.

[25] Hensel M, Shea JE, Waterman SR, et al. Genes encoding putative effector proteins of the type III secretion system of Salmonella pathogenicity island 2 are required for bacterial virulence and proliferation in macrophages. Mol Microbiol 1998;30(1):163–74.

[26] Chiu CH, Chu C, Ou JT. Lack of evidence of an association between the carriage of virulence plasmid and the bacteremia of Salmonella typhimurium in humans. Microbiol Immunol 2000;44(9):741–8.

[27] MacLennan CA, Gilchrist JJ, Gordon MA, et al. Dysregulated humoral immunity to nontyphoidal Salmonella in HIV-infected African adults. Science 2010;328(5977):508–12.

[28] Kops SK, Lowe DK, Bement WM, et al. Migration of Salmonella typhi through intestinal epithelial monolayers: an in vitro study. Microbiol Immunol 1996;40(11):799–811.

[29] Tartera C, Metcalf ES. Osmolarity and growth phase overlap in regulation of Salmonella typhi adherence to and invasion of human intestinal cells. Infect Immun 1993;61(7):3084–9.

[30] van de Vosse E, de Visser AW, Al-Attar S, et al. Distribution of CFTR variations in an Indonesian enteric fever cohort. Clin Infect Dis 2010;50(9):1231–7.

[31] House D, Bishop A, Parry C, et al. Typhoid fever: pathogenesis and disease. Curr Opin Infect Dis 2001;14(5):573–8.

[32] Wain J, Pham VB, Ha V, et al. Quantitation of bacteria in bone marrow from patients with typhoid fever: relationship between counts and clinical features. J Clin Microbiol 2001;39(4):1571–6.

[33] Gasem MH, Dolmans WM, Isbandrio BB, et al. Culture of Salmonella typhi and Salmonella paratyphi from blood and bone marrow in suspected typhoid fever. Trop Geogr Med 1995;47(4):164–7.

[34] Vidal S, Tremblay ML, Govoni G, et al. The Ity/Lsh/Bcg locus: natural resistance to infection with intracellular parasites is abrogated by disruption of the Nramp1 gene. J Exp Med 1995;182(3):655–66.

[35] Monack DM, Bouley DM, Falkow S. Salmonella typhimurium persists within macrophages in the mesenteric lymph nodes of chronically infected Nramp1+/+ mice and can be reactivated by IFNgamma neutralization. J Exp Med 2004;199(2):231–41.

[36] Sirinavin S, Jayanetra P, Lolekha S, et al. Predictors for extraintestinal infection in Salmonella enteritis in Thailand. Pediatr Infect Dis J 1988;7(1):44–8.

[37] Mandal BK, Brennand J. Bacteraemia in salmonellosis: a 15 year retrospective study from a regional infectious diseases unit. BMJ 1988;297(6658):1242–3.

[38] Jones TF, Ingram LA, Cieslak PR, et al. Salmonellosis outcomes differ substantially by serotype. J Infect Dis 2008;198(1):109–14.

[39] Varma JK, Molbak K, Barrett TJ, et al. Antimicrobial-resistant nontyphoidal Salmonella is associated with excess bloodstream infections and hospitalizations. J Infect Dis 2005;191(4):554–61.

[40] Hyams JS, Durbin WA, Grand RJ, et al. Salmonella bacteremia in the first year of life. J Pediatr 1980;96(1):57–9.

[41] Meadow WL, Schneider H, Beem MO. Salmonella enteritidis bacteremia in childhood. J Infect Dis 1985;152(1):185–9.

[42] Rice PA, Craven C, Wells JG. Salmonella heidelberg enteritis and bacteremia. An epidemic on two pediatric wards. Am J Med 1976;60(4):509–16.

[43] Vugia DJ, Samuel M, Farley MM, et al. Invasive Salmonella infections in the United States, FoodNet, 1996-1999: incidence, serotype distribution, and outcome. Clin Infect Dis 2004;38(Suppl 3):S149–56.

[44] Graham SM. Nontyphoidal salmonellosis in Africa. Curr Opin Infect Dis 2010;23(5): 409–14.

[45] Gordon MA. Invasive nontyphoidal Salmonella disease: epidemiology, pathogenesis and diagnosis. Curr Opin Infect Dis 2011;24(5):484–9.

[46] Appelbaum PC, Scragg J. Salmonella meningitis in infants. Lancet 1977;309(8020): 1052–3.

[47] Haeusler GM, Curtis N. Non-typhoidal Salmonella in children: microbiology, epidemiology and treatment. Adv Exp Med Biol 2013;764:13–26.

[48] Buchwald DS, Blaser MJ. A review of human salmonellosis: II. Duration of excretion following infection with nontyphi Salmonella. Rev Infect Dis 1984;6(3):345–56.

[49] Nelson JD, Kusmiesz H, Jackson LH, et al. Treatment of Salmonella gastroenteritis with ampicillin, amoxicillin, or placebo. Pediatrics 1980;65(6):1125–30.

[50] Davis TM, Makepeace AE, Dallimore EA, et al. Relative bradycardia is not a feature of enteric fever in children. Clin Infect Dis 1999;28(3):582–6.

[51] Huang DB, DuPont HL. Problem pathogens: extra-intestinal complications of Salmonella enterica serotype Typhi infection. Lancet Infect Dis 2005;5(6):341–8.

[52] Butler T, Islam A, Kabir I, et al. Patterns of morbidity and mortality in typhoid fever dependent on age and gender: review of 552 hospitalized patients with diarrhea. Rev Infect Dis 1991;13(1):85–90.

[53] Edelman R, Levine MM. Summary of an international workshop on typhoid fever. Rev Infect Dis 1986;8(3):329–49.

[54] Siddiqui FJ, Rabbani F, Hasan R, et al. Typhoid fever in children: some epidemiological considerations from Karachi, Pakistan. Int J Infect Dis 2006;10(3):215–22.

[55] Lanata CF, Levine MM, Ristori C, et al. Vi serology in detection of chronic Salmonella typhi carriers in an endemic area. Lancet 1983;2(8347):441–3.

[56] Parry CM, Hien TT, Dougan G, et al. Typhoid fever. N Engl J Med 2002;347(22): 1770–82.

[57] Onwuezobe IA, Oshun PO, Odigwe CC. Antimicrobials for treating symptomatic nontyphoidal Salmonella infection. Cochrane Database Syst Rev 2012;(11):CD001167.

[58] Committee on Infectious Diseases. Salmonella infections. In: Pickering L, Baker C, Kimberlin D, et al, editors. Red book: 2012 report of the committe on infectious diseases. 29th edition. Elkgrove Village (IL): American Academy of Pediatrics; 2012. p. 634–40.

[59] Geme J, Hodes H, Marcy S, et al. Consensus: management of Salmonella infection in the first year of life. Pediatr Infect Dis J 1988;7(9):615–22, (11/23/2014).

[60] Christenson JC. Salmonella infections. Pediatr Rev 2013;34(9):375–83.

[61] Stephens I, Levine MM. Management of typhoid fever in children. Pediatr Infect Dis J 2002;21(2):157–8.

[62] Meltzer E, Stienlauf S, Leshem E, et al. A large outbreak of Salmonella Paratyphi A infection among israeli travelers to Nepal. Clin Infect Dis 2014;58(3):359–64.

[63] Frenck RW Jr, Nakhla I, Sultan Y, et al. Azithromycin versus ceftriaxone for the treatment of uncomplicated typhoid fever in children. Clin Infect Dis 2000;31(5):1134–8.

[64] Bethell DB, Hien TT, Phi LT, et al. Effects on growth of single short courses of fluoroquinolones. Arch Dis Child 1996;74(1):44–6.

[65] White NJ, Dung NM, Vinh H, et al. Fluoroquinolone antibiotics in children with multidrug resistant typhoid. Lancet 1996;348(9026):547.

[66] Humphries RM, Fang FC, Aarestrup FM, et al. In vitro susceptibility testing of fluoroquinolone activity against Salmonella: recent changes to CLSI standards. Clin Infect Dis 2012;55(8):1107–13.

[67] Hoffman SL, Punjabi NH, Kumala S, et al. Reduction of mortality in chloramphenicol-treated severe typhoid fever by high-dose dexamethasone. N Engl J Med 1984;310(2):82–8.

[68] McGowan J, Chesney P, Crossley K, et al. Guidelines for the use of systemic glucocorticosteroids in the management of selected infections. J Infect Dis 1992;165(1):1–13.

[69] Punjabi NH, Hoffman SL, Edman DC, et al. Treatment of severe typhoid fever in children with high dose dexamethasone. Pediatr Infect Dis J 1988;7(8):598–600.

[70] Girgis NI, Sultan Y, Hammad O, et al. Comparison of the efficacy, safety and cost of cefixime, ceftriaxone and aztreonam in the treatment of multidrug-resistant Salmonella typhi septicemia in children. Pediatr Infect Dis J 1995;14(7):603–5.

[71] France GL, Marmer DJ, Steele RW. Breast-feeding and Salmonella infection. Am J Dis Child 1980;134(2):147–52.

[72] Anwar E, Goldberg E, Fraser A, et al. Vaccines for preventing typhoid fever. Cochrane Database Syst Rev 2014;(1):CD001261.

[73] World Health Organization. WHO. 2003. WHO Technical Report Series/Immunizations, Vaccines and Biologicals. Report No.: V&B/03.07.

[74] von Seidlein L. The need for another typhoid fever vaccine. J Infect Dis 2005;192(3):357–9.

Advances in Pediatrics 62 (2015) 59–90

ELSEVIER
MOSBY

ADVANCES IN PEDIATRICS

Childhood Tuberculosis
An Overview

Diala Faddoul, MD

Descanso Pediatrics, Huntington Medical Foundation, 1346 Foothill Boulevard Suite 201,
La Canada, CA 91011, USA

Keywords
- Childhood tuberculosis • *Mycobacterium tuberculosis* • Tuberculin skin test
- Interferon-γ release assay

Key points
- Tuberculosis (TB) is one of the oldest diseases known to mankind and still ranks as the second leading cause of death from infection worldwide.
- Transmission of *Mycobacterium tuberculosis* occurs person to person via inhalation of mucous droplets that become airborne when an individual with pulmonary or laryngeal TB coughs, sneezes, speaks, laughs, or sings.
- Even though TB incidence in the United States is low, pediatricians in this country should always consider TB as cause of a child's symptoms, especially those who traveled to endemic areas.
- The Centers for Disease Control and Prevention guidelines indicate that a tuberculin skin test (TST) or an interferon-γ release assay (IGRA) may be used to test for latent TB infection. An IGRA is preferred over the TST when testing people who are Bacille-Calmette-Guérin (BCG) vaccinated or are unlikely to return for TST reading.
- Multidrug-resistant TB strains are resistant to isoniazid and rifampin, while extensively drug-resistant TB is also resistant to fluoroquinolones and at least one of the second-line injectable drugs (amikacin, kanamycin, and capreomycin).
- BCG vaccine protects young children against severe forms of the disease (eg, TB meningitis) and disseminated TB. It has variable efficacy against pulmonary TB.

INTRODUCTION

Is it tuberculosis (TB) or another pulmonary process? Is it latent or active TB? If it is active TB, is it due to a susceptible or resistant strain? Will my pediatric patient tolerate the drug regimen that was prescribed without having side effects? How did this bacillus manage to survive millions of years in nature and thousands of years in our bodies and make best use of our immune

E-mail address: dalo_dadoy@hotmail.com

0065-3101/15/$ – see front matter
http://dx.doi.org/10.1016/j.yapd.2015.04.001

system? Will there ever be a vaccine as good as the polio vaccine to eradicate TB? All these and more questions are addressed in this article, starting with a brief historical overview, then moving to the most recent World Health Organization (WHO) report that was released in 2014. Next is the pathogenesis section, with reference to Tobin's work and the utilization of the zebrafish model in trying to elucidate how this organism takes over our immune system in the smartest of ways to survive. This article then addresses the challenges that clinicians face in trying to make the correct diagnosis and choosing the right drug regimen in light of the finding that techniques to diagnose and check drug susceptibilities have been lacking in sensitivity. The emerging concern of multidrug-resistant (MDR) and extensively drug-resistant (XDR) TB is discussed as well. Finally, this article addresses what the future holds in regards to new vaccines in clinical trials.

HISTORY

TB is one of the oldest diseases known to mankind [1]. It is possible that the genus Mycobacterium originated more than 150 million years ago and that a progenitor of *Mycobacterium tuberculosis* (Mtb) was present in East Africa as early as 3 million years ago. It is likely that all modern members of the *Mycobacterium tuberculosis* complex (MTBC), including not only Mtb but also its African variants *M africanum* and *M canettii* as well as *M bovis* had a common African ancestor about 35,000 to 15,000 years ago [2]. Recent work based on phylogenetic analysis of Mtb strains goes further to suggest that Mtb has been infecting humans for more than 70,000 years [3].

Given the long historical relationship between TB and humans, it may seem surprising that TB still ranks as the second leading cause of death from infection worldwide. However, the long coevolution of the human immune system with Mtb may also explain the remarkable ability of this bacterium to evade the immune response.

In Egypt, TB was documented more than 5000 years ago with evidence of Pott deformities in Egyptian mummies in early Egyptian art. There are written texts as well describing TB in India and China 3300 and 2300 years ago, respectively [2]. In Greece, it was called phthisis, and Hippocrates wrote in his *Book I, Of the Epidemics*: "Consumption was the most considerable of the diseases which then prevailed, and the only one which proved fatal to many persons" [2]. In the middle ages, scrofula was treated with the "royal touch" by monarchs in Europe [2,4]. TB has claimed its victims throughout much of known human history. It reached epidemic proportions in Europe and North America during the eighteenth and nineteenth centuries.

It was René Théophile Hyacinthe Laennec who clearly elucidated the pathogenesis of TB early in the nineteenth century. Jean-Antoine Villemin demonstrated the infectious nature of TB in 1865 after inoculating a rabbit with pus taken from a tuberculous cavity [2]. On March 24, 1882, Hermann Heinrich Robert Koch made his famous presentation, *Die Aetiologie der Tuberculose*, demonstrating that the tubercle bacillus was the causative agent of TB [5].

From 1907 onward, a series of experiments led to the discovery of the tuberculin skin test (TST) with the initiation of Clemens Freiherr Von Pirquet, with Charles Mantoux then improving the technique and Florence Seibers developing the purified protein derivative (PPD) [2].

Treatment of TB started with rest, fresh air, and home remedies. In the late nineteenth and early twentieth centuries, sanatoriums developed for the treatment of patients with TB. Then, the treatment was pulmonary collapse therapy and therapeutic pneumothorax, especially for treatment of cavitary disease. Streptomycin, the first antibiotic and first bactericidal agent effective against Mtb, was isolated in 1944. It was unlucky that the great writer George Orwell could not tolerate this drug and died of TB [4]. Isoniazid (INH), the first oral mycobactericidal drug, followed in 1952 and rifamycins in 1957. A new era of TB treatment had started with closure of the sanatoriums and implementation of effective public health measures [2].

EPIDEMIOLOGY

"Clearly we are still some distance from a world without tuberculosis" [6]. TB remains a major global health problem and ranks second as leading cause of death from an infectious disease worldwide, after the human immunodeficiency virus (HIV). There were 9.0 million new TB cases in 2013 and 1.5 million TB deaths (1.1 million among HIV-negative people and 0.4 million among HIV-positive people). The estimates in children are 550,000 cases and 80,000 deaths [7]. In comparison with the most recent estimates, in 1989 there were 1.3 million new cases of childhood TB reported with 450,000 deaths. Although childhood TB usually represents less than 5% of disease in industrialized countries, the burden of disease borne by children in less developed, resource-poor countries may be as high as 39% [8,9]. Approximately one-third of the human population can be demonstrated to have immunologic evidence of current or past infection with Mtb [10].

In the United States, there were less than 10,000 cases reported in 2012 with an incidence rate of 3.2 new cases per 100,000 population in 2012 (as opposed to 122 globally). Sixty-three percent of TB cases and 88% of MDR-TB cases were foreign-born from countries where TB prevalence and drug-resistance rates are high [10].

With the emergence of drug-resistant TB, a new threat to the control of TB occurred. Globally, it is estimated that 3.5% of new cases and 20.5% of previously treated cases have MDR TB [11]. In 2013, there were an estimated 480,000 new cases of MDR-TB worldwide, and approximately 210,000 deaths from MDR-TB. XDR-TB has been reported by 100 countries. On average, an estimated 9.0% of people with MDR-TB have XDR-TB [7].

TB in children is common wherever TB is common in adults (ie, TB endemic settings). Studies done in child contacts in African communities have shown that one-third to two-thirds of child household contacts of TB cases have evidence of TB infection (ie, TST-positive) [12,13]. Of children with TB, 70% to 80% have the disease in their lungs (pulmonary TB, PTB).

The rest are affected by TB disease in other parts of the body (extrapulmonary TB). The HIV epidemic has increased the burden of childhood TB and made it more difficult to diagnose and treat [14].

In North America and Europe, childhood TB cases occurred mostly in high-risk populations, including immigrants and racial/ethnic minorities. Studies from low-income and middle-income countries have confirmed the long-recognized association of childhood TB with poverty, crowding, and malnutrition [8].

Risk factors for TB infection in children include closeness to a TB case and duration of the contact. Another risk factor is the smear positivity and presence of cavities on chest radiograph (CXR) of the source case. The first 2 years of life infer the greatest risk for developing TB disease in addition to HIV infection, immunosuppression, malnutrition, and other diseases. Most disease occurs within 2 years after exposure.

There has been much progress in the 15 years since 1995 with the Stop TB Strategy, whereby 36 million patients were cured. Case fatality rate halved from 7.6% to 4%. TB incidence, however, is declining much more slowly than predicted [14]. The rate of decline in TB approaches 2% per year, a number much lower than what is needed to eliminate TB by 2050. The HIV epidemic and the spread of MDR-TB and XDR-TB have slowed this decline. An estimated one-third of new TB cases are still being missed each year, and the unavailability of a rapid, low-cost, accurate diagnostic assay that can be used at the point of care is a major hindrance [15].

Children rarely develop sputum smear-positive TB and therefore they are often excluded from being reported; hence, the burden of disease in this population is underestimated [16,17]. In most settings, children with TB continue to be given low priority by National TB Control Programmes because they are less likely to transmit disease. Despite being a major contributor to childhood morbidity and mortality, childhood TB has been largely absent from the global public health agenda. In addition, scientific progress has been lagging [16].

National programs in low-income and middle-income countries are underfunded by about US $2 billion for both 2014 and 2015. "Tuberculosis suffers because it is a disease of poverty–there is very little interest in big pharma in diseases of this type because they know that since the big sales are going to be in developing countries, there is no income generation," explained Mario Raviglione of the WHO [18].

TRANSMISSION

Transmission of Mtb occurs person to person via inhalation of mucous droplets that become airborne when an individual with pulmonary or laryngeal TB coughs, sneezes, speaks, laughs, or sings. After drying, the droplet nuclei can remain suspended in the air for hours. Only small droplets (<10 μm in diameter) can reach alveoli. Droplet nuclei can also be produced by aerosol treatments, by sputum induction, and through manipulation of lesions [8].

Numerous factors are associated with the risk of acquiring Mtb infection, including the extent of contact with the index case, the burden of organisms in the sputum, and the frequency of cough in the index case. Urban living, overcrowding, and lower socioeconomic status all are correlated with the acquisition of infection. An increased risk of developing infection has been demonstrated in multiple institutional settings, including nursing homes, correctional institutions, homeless shelters, as well as in refugee and orphanage settings [8].

PATHOGENESIS

The MTBC includes Mtb, *Mycobacterium bovis*, *Mycobacterium africanum*, *Mycobacterium canettii*, *Mycobacterium caprae*, *Mycobacterium microti*, and *Mycobacterium pinnipedii*. Mtb causes around 98% and *M bovis* causes around 1% to 2% of human TB. MTBC's complex cell wall contains mycolic acid that retains the stain with carbol fuchsin or auramine when decolorized by acid alcohol, hence the term acid-fast bacilli. The MTB genome contains 4,411,529 base-pairs with high guanine cytosine content (>65%) [10].

TB's varied clinical manifestations are due to the spectrum of immune responses in different human subjects; this can be asymptomatic with a positive TST to severe and fatal disease. Some studies have looked into the factors that influence development of TB. The highest risk of acquiring disease is greatest shortly after initial infection and is associated inversely with age from birth to 8 years of age. A second peak in the risk of developing disease occurs during late adolescence and early adult life. Exposure to a large infecting dose and immunosuppression are other risk factors. Children 0 to 5 years of age with recent infection have significant annual risk of developing disease [8].

A fundamental question in TB is the extent to which pathogenesis is a function of the pathogen, and to what extent it is a consequence of the immune responses of the host [19]. By evolving inside the macrophage, Mtb learned to take advantage of its inflammatory response. The initial phase is a silent infection; then, it is the formation of a granuloma in which the Mtb survives, and finally, the rearrangement of immunity between latent TB infection (LTBI) and active infection. During dormancy, no damage is done to the host; however, when immune disbalance occurs, Mtb becomes metabolically active, replicates to billions of organisms, damages the host, and gets transmitted to other subjects [20]. In approximately 90% of patients, the disease is controlled as LTBI; TB bacilli may remain viable within dormant lesions over many years and can be reactivated when the host immune system weakens [10,21].

The first checkpoint that Mtb has to overcome is the oxidative and nitrosative burst of the host. Mtb actively avoids the detrimental effects of the transient superoxide burst using its superoxide dismutase and cell surface glycolipids that possibly scavenge oxygen radicals [22].

Much of the understanding of TB's pathogenesis in recent years came from the zebrafish model (with similar immune system to that of humans). That model used *Mycobacteriummarinum*, Mtb's closest species. Cronan and Tobin provide a nice review of how both host and bacterial factors contribute to Mtb's pathogenesis. They also challenge the old understanding of the granuloma. During infection, Mtb is phagocytosed by macrophages; then other immune cells (T cells, B cells, neutrophils) are recruited, forming the granuloma. Necrosis and then hypoxia result in caseum formation in the granuloma's inner core. Bacteria persist inside this granuloma and eventually are released when this granuloma ruptures [23]. Mtb binds to receptors on macrophages, including Toll-like receptors, Nod-like receptors, C-type lectin receptors, mannose receptor, DC-SIGN (dendritic cell-specific intracellular adhesion molecule 3–grabbing nonintegrin), complement receptors, Fc receptors, and DNA sensors. Once inside the macrophage, Mtb enters and inhibits maturation and fusion with lysosome of the phagocytic vacuole. At certain times and under certain conditions, phagolysosomal fusion and secretion of various cytokines (tumor necrosis factor, interferon [IFN], and interleukin-6 [IL-6]) occur, in addition to production of reactive nitrogen/oxygen species that aid in killing of the bacilli. Mtb-infected cells migrate to pulmonary lymph nodes, where an adaptive immune response is mounted with T-cell production of IFN and B-cell production of antibodies. Successful killing of Mtb occurs with activation of more macrophages by T cells through IFN release [24]. When partial success occurs, activated macrophages and other host cells (T cells, B cells, and fibroblasts) surround the Mtb-infected cells in an organized display, a granuloma, creating hypoxic, acidic, nutrient-poor conditions that are less permissive for Mtb replication. However, the lesions are not always sterilized, as Mtb uses several strategies to ensure its survival, including resisting toxic molecules produced by the host, modifying phagosome biogenesis to create an environment suitable for survival and growth, co-opting the trafficking of cells within the granuloma to expand the number of infected cells, and inhibiting macrophage apoptosis to preserve its host niche. Although the immune response in the lung is directed at eliminating the bacillus, activation of pathways that damage lung tissue results in fibrosis, scar formation, and impaired lung function. Hence, mycobacterial phagocytosis is not exclusively host driven; instead, it is a process tuned by the mycobacteria themselves to establish a productive niche for their growth and dissemination [23].

The idea that the granuloma is exclusively host-driven and static was challenged again using the zebrafish, M marinum model. In fact, the granuloma is a dynamic structure with cells moving into and within it. The granuloma is essential for mycobacterial survival. M marinum species lacking the RD1 virulence locus were found to be less virulent because of inefficient granuloma formation. In addition, multiple secretion systems were identified (ESX-1 system, which ESAT-6 is part of, and SecA2 system) and found to facilitate granuloma formation and lead to macrophage death and recruitment of more macrophages. ESAT-6 induces the inflammatory matrix metalloprotease, MMP-9, in adjacent epithelial cells, acting as a guidance cue for nearby macrophages, leading to further bacterial expansion and granuloma formation [23].

When the body's defense system fails, Mtb continues to grow intracellularly until it lyses the cell and either reinfects new cells or replicates extracellularly. Extracellular TB can be associated with high numbers of bacteria (eg, in lung cavities), which, due to their growth rate and metabolic state, likely have varying susceptibilities to TB drugs in comparison with intracellular bacilli. In addition, the extracellular niche can be a source of drug-resistant organisms due to the high bacterial burden and known ability of Mtb to develop drug resistance [24].

One of the mechanisms by which Mtb survives is that it leads to macrophage necrosis rather than apoptosis. Apoptosis is associated with a reduction in the viability of intracellular Mtb and provides an important link to the establishment of T-cell immunity. The mechanisms by which virulent Mtb leads to macrophage necrosis are inhibition of plasma membrane repair, damage of inner mitochondrial membrane, and inhibition of formation of apoptotic cellular envelope [25]. Another process that aids Mtb's persistence is biofilm formation through the production of the *pks1* gene. This characteristic is common among TB isolates throughout the world [26].

Only a small fraction of individuals exposed to Mtb develop clinical TB. Over the past century, epidemiologic studies have shown that human genetic factors contribute significantly to this interindividual variability [27]. Studies have shown that certain genes affect susceptibility to TB. One of those is the STAT 4 promoter-region polymorphism found in a Moroccan population that may impact STAT 4 expression [28]. In the zebrafish model, Tobin and colleagues [29] found that mutations in the gene leukotriene A4 hydrolase (LTA4H), which catalyzes the production of the pro-inflammatory eicosanoid LTB4, were associated with hypersusceptibility to *M marinum*. Reduced LTA4H activity confers hypersusceptibility via an excess production of anti-inflammatory lipoxins. In humans, 2 intronic single-nucleotide polymorphisms (SNPs) at the LTA4H locus were associated with TB. Heterozygosity for the 2 SNPs was protective, while both homozygous states corresponded to increased disease severity. Tobin explains that therapies for TB must be directed against the host rather than the bacillus. Susceptibility to TB can be due to hypo-inflammatory or hyperinflammatory states, both ruled by the patient's genotype and causing either an increase or a decrease in LTA4H and both leading to macrophage lysis.

Because of the difference in their immune system, children are more susceptible than adults to progress from Mtb exposure to infection and disease [16]. In addition, children have a higher risk of extrapulmonary dissemination and death. Because of immaturity in their immune response, infants have a particularly high morbidity and mortality from TB [30].

Most patients with disseminated TB, whether children or adults, especially in endemic countries, have no known underlying immunodeficiency, inherited or acquired. However, a category of primary immunodeficiency that leads to disseminated mycobacterial disease is Mendelian susceptibility to mycobacterial diseases (MSMD), which is primarily seen in children. Cases of disseminated TB have been reported among children with MSMD, particularly in those presenting with IL-12Rβ1 deficiency, the most common known genetic cause of MSMD [31]. In addition to infecting the lungs, TB has the capability to disseminate to other organs. On Mtb infection, human macrophages express numerous factors including vascular endothelial growth factor that controls the formation of new blood vessels. It was found that inhibiting angiogenesis in a murine model strongly decreased the spread of bacteria [6].

Description of the natural history of TB was documented before anti-TB drugs were introduced, and it gave an important description of disease progression. After inhalation of the bacilli, those reach a terminal airway, where a localized pneumonic inflammatory process occurs; this is called the parenchymal (Ghon) focus. From this focus, bacilli drain to regional lymph nodes and both the Ghon focus and the lymph nodes involved are termed the primary complex. During the incubation period and before adequate immune response, these bacilli disseminate systemically and infect other organs. Five phases of TB infection were described. Phase 1 occurred 3 to 8 weeks after primary infection with fever and formation of the primary complex. Phase 2 occurred 1 to 3 months after the primary infection, following the hematogenous spread with high risk for TB meningitis (TBM) or military TB. Phase 3 occurred 3 to 7 months after the primary infection, when pleural effusions in children older than 5 years or bronchial disease in children younger than 5 years occurred. The calcification of the primary complex occurred 1 to 3 years later, during phase 4. It is during this phase that osteoarticular TB in children younger than 5 years of age and adult-type disease in adolescents occur. Finally, during phase 5, which occurs after the age of 3 years, late manifestations of TB, including pulmonary reactivation, develop [32].

CLINICAL MANIFESTATIONS

Persistent cough, associated with weight loss/failure to thrive, fever, fatigue, and reduced playfulness without improvement following other therapies, including antibiotics, antimalarial treatment, and nutritional support, should make a pediatrician highly suspicious of PTB. Specificity of these symptoms is highest in children 3 years of age or older (98.9%), decreases to 82.6% in those less than 3 years, and performs poorly in HIV-infected children [14]. Extrapulmonary TB occurs in 10% to 42% of patients, depending on race or ethnic background, age, presence or absence of underlying disease, genotype of the Mtb strain, and immune status. Extrapulmonary TB can affect any organ in the body, has varied and protean clinical manifestations, and therefore, requires a high index of clinical suspicion [33].

HIV coinfection poses special challenges to clinical management in patients with active TB. The risk of active TB increases soon after infection with HIV, and the manifestations of PTB at this stage are similar to those in HIV-negative persons. At CD4 counts of less than 200 per cubic millimeter, the presentation of TB may be atypical, with subtle infiltrates, pleural effusions, hilar lymphadenopathy, and other forms of extrapulmonary TB in as many as 50% of patients. At CD4 counts of less than 75 per cubic millimeter, pulmonary findings may be absent, and disseminated TB, manifested as a nonspecific, chronic febrile illness with widespread organ involvement and mycobacteremia, is more frequent, with high early mortality; polyclonal disease has also been described. Such cases may be mistakenly diagnosed as other infectious diseases and are often identified only on autopsy [33]. Up to 25% of patients presenting for HIV care in endemic regions have undiagnosed active TB. Therefore, screening for TB is recommended for all patients with HIV infection to identify patients with active disease and before instituting INH preventive therapy (IPT) in the remainder [33]. Although an exuberant immune response in immunocompetent adolescents tends to result in adult-type, cavitating disease, in young children or individuals with HIV coinfection, poor cell-mediated immunity is thought to allow unrestrained proliferation of bacilli with progressive parenchymal lung damage (with or without cavity formation) and dissemination [30].

The following describes the disease classifications of PTB in childhood. The prechemotherapy literature documented the natural history of TB in childhood. These disease descriptions remain invaluable for guiding public health policy and research, because the introduction of effective chemotherapy radically changed the history of disease [32].

Pulmonary infection without progression to disease implies an effective immune response that has contained the tubercle bacilli and is characterized by infection with Mtb that is uncomplicated by clinical symptoms (other than self-limited, virallike illness) or radiological abnormalities (other than the primary complex). In pulmonary infection, the child has a positive TST, nonspecific viral respiratory symptoms, and enlarged lymph nodes on CXR. Over time, the lesions either disappear or calcify, indicating clinical quiescence. The prognosis of pulmonary infection was favorable, with the associated risk mainly dependent on the age at the time of primary infection.

Pulmonary disease is characterized by infection with Mtb that is complicated by marked clinical symptoms or additional radiological abnormalities apart from the primary complex. Approximately 70% of the primary foci are subpleural. Lobes are affected equally. Twenty-five percent of cases have multiple parenchymal foci. Pulmonary disease may be associated with a diverse spectrum of pathologic abnormality. Bronchial disease predominated in children aged less than 5 years with a range of bronchoscopic findings: no visible involvement, obstruction from external nodal compression, endobronchial nodal breakthrough with caseous drainage, granulation tissue with polyps, and fistula formation. Symptoms varied according to the degree of airway irritation and obstruction. Pleural effusions increased in incidence from 5 years of age onward. Pleural effusions varied in size from small to massive and had a characteristic clinical course, starting with an acute pleuritic pain in the chest, accompanied by a high fever in the absence of acute illness, an ill-defined loss of vigor, and a dry cough.

A Ghon focus with cavitation was rare. It occurred predominantly in black children aged less than 2 years. Clinical symptoms of Ghon focus cavitation included weight loss, fatigue, fever, and chronic cough. In those with cavitation, disease progressed to death within 1 year in most cases. Healing was rare, and even those that survived the initial illness ultimately died of TB or associated complications. Cavitation following primary infection occurred frequently during adolescence, but in this age group, parenchymal breakdown probably reflected excessive rather than poor disease containment.

Enlarged regional lymph nodes on CXR rarely caused symptoms except when they were associated with bronchial disease, or when excessive nodal caseation caused persistent fever and weight loss. The subcarinal nodes were most commonly involved, and rarely, pericardial effusion developed following nodal erosion with caseous discharge into the pericardial space.

Adult-type disease resulted from primary infection, endogenous reactivation, or exogenous reinfection. Adult-type disease was most common after recent primary infection in children older than 10 years of age. The interval from primary infection to adult-type disease was widely variable (3 months to 20 years), mostly dependent on the age at primary infection. The shortest time intervals and highest risk followed primary infection during adolescence, especially in girls of perimenarchal age. The disease started off with minimal symptoms, such as cough, loss of appetite, and fatigue. With disease progression, typical TB symptoms of chronic cough, chest pain, lethargy, anorexia, and weight loss became evident. Children with advanced disease became anemic, developing an oscillating fever and hemoptysis. A frequent complaint, even in the absence of fever, was night sweats. The prognosis of adult-type disease was poor, with 50% to 60% mortality within 5 to 10 years. These children were sputum smear-positive and able to transmit infection.

With hematogenous spread, bacilli seed to susceptible organs, especially the spleen, bone, kidney, and cerebral cortex, and possibly to the lung apices (Simon foci). Infection in a child less than 2 years of age carried a significant risk of serious disease. TBM was present in more than 30% of children who presented with TB before 2 years of age. The risk of TBM after 3 years of age was extremely low, and those who did develop TBM had significant preceding symptoms. Infants were most vulnerable to developing miliary disease. The symptoms included prolonged pyrexia, lassitude, anorexia, and weight loss. Children appeared acutely ill, with minimal physical signs apart from possible tachypnea and hepatosplenomegaly. Radiological mottling followed 7 to 21 days after febrile onset, starting as barely visible nodules that slowly progressed to large, poorly defined patches. The initial miliary lesions were often difficult to visualize, with 30% to 40% of autopsy-proven miliary lesions missed on CXR before death. Bone marrow biopsy and ophthalmoscopy were useful diagnostic aids. The prognosis of miliary disease was poor. Clinical progression with persistent fever, increased irritability, and weight loss frequently terminated in TBM. The majority died within 6 months, but chronic forms were occasionally seen whereby children eventually died from toxemia, malnutrition, or amyloidosis [32].

DIAGNOSIS

Even though TB incidence in the United States is low, pediatricians in this country should always consider TB as cause of a child's symptoms, especially if there's a history of TB exposure. Those who traveled from endemic areas should be routinely screened for TB on arrival [34].

In making the diagnosis of TB, a pediatrician should pay careful attention to history of TB contact in addition to symptoms suggestive of TB as described in the previous section. Assessment of growth is extremely important. Then, TST, bacteriologic confirmation whenever possible, and HIV testing must be done [14]. Unfortunately, in many countries, TST and culture may not be readily available; however, neither is required to make a decision to treat.

While taking history, it is important to note the closeness of contact with a TB patient as well as duration of this contact. If the pediatrician is unable to identify a confirmed contact, then he or she should always ask if anyone in the household has been coughing and request immediate assessment of that person for possible TB.

The following sections discuss the proper up-to-date recommendations in making diagnosis of LTBI and active TB.

Latent tuberculosis

Testing for LTBI should be targeted and restricted to persons at high risk for LTBI and progression to active TB disease. It is indicated for groups in which the prevalence of latent infection is high (eg, foreign-born persons from regions in which TB is endemic), those in whom the risk of reactivated disease is high (eg, patients with HIV infection or diabetes, and patients receiving immunosuppressive therapy), and recent contacts of patients with TB [33]. Two tests exist for making the diagnosis of LTBI, namely, the TST and IFN-γ release assay (IGRA).

A major obstacle to the development and assessment of LTBI tests is the lack of a gold standard to measure sensitivity and specificity [35].

Active TB should be ruled out in patients with a positive diagnostic test for LTBI before the initiation of therapy for the treatment of LTBI [36].

Before 2001, the TST was the only test for TB. TST requires proper administration by the Mantoux method with intradermal injection of 0.1 mL of tuberculin-PPD into the volar surface of the forearm. False-positive TSTs can result from contact with nontuberculous mycobacteria (NTM) or Bacille-Calmette-Guérin (BCG) vaccine [37]. The degree of BCG cross-reactivity depends on many factors, including the strain of BCG used, the patient's age and nutritional status at the time of vaccination, frequency of skin testing, and years since the vaccination was given. In most studies of children vaccinated with BCG during the newborn period, only 5% react to tuberculin testing at 12 months and 80% to 90 % lose such reactivity within 2 to 3 years. Although BCG vaccination of older children or adults results in greater initial and more persistent cross-reactivity, most of these individuals lose cross-reactivity within 10 years of receiving the vaccination. Exposure to NTM varies geographically and generally results in smaller, transient indurations than those of TB [8].

The reaction to tuberculin typically begins 5 to 6 hours after the patient receives the injection and reaches maximal induration at 48 to 72 hours. In some individuals, the reaction may peak after 72 hours. In these instances, the TST should be measured again and interpretation of the test should be based on the larger, later reading. Rarely, vesiculation and necrosis may occur. In these cases, repeat tuberculin testing should be avoided. Forty-eight to 72 hours after the injection is given, the diameter of induration should be measured transversely to the long axis of the forearm and recorded in millimeters. A trained health care professional should read all skin tests. A nonreactive TST does not exclude LTBI or TB [8].

Cutoff values for TST exist. The test is considered positive depending on the risk factors present (Table 1) [8]. There are factors that might lead to false negative TST results, including viral infections (measles, mumps, chicken pox, HIV), bacterial infections (typhoid fever, brucellosis, typhus, leprosy, pertussis, overwhelming TB, TB pleurisy), fungal infections (South American blastomycosis), live virus vaccines (measles, mumps, polio, varicella; TST can be performed either on the same day that the vaccination with live virus is given or 4–6 weeks later), metabolic derangements (chronic renal failure), low protein states (severe protein depletion, afibrinogenemia), diseases affecting lymphoid organs (Hodgkin disease, lymphoma, chronic leukemia, sarcoidosis), drugs (corticosteroids and other immunosuppressive agents), age (newborns, elderly patients with "waned" sensitivity), stress (surgery, burns, mental illness, graft-versus-host reactions), improper storage of tuberculin, contamination, improper administration such as subcutaneous injection, or error in reading the test [8].

IGRAs detect sensitization to Mtb by measuring IFN-γ release in response to antigens representing Mtb. In 2001, the QuantiFERON-TB test (QFT; Cellestis Inc, Valencia, CA, USA) became the first IGRA approved by the US Food and

Table 1
Definitions of a positive tuberculin skin test results in infants, children, and adolescents

Induration	Risk Factors
>5 mm	Children close to a known or suspected contagious TB case
	Children with CXR findings consistent with active with active or previously active TB
	Children with symptoms suggestive of TB disease
	Immunocompromised children
>10 mm	Children at increased risk of disseminated disease:
	Children less than 4 years of age
	Children with diseases including Hodgkin's disease, lymphoma, diabetes mellitus, chronic renal failure, or malnutrition
	Children with increased exposure to TB disease based on country of birth, exposure to high-risk adults (including drug users, HIV-infected adults)
	Children who traveled to high-prevalence regions of the world
>15 mm	Children who are 4 years or older who do not have any other risk factors

Data from Mandalakas AM, Starke JR. Current concepts of childhood tuberculosis. Semin Pediatr Infect Dis 2005;16:93–104.

Drug Administration (FDA). It used the PPD, was found to be less specific than TST, and was subsequently removed in 2005. In 2005, the QuantiFERON-TB Gold test (QFT-G) was introduced and in 2007 the QuantiFERON-TB Gold In-Tube test (QFT-GIT) was introduced. In July 2008, T-Spot became the fourth IGRA to be approved by the FDA. With the newer IGRAs, there was improved specificity as they assessed MTB-specific peptides (ESAT-6) and (CFP-10). However, ESAT-6 and CFP-10 are present in *M kansasii, M szulgai,* and *M marinum* [37].

Several studies have been done trying to assess the sensitivity and specificity of IGRAs. In a meta-analysis published in *The Pediatric Infectious Disease Journal,* the investigators found that there was not enough evidence to support the use of IGRAs over TST for LTBI in children. They even concluded that IGRA sensitivity was low in high-burden TB settings compared with low-burden TB settings [38].

In a small French study where TB incidence is low, the sensitivity of IGRA in immunocompetent children older than 2 years of age was high [39].

In a study conducted in the United States on immigrant children (Mexico, the Philippines, and Vietnam), it was found that IGRA should be used for screening children 2 years and older instead of TST because most of these children are BCG vaccinated. The benefits of such practice whereby fewer children are QFT-positive include decreasing radiation exposure, lowering cost, and decreasing LTBI treatment [35].

Studies on the utility of IGRA in children less than 5 years of age are scarce and only recently published. One of these studies showed good sensitivity and specificity of IGRA and a low rate of indeterminate results in the first 2 years of life, supporting its use at this age [40]. Another study was done in children less than 5 years of age that showed that IGRA performed well in this age group; however, in this study, there was discordance between IGRA and TST, which led the authors to conclude that both tests should be considered in high-risk populations [41].

Now that it is known that IGRA is more specific than TST, a study done in US college students who have been in TB-endemic areas showed that IGRA was not superior to TST in that population and was actually less specific. The investigators recommended adopting a higher cutoff value of 1.0 IU/mL or higher for those at lower risk of exposure to TB, such as matriculating health care professional students from low prevalence countries such as the United States, and the current manufacturer's recommended cut point of TB-nil 0.35 IU/mL or higher for those at higher risk of exposure, such as students coming from countries with high TB burden [42].

The Centers for Disease Control and Prevention guidelines indicate that a TST or an IGRA may be used to test for LTBI. An IGRA is preferred over the TST when testing people who are BCG vaccinated or are unlikely to return for TST reading. The TST is preferred for serial testing programs, such as those involving health care workers, because the IGRA has a high false positive rate in this setting in the United States [36]. The TST is less expensive and is therefore preferred in low-income regions [33].

The American Academy of Pediatrics has also published in its Red Book recommendations on the use of TST versus IGRA in children (Table 2).

Newer concerns have also emerged about IGRAs. Considerable fluctuations with serial testing in individual patients have been reported; some might be attributed to new infection, to boosting following a TST, or response to antimycobacterial treatment. Most of these fluctuations, however, remain unexplained. Hence, well-controlled studies are needed to define the causes of individual variations in IFN-γ response and to develop criteria to differentiate nonspecific variation from that associated with new or resolving infection [43,44].

One must conclude with the WHO 2011 report on use of IGRA in high-TB endemic areas. In this report, the WHO recommends against use of IGRAs instead of TST in low- and middle-income countries for the diagnosis of LTBI in children (irrespective of HIV status) [45].

Active tuberculosis

Diagnosing TB in children can be challenging because it can mimic many common childhood diseases like pneumonia, malnutrition, and HIV. In attempting to reach a definite diagnosis after TB is considered, clinicians are faced with another challenge of the paucibacillary nature of the disease in this age group. Sputum production is often faint and mostly swallowed rather than expectorated. Gastric samples require that children be hospitalized and fasting for 3 nights. Even when a good sample is produced, only in 10% to 15% of the samples is the acid-fast bacilli smear positive and in 30% the culture is positive. Ways to improve sputum production include use of nebulized hypertonic saline that yields more TB compared with gastric washings [30].

Table 2
Use of interferon-γ release assay and tuberculin skin test in children

TST preferred, IGRA acceptable	• Children who are younger than five years of age
IGRA preferred, TST acceptable	• Children older than five years who had the BCG vaccine or those unlikely to return for TST reading
TST and IGRA should be considered when	• T The initial and repeat IGRA are indeterminate
	• The initial TST or IGRA is *negative* and:
	○ There is moderate to high clinical suspicion for TB disease
	○ There is high risk of progression and poor outcome
	• The initial TST is *positive* and:
	○ History of BCG vaccination in a child older than five years of age
	○ The additional evidence is needed to increase compliance
	○ Nontuberculous mycobacterial disease is suspected

Data from Daley CL, Reves RR, Beard MA, et al. A summary of meeting proceedings on addressing variability around the cut point in serial interferon-gamma release assay testing. Infect Control Hosp Epidemiol 2013;34:625–30.

In the absence of bacteriologic confirmation, the diagnosis of childhood TB is often based on the triad of (1) close contact with an infectious index case, (2) a positive TST result, and (3) observation of suggestive signs on a CXR. This triad is less helpful in areas of endemicity, whereby a positive TST result is not uncommon and where exposure to Mtb is often undocumented. In TB-endemic countries, the diagnosis of childhood TB depends mainly on clinical characteristics and the subjective interpretation of the CXR; however, CXR has well-recognized limitations and is unavailable in many resource-limited countries.

Clinical scoring systems designed to aid diagnosis have not been validated against the standard of culture-confirmed diagnosis, and the diagnostic accuracy of these systems varies markedly [46]. It is important to emphasize that neither IGRAs nor the TST have high accuracy for the prediction of active TB [47].

Since declaration of TB as a public health emergency in 1983, the diagnostic tests developed have shown improvement in sensitivity and specificity. The initial tests used had many limitations: direct-smear microscopy was insensitive; TST did not distinguish latent from active disease; solid culture was slow with results arriving too late to influence clinical decisions; and CXRs were unable to differentiate between TB and other pulmonary pathologic conditions [48]. Acid-fast stain with microscopic examination is the easiest, quickest, and least expensive diagnostic procedure. However, this method cannot differentiate TB and NTM. There must be 5000 to 10,000 bacilli per millimeter of specimen present to allow detection of the bacteria in stained smears, resulting in only moderate sensitivity in children. Thus, negative smears do not preclude the presence of TB in children [8].

Newer tests are found in later discussion.

Culture

Traditional culture media often require 4 to 6 weeks for positivity and another 2 to 4 weeks for susceptibility testing [8]. The microscopic-observation drug-susceptibility assay (MODS) and the automated liquid culture methods have increased the sensitivity of culture and are faster than Lowenstein–Jensen and other solid media, with the added advantage of obtaining drug-sensitivity information. Both MODS and liquid culture have lower sensitivity in gastric aspirates than in sputum. The results for all culture methods are rarely obtained before 1 week of incubation [48].

Improvement in the protocol to expedite culture results has been published but not yet implemented. These improvements include a new medium, micro-aerophilic atmosphere or ascorbic-acid supplement, and autofluorescence detection [49].

Nucleic acid amplification tests

Nucleic acid amplification tests (NAAT) are technologies that vary from in-house assays to fully automated, self-contained kits. Data on their performance in children are limited. These tests are usually expensive [48] and are mostly intended for use at reference laboratory level only, requiring dedicated infrastructure and experienced staff [7]. The Xpert MTB/Rif test is a cartridge-based fully automated NAAT and is discussed later.

Among the first FDA-approved NAAT was the *M tuberculosis* direct test (Hologic Gen-Probe, San Diego, CA, USA) for detection of MTBC from *N*-acetyl-L-cysteine–NaOH concentrated specimens, either smear-positive or smear-negative. The test marked a successful beginning of the molecular era in the United States for TB diagnosis with high sensitivity and specificity, and remarkably shortened the turnaround time with cost savings [10].

Loop-mediated isothermal amplification

The loop-mediated isothermal amplification (LAMP) assay is a rapid, easy-to-perform technology that has recently been used to develop diagnostic tests for several pathogens such as *Staphylococcus aureus*, foot and-mouth disease virus, and salmonella. Some of these assays can be performed in specimens collected on swabs and are completed within 1 to 2 hours, requiring only a water bath or heat block for reaction. Results of initial studies reporting the performance of LAMP amplification assays of Mtb-specific DNA in clinical specimens, including specimens of patients with extra PTB, have been promising, as opposed to conventional polymerase chain reaction (PCR), in which LAMP is isothermal and eradicates the need for expensive thermocyclers. LAMP assays for TB have reported sensitivity ranging from 88% to 100% and specificity between 94% and 99% in sputum. The most recent prototypes perform better than conventional PCR. The low cost and technology requirements of these assays, their performance in nonsputum specimens, and the potential to develop tests for a large number of pathogens make the technique promising for children [48]. Because of insufficient evidence, this platform has not yet been endorsed by the WHO. FIND (Foundation for Innovative New Diagnostics) has subsequently re-evaluated TB LAMP in multiple country settings in comparison with fluorescent smear microscopy, Xpert MTB/RIF, and culture and plans to submit a dossier of performance characteristics and diagnostic accuracy to WHO for review in 2015 [7].

BlaC-specific fluorogenic probe

The BlaC-specific fluorogenic probe approach uses BlaC, a highly conserved class A β-lactamase enzyme, which is naturally expressed and secreted by the tubercle bacilli. The fluorogenic substrates then enhance the natural fluorescence, facilitating detection, and increasing the specificity of the reaction. The light emitted can be detected by a camera built on a mobile phone. As the probe would not require laboratory infrastructure, it has the potential to be developed as a rapid, low-cost TB diagnostic tool that might be suitable for children [48].

Xpert MTB/RIF

Even though the author of "Xpert MTB/RIF: a game changer for the diagnosis of pulmonary tuberculosis in children?" [50] has concluded that this test will not be a crucial diagnostic tool in high burden countries, the WHO endorsed its use in children in 2013. Several studies published on its use in the pediatric population have shown promising results be it in gastric lavage [51,52], sputum [53–59], bronchoalveolar lavage specimens [60], or stool in HIV-infected patients [61].

In 2010, WHO endorsed the Xpert MTB/RIF assay, a cartridge-based fully automated molecular diagnostic assay that uses real-time PCR to identify MTBC DNA and the mutations associated with rifampicin resistance directly from sputum specimens, in less than 2 hours. The assay has similar sensitivity, specificity, and accuracy as culture on solid media. A policy update was issued at the end of 2013 to include its use in children.

a. Xpert MTB/RIF should be used rather than conventional microscopy, culture, and DST as the initial diagnostic test in adults and children suspected of having MDR-TB or HIV-associated TB.
b. Xpert MTB/RIF may be used rather than conventional microscopy and culture as the initial diagnostic test in all children suspected of having TB.
c. Xpert MTB/RIF may be used as a follow-on test to microscopy in adults and children, where MDR-TB and HIV is of lesser concern, especially in further testing of smear-negative specimens [62].

Children suspected of having PTB but with a single Xpert MTB/RIF-negative result should undergo further diagnostic testing, and a child with high clinical suspicion for TB should be treated even if an Xpert MTB/RIF result is negative or if the test is not available.

Another benefit was demonstrated in a study that showed that Xpert significantly reduced duration of airborne isolation [63].

A few of Xpert's strengths include simplicity of use, accuracy, rapidity of result, and ability to use on a variety of samples, including lymph node aspirates, cerebrospinal fluid (CSF), and other areas. On the other hand, it is expensive; needs calibration, maintenance, and linkage to a computer and secured premises; needs continuous electrical power supply and air conditioning; cannot differentiate between live and dead Mtb; and thus, cannot be used to monitor treatment success, failure, or relapse [15]. Use of Xpert MTB/RIF was not supported in a study done in malnourished children from a high TB area in Malawi [64].

Difficulty in acquiring sputum samples from children has led researchers to test new blood assays: the T-cell activation marker–tuberculosis, which is a flow cytometric analysis test of the CD27 on circulating Mtb-specific T cells that can discriminate active TB from latent TB [65] and transcriptome signatures [46]. The first study was published in *Lancet* as a proof of concept and the second in *New England Journal of Medicine*. Although these seem to be promising new tests, there is always the challenge of their use in poor countries because of their high cost and technical complexity. Also, more validation studies are needed to confirm their accuracy in diagnosing active TB in children. Both of these tests do not address the issue of resistance, which is becoming a crucial element in giving the right treatment for patients with confirmed active TB.

Urine lipoarabinomannan has shown little value in diagnosing children with tuberculous meningitis [66] or PTB [67].

Imaging

CXR remains an important tool for the diagnosis of PTB in children. The commonest abnormality is due to lymphadenopathy and tends to be asymmetrical. CXR does have limitations, especially as quality of CXR is often poor. The diagnostic accuracy of experienced specialist pediatricians and primary level practitioners in detecting radiographic lymphadenopathy was low [68].

Computed tomography (CT) scan is more sensitive than CXR and can help distinguish between an active and an inactive form of TB. In one study aimed at finding the relationship between high-resolution CT findings and smear positivity, the investigators concluded that cavity, tree-in-bud pattern, and upper lobe nodular infiltration were highly associated with smear positivity in children. Conversely, lymphadenopathy and collapse had significant association with a negative smear [69].

Diagnostic problems are more pronounced in HIV-infected children. HIV-infected children who live with HIV-infected adults are more likely to be exposed to an adult TB index case at home. However, HIV-infected adults often have sputum smear–negative TB, and, therefore, the risk of infection posed by this exposure is often not appreciated. TST is much less sensitive in HIV-infected children than in HIV-uninfected children. Chronic pulmonary symptoms may be related to other HIV-related conditions, such as gastroesophageal reflux and bronchiectasis, thus reducing the specificity of symptom-based diagnostic approaches. Weight loss and failure to thrive are typical characteristics of both TB and HIV infection. Rapid TB disease progression is more likely to occur in HIV-infected children, reducing the sensitivity of diagnostic approaches that focus on persistent, non-remitting symptoms. Interpretation of CXRs is complicated by HIV-related comorbidities, such as bacterial pneumonia, lymphocytic interstitial pneumonitis, bronchiectasis, pulmonary Kaposi sarcoma, and the atypical presentation of TB in immunocompromised children [17].

EXTRAPULMONARY TUBERCULOSIS

TBM is the most common form of extrapulmonary TB, developing 3 to 6 months after primary infection. TBM is the most severe form of childhood TB [30]. The pathologic abnormality in TBM includes an increase in intracranial pressure, cerebral infarction, and severe hydrocephalus. Infants and young children are more likely to experience a rapid progression to hydrocephalus, seizures, and cerebral edema. In older children, signs and symptoms progress slowly over the course of several weeks, with symptoms of fever, headache, and drowsiness, which then proceed to vomiting, seizures, and then finally, to a comatose state. TST may be nonreactive in 40% of cases. TB therapy should be initiated in any child with basilar meningitis and hydrocephalus or cranial nerve involvement that has no other apparent cause [8,70].

Patients with pericardial TB disease experience cardiac tamponade or severe pericardial constriction that can be fatal in those patients with pericardial TB [71].

Other forms of extrapulmonary TB include superficial lymph node infection (scrofula), osteoarticular, abdominal, gastrointestinal, genitourinary, cutaneous, and congenital disease.

TB of the superficial lymph nodes can be associated with drinking unpasteurized cow's milk or can be caused by extension of primary lesions of the upper lung fields or abdomen leading to involvement of the supraclavicular, anterior cervical, tonsillar, and submandibular nodes. Although spontaneous resolution may occur, untreated lymphadenitis frequently progresses to caseating necrosis and capsular rupture and spreads to adjacent nodes and overlying skin, resulting in a draining sinus tract that may require surgical removal [8].

TB adenitis is most common in the cervical region. Lymph node enlargement is painless and asymmetrical, often multiple, discreet, or matted. Nodes are typically large (>2 × 2 cm; ie, visibly enlarged, not just palpable). Lymph node enlargement is persistent (>1 month) and not responsive to other treatment such as antibiotics. Sinus and discharge may develop. Usual age is 2 to 10 years.

Osteoarticular TB is not uncommon in children. Spinal TB causes destruction of vertebral bodies leading to typical spinal deformity and possibly paralysis. Hips and knees are the other typical site, usually mono-articular with painless effusion.

TB pleural effusion is common and tends to occur in school-aged children. Pleural tap is safe and very useful to differentiate TB from suppurative empyema. Other less common sites for effusion, usually painless, include peritoneal and pericardial spaces, also usually in school-aged children. Ultrasound and tap of effusion for microscopy and protein are very useful [14].

Newborn babies acquire TB from mothers who develop disseminated TB through placenta and into the liver or by aspirating infected amniotic fluid. Early diagnosis and treatment are crucial to prevent rapid disease progression [70].

TREATMENT

Children with TB, even those with drug-resistant disease, usually have an excellent clinical outcome if diagnosed in a timely fashion and treated appropriately [70]. However, it is very difficult to assess the outcome and efficacy of any regimen for treatment of TB in children because they rarely have positive sputum and gastric washings and hence scientific studies are scarce. Treatment should be guided by culture and susceptibilities when available [16].

The effective treatment of TB using current antibiotics faces obstacles that include a lengthy duration of treatment, potential drug toxicity, drug interactions with HIV medications, and increasing rates of drug resistance [24]. Therefore, local TB control programs should take responsibility of ensuring that all persons with suspected TB are identified and evaluated promptly. Unfortunately, when resources are limited, children receive lower priority [8].

Latent infection

After infection with Mtb, children may take up to 3 months to develop an immune response sufficient to produce a positive TST. Children younger than 5 years of age have a short incubation period and may develop severe disease before developing skin test reactivity. As the result of this risk, children with a negative TST and known or suspected exposure to an adult with contagious TB benefit from INH therapy. TST should be repeated 3 months after the initial exposure. If the second TST is negative, therapy may be discontinued. If skin test conversion occurs, therapy should be continued for the full duration. Although this strategy is considered standard of care in many industrialized countries, resource-poor countries frequently neglect to implement this WHO recommended strategy [8].

Most children with Mtb infection will have LTBI. These children have a reactive TST, normal CXR, no clinical evidence of TB, and presumed infection with low numbers of viable tubercle bacilli that are dormant. The treatment of children with LTBI should be considered a public health priority for numerous reasons: infants and children younger than 5 years of age have been infected recently, risk of progression to active disease is high, risk of developing severe disease is inversely related to age, children with LTBI have more years at risk for the development of active disease later in life, and children with LTBI become adults who may spread disease. Several large clinical trials conducted during the 1950s and 1960s demonstrated the efficacy of INH to reduce the risk of TB developing in children with LTBI. Secondary analysis of 2 large household contact studies suggested that the efficacy of INH treatment of LTBI plateaus at 9 to 10 months of therapy. Other studies demonstrated that a second year of treatment with INH did not result in additional benefit beyond that conferred by the first year of treatment. Treatment of LTBI should be tailored according to host immune factors, drug-susceptibility, tolerance, and compliance. In most cases, treatment may be given daily without observation. If adherence is inadequate, intermittent directly observed therapy (DOT) may be instituted. Treatment of latent MDR-TB should be delivered via DOT [8].

The diagnosis of LTBI in HIV-infected children is important because of the high risk of disease progression. IPT is recommended for any HIV-infected child with TB risk factors even when the TST is negative and when active TB has been excluded. The beneficial effect of IPT, however, wanes in 2 to 3 years and there is limited protection to future reinfection [17].

The preferred regimen for treatment of LTBI is INH for 9 months or for a longer duration in HIV-infected persons in areas with a high prevalence of TB. DOT with weekly administration of INH and rifapentine for 12 weeks has been shown to be as effective as INH alone in adults without HIV infection in countries with a low burden of TB [72]. The trial is continuing to assess safety and effectiveness in children and HIV-infected persons. HIV patients with a positive TST who are receiving preventive therapy with INH have decreased rates of active TB and death, but protection against TB wanes within a few months after cessation of INH therapy. A trial in Botswana recently showed that 36 months of preventive therapy with INH, as compared with 6 months of therapy, reduced the subsequent rate of TB by 43%. However, compliance with such a long-term regimen may be poor [33].

A phase III randomized noninferiority study comparing 3 months of directly observed once-weekly therapy with rifapentine (900 mg) plus INH (900 mg) (combination-therapy group) with 9 months of self-administered daily INH (300 mg) (INH-only group) in subjects at high risk for TB was published. Follow-up was for 33 months. This regimen was as effective as the 9 months INH-alone regimen in preventing TB and had a higher completion rate [72].

The pharmacokinetics of rifapentine was also studied in children and it was found that a higher dose per weight was needed to achieve comparable adult serum concentration of a 900-mg dose [73].

It is very important that before starting preventive therapy that active TB be excluded; this will prevent development of resistance, especially in adolescents and adults, who have a high organism load [17].

Active tuberculosis

Once active TB is diagnosed, effective treatment should be started. Close monitoring for relapse is crucial and its risk factors include cavitation, extensive disease, immunosuppression, and a sputum culture that remains positive at 8 weeks. If any of these risk factors is present, therapy may be extended for up to 9 months [33].

Challenges with current therapy include inconsistent drug quality, the need to ensure that drug administration is directly observed and that other support is provided to patients, treatment interruptions and changes in regimen because of side effects, toxic effects, pharmacokinetic interactions (particularly with antiretroviral therapy in patients with HIV coinfection), and compliance issues owing to the lengthy treatment period. Several trials in progress are adding or substituting fluoroquinolones in an attempt to shorten standard therapy to 4 months (eg, Remox-TB trial). None of these trials have showed noninferiority so far [33,74].

Young children with uncomplicated disease who are from areas with a low prevalence of INH resistance can be treated with 3 drugs (INH, rifampin [RMP], and pyrazinamide) during the 2-month intensive phase of treatment, followed by INH and RMP only during the 4-month continuation phase. Combination therapy is important to prevent emergence of resistant organisms. This regimen is successful with a 95% cure rate and is well-tolerated. However, children who have extensive or cavitary lung disease (either of which suggests a high bacillary load) or who are from areas with a high prevalence of INH resistance should receive a fourth drug (ethambutol, which is safe in children of all ages) during the 2-month intensive phase of treatment [8,9].

The 3 main categories of intrathoracic TB in children and appropriate drug regimens are as follows:

1. Sputum smear–negative paucibacillary TB: The success of the standard regimen of 3 drugs (RMP, INH, and pyrazinamide for 2 months) during the intensive treatment phase and of 2 drugs (RMP and INH for 4 months) for the continuation phase is well established, and the risk of acquired drug resistance is low.
2. Sputum smear–positive TB with a high organism load: Older children—especially adolescents—are more prone to sputum smear–positive paucibacillary TB and

may contribute to disease transmission in congregate settings, such as schools. Four drugs (RMP, INH, pyrazinamide, and ethambutol for 2 months) are warranted during the intensive treatment phase because of a higher risk for acquired drug resistance.

3. Disseminated/miliary TB occurs predominantly in very young (with an immature immune system) or immunocompromised children. It is frequently associated with tuberculous meningitis, and it is important to consider the CSF penetration of drugs used in the treatment of these children [17].

Poorer response to treatment and higher mortality are seen among HIV-infected children with TB. Possible reasons include higher incidence of coinfections with other pathogens, poorer absorption and low levels of anti-TB drugs, presence of underlying chronic lung disease resulting in poor penetration of drugs into fibrotic or bronchiectatic areas, poor adherence to treatment because of chronic illness or the death of the parent responsible for the child's treatment, and advanced immunosuppression and severe malnutrition [17].

In children with HIV and severe immunosuppression, WHO recommends starting HIV therapy after 2 to 8 weeks of TB treatment to prevent immune reconstitution inflammatory syndrome [30].

Although therapeutic trials have not been completed in children with extrapulmonary TB, duration of therapy depends on the site of infection and is generally extended for miliary TB and TBM [8].

Adjunctive therapy

Pyridoxine (25–50 mg/d) is recommended for infants, children, and adolescents treated with INH who have nutritional deficiencies, symptomatic HIV infection, or diets low in milk or meat products, and for breast-feeding infants. The administration of corticosteroids is beneficial in the management of children when the host inflammatory reaction contributes significantly to tissue damage or impaired function. The administration of corticosteroids decreases mortality and morbidity in patients with TBM by reducing vasculitis, inflammation, and intracranial pressure. The administration of corticosteroids may reduce significantly compression of the tracheobronchial tree caused by hilar lymphadenopathy and alveolar-capillary block, pleural effusion, and pericardial effusion associated with miliary disease. Prednisone (1–2 mg/kg/d for 4–6 weeks) usually is used [71,75,76].

A systemic review and meta-analysis on the effectiveness of steroids in all forms of TB was published in *Lancet*. The investigator's conclusion was that steroids reduced mortality in all forms of TB, including PTB. The results of this review are to be interpreted with caution because most of the cases were in patients with TBM and pericardial disease [71,77].

Monitoring for adverse effects

Among children, rates of adverse reactions secondary to antituberculous medication are low. INH and RMP treatment are associated infrequently with elevated levels of serum alanine aminotransferase that generally are less than 3 times the normal values, are not predictive of hepatotoxicity, and are not indications for discontinuing treatment. Education of caregivers relative to potential adverse events and clinical symptoms necessitating medical evaluation and discontinuation of medication is preferable to routine laboratory screening [8].

Monitoring response
Because of the lack of culture positivity in the pediatric population, monitoring of treatment response is mostly done by measuring weight gain, monitoring for persistent fever, and checking radiological findings. The role of IGRA in monitoring response to anti-TB therapy seems promising, but requires further evaluation. The TST is unsuitable for monitoring response to anti-TB treatment because of the boosting effect through repeated injections [78].

ALTERNATIVE TREATMENTS
In children, the primary tuberculous lymph node complex is directly or indirectly the predominant etiologic factor for surgical intervention. The predominant role of thoracic surgery in children following tuberculous infection lies in relieving airway obstruction to restore lung function and to prevent future irreversible lung damage. Later pulmonary resections during childhood are required for both the sequelae of airway obstruction and the chronic secondary PTB infection [79].

Acute or chronic obstruction of the major airways was the indication for 38% (64/168) of the procedures done for childhood TB during a 15-year review. Surgical decompression of tuberculous lymph nodes causing extraluminal compression made up 56% of these 64 procedures [79].

Collapse therapy in the form of artificial pneumothorax or pneumoperitoneum was used in the past. Some of the indications for this form of therapy were primary cavitation, caseating tuberculous pneumonia, not responding to conservative treatment, lesions involving a whole lung, pleural thickening after effusion, and causing gross interference with the function of the affected lung [80].

Ibuprofen was studied in mice infected with TB. No other treatment was given. Animals treated with ibuprofen had a statistically significant decrease in the size and number of lung lesions, decrease in the bacillary load, and improvement in survival, compared with findings for untreated animals. Because ibuprofen is already known to be safe in children, it might be an attractive adjunctive therapy that will not need a long development process [81].

Experiments are also being conducted in mice to test the usefulness of host-directed therapies. Therapeutic small molecules that could inhibit Th2 cells and Tregs, Suplatast tosylate, have been shown to disrupt production of IL-4 and other Th2-type cytokines without impeding IFN-γ production. During progression of TB, Mtb elicits Th2 and Treg cell responses in susceptible hosts, which facilitates disease progression by antagonizing host protective immune responses [82]. Another study established proof of concept for host-directed treatment strategies that manipulate the host eicosanoid network. IL-1 confers host resistance through the induction of eicosanoids that limit excessive type I IFN production and foster bacterial containment. Host-directed immunotherapy with clinically approved drugs that augment prostaglandin E2 levels in these settings prevented acute mortality of Mtb-infected mice [83].

MULTIDRUG-RESISTANT TUBERCULOSIS

Drug-resistant TB is a serious and growing problem and encompasses MDR-TB and XDR-TB. MDR-TB strains are resistant to INH and RMP, whereas XDR-TB is also resistant to fluoroquinolones and at least one of the second-line injectable drugs (amikacin, kanamycin, and capreomycin) [84]. XDR strains were first reported in 2006 [62].

Despite progress in the detection of MDR-TB cases, a major diagnostic gap remains: 55% of reported TB patients estimated to have MDR-TB were not detected in 2013 [7]. The WHO estimates that 3.7% of new cases and 20% of previously TB treated cases, or greater than 500,000 TB cases each year, are due to MDR strains [11]. Nearly half a million cases of MDR TB are diagnosed worldwide every year and a third of patients with this disease will die because of failure of diagnosis or unavailability of appropriate treatment. Drug resistance beyond XDR-TB is increasingly being reported. In certain settings, patients were infected with TB strains that required all available drugs [62,85]. Rates of MDR-TB and XDR-TB are increasing in southern Africa and the former Soviet Union with immigration leading to an increase in resistant strains in developed countries.

Epidemiologic studies on the prevalence of resistant TB in children are scarce. As in susceptible TB cases, the paucibacillary nature of the disease in the pediatric population makes the diagnosis and reporting of MDR/XDR incidence difficult [86–89]. A high index of suspicion is required in pediatric patients especially if there is a known resistant TB contact, and if the child shows no response to or deteriorates after the TB regimen is prescribed [30].

Resistance might occur because of any of the following: alterations of the binding site of drug-target molecules; loss of enzymes activating drug molecules; permeability changes to the drug, including efflux; and production of drug-inactivating enzymes, such as β-lactamase [90].

Resistance may be primary or acquired. In the case of primary drug resistance, the patient acquires a resistant strain and may transmit it to others. Poor infection control practices lead to the spread of resistant TB strains. On the other hand, acquired drug resistance results from inadequate treatment that leads to the selection of resistant strains. One example that leads to resistance is the stepwise addition of drugs or early discontinuation of proper therapy [33,62,89,90]. Drug-resistant strains of Mtb arise from spontaneous chromosomal mutations at a predictable low frequency. Outbreaks of highly fatal drug-resistant infection have been documented in several settings, especially those in which the prevalence of HIV infection is high [33]. In children, primary resistance is more common than acquired resistance, but the latter occurs mostly in children infected with HIV [30,89].

It is important to detect drug resistance and start proper treatment as early as possible to prevent spread of resistant strains. However, lack of appropriate tools is a major obstacle in achieving this goal [33]. Culture and drug susceptibility testing (DST) methods require prolonged lengths of time to confirm mycobacterial growth and detect drug resistance, during which period patients may be inappropriately treated, drug-resistant strains may continue to spread, and amplification of resistance may occur. Early and rapid diagnosis of TB and drug resistance will therefore have obvious benefits for patient and public health, including better prognosis, increased survival, prevention of acquisition of further drug resistance, and reduced spread of drug-resistant strains to vulnerable populations.

Drug resistance should be considered in children from areas with a high prevalence of drug-resistant TB and in those who have had documented contact with a person with drug-resistant disease, with someone who died during treatment of TB or who is not adhering to therapy, or with someone who is undergoing re-treatment of TB [9].

Treatment must be based on DST for first- and second-line drugs; however, in most cases, DST is not performed. In addition, second-line drug tests are not reliable [11]. Second-line drugs have limited efficacy and toxicity. After thorough diagnostic testing, if Xpert MTB/RIF and culture results are negative, children with active TB who are close contacts of patients with MDR-TB can be started on MDR regimens [62].

The first evidence that mutations in Kat G encoding catalase-peroxidase were associated with INH resistance was reported in 1992. This evidence led to increased efforts in advancing molecular assays to detect drug resistance. These tests are not 100% sensitive and therefore culture-based susceptibility still plays an integral role in confirming the molecular assays [10].

The current standard for first-line DST is an automated liquid culture system, which requires 4 to 13 days for results [33]. Molecular methods used to detect drug resistance include Cepheid GeneXpert MTB/RIF with 2-hour testing time and detecting resistance to rifampicin [10]. Ninety-five percent of all rifampicin-resistant strains have mutations localized to the 81-bp core region of the bacterial RNA polymerase β subunit (*rpoB*) gene, which encodes the active site of the enzyme and therefore molecular detection is reliable [15]. Line probes detect resistance within 6 to 7 hours, pyrosequencing within 5 to 6 hours, and Sanger sequencing within 1 to 2 days. The latter 3 detect resistance to INH, RMP, ethambutol, fluoroquinolones, amikacin, capreomycin, and kanamycin [10]. With molecular DST's excellent turnaround time, management of TB patients has improved. One should realize though that mutations do not always confer resistance, and therefore, a sequence-based method is recommended whenever available [10,91,92].

Benefit of prophylactic treatment of asymptomatic children exposed to MDR-TB has not been well studied and is not yet endorsed by the WHO [7,34,89].

There is a paucity of studies on the treatment of MDR/XDR-TB in children. Case-by-case management is needed with involvement of a childhood TB expert. Every child should be evaluated with history taking, physical examination, CXR, TST, sputum testing (with Xpert MTB/RIF if available or sputum smear microscopy, culture, and DST), and HIV testing [62]. Cure and probable cure rates in children are 80% to 90% compared with successful treatment in adults of 48% to 62% [86,89,93]. In these studies, it was not possible to judge the optimal treatment duration. It is recommended that children be given drugs based on the index case strain's susceptibility profile, especially in those where bacteriologic confirmation is not possible or delayed [89]. "A second-line injectable drug, a fluoroquinolone and at least two other drugs to which the index case strain or the strain isolated from the child is sensitive by DST should be included in the initial drug regimen. Pyrazinamide should be added to these four drugs for the whole course of treatment but should not be counted among the active drugs, providing that DST suggests susceptibility of the causative Mtb strain to pyrazinamide. Parenteral treatment with the second-line injectable drugs (SLID) should be continued for at least 4–6 months, or sometimes longer, depending on disease severity. When treatment with the SLID is discontinued, treatment should be continued orally with at least three active drugs, not counting pyrazinamide. The optimal duration of MDR/XDR-TB treatment in children is unclear and may be very variable from case to case. Depending on the extent of the disease, the DST pattern of the causative bacteria and the immune status of the child, a total duration of treatment between 12 and 18 months following culture conversion could be reasonable and treatment may have to be prolonged in some cases to avoid the risk of relapse. Finally, the decision on the exact number of drugs and length of therapy also depend on extent and site of disease, penetration of the chosen drugs and treatment response" [30,89]. It is important not to add a single drug to a failing regimen and to use daily treatment regimen with DOT whenever possible. Advice about side effects and importance of adherence should be discussed at every visit [84]. In addition to providing a proper drug regimen, the pediatrician should provide psychosocial support and assess for child and caretakers' risk factors that might lead to nonadherence. Pain management, hearing tests, and nutritional support are also important [94].

There are limited data on the safety of second-line drugs in TB, but their use with intense monitoring might be warranted in life-threatening situations. Children who have received treatment of drug-resistant TB have generally tolerated the second-line drugs well. The benefit of fluoroquinolones in treating drug-resistant TB in children has been shown to outweigh any risk.

In addition, ethionamide, para-aminosalicylic acid, and cycloserine have been used effectively in children and are well tolerated. Linezolid for XDR-TB has been studied in children with little adverse effects documented. When it occurred, peripheral neuropathy, previously reported to be irreversible, resolved in all children [86].

In general, anti-TB drugs should be dosed according to body-weight dosing. Expert opinion is that all drugs, including fluoroquinolones, should be dosed at the higher end of the recommended ranges whenever possible, except ethambutol. Ethambutol should be dosed at 15 mg/kg, and not at 25 mg/kg as sometimes used in adults with drug-resistant TB, because it is more difficult to monitor optic neuritis in children.

Many new TB drugs are being tested in phase 2 trials. Most of these studies, however, are conducted in the adult population [18]. Thankfully, Delamanid, a new nitro-dihydro-imidazooxazole derivative active against Mtb, is the first new drug to enter phase I/II trials in children with MDR-TB (expected completion is in 2017), and bedaquiline, a diarylquinoline (recommended for adult patients), will soon follow [7,86]. Table 3 lists the 5 different groups of TB medications.

VACCINES

The TB vaccine BCG was first developed in 1921 and remains the only licensed TB vaccine to date. It is well tolerated with an 80-year safety record with 100 million doses administered every year [4]. This vaccine protects young children against severe forms of the disease (eg, TBM) and disseminated TB. It has variable efficacy against PTB. It is not recommended in HIV-infected infants because of a high risk of disseminated BCG disease and the possible acceleration of HIV disease [16,33]. In practice, this has had little effect in HIV-endemic countries, where the HIV status of the baby is rarely established at birth, which is the usual time of BCG vaccination. The BCG is administered in infants at birth in most regions where TB is endemic. Its efficacy for preventing TB is around 50% and ranges from 0% to 80% worldwide [30]. The BCG is not routinely used in the United States, but can be given to adults planning to travel to endemic areas. In light of MDR-TB and XDR-TB becoming more prevalent, there is an urgent need for a more effective vaccine for children [16]. More than 30 vaccines are being studied [33]. Unfortunately, the lack of reliable correlates of protective immunity remains a major obstacle for predicting vaccine efficacy in all TB vaccine trials in adults and children [30]. The WHO advises that all asymptomatic HIV-exposed infants in

Table 3
Different tuberculosis therapy groups

Group name	Anti-TB medications
1. Oral agents	INH, Rifampicin, Ethambutol, Pyrazinamide, Rifabutin, Rifapentine
2. Intravenous or injectable medications	Streptomycin, Kanamycin, Amikacin, Capreomycin
3. Quinolones	Levofloxacin, Moxifloxacin, Gatifloxacin
4. Second-line medications	Ethionamide, Cycloserine, Para-aminosalicylic acid, Terizidone, Prothionamide
5. New anti-TB medications	Bedaquiline, Delamanid, Linezolid, Clofazimine, Amoxicillin-clavulonic acid, Imipenem-cilastatin, Meropenem, Clarithromycin, Thioacetazone, high-dose isoniazid

TB-endemic areas receive BCG vaccination as well as careful monitoring for the development of BCG-related disease [33].

Factors leading to the large variability of BCG's efficacy include strain-specific immunogenicity, technique of vaccine administration age at vaccination, genetic differences between populations, host nutritional factors, host coinfection by parasites, exposure to environmental mycobacteria, and genetic variation in Mtb strains. The longevity of protection is not very clear. A meta-analysis of recent data suggests protection could persist for 50 to 60 years. Additional protection by revaccination with BCG has not been shown [30].

Early in 2013, the long-awaited outcome of the efficacy trial of the first TB vaccine candidate for almost a century, MVA85A, was released. Safety data were encouraging; however, efficacy data were highly disappointing. Because MVA85A induced a large spectrum of IFN-γ responses without protection, these findings emphasize the urgent need for more appropriate biomarkers to determine, and ideally predict, vaccine efficacy [20].

References

[1] Ritz N, Curtis N. Novel concepts in the epidemiology, diagnosis and prevention of childhood tuberculosis. Swiss Med Wkly 2014;144:w14000.

[2] Daniel TM. The history of tuberculosis. Respir Med 2006;100:1862–70.

[3] Comas I, Coscolla M, Luo T, et al. Out-of-Africa migration and Neolithic coexpansion of Mycobacterium tuberculosis with modern humans. Nat Genet 2013;45:1176–82.

[4] Bynum H. Getting it in the neck: the special case of scrofula. In: Spitting blood. United Kingdom: Oxford University Press; 2012. p. 33–9.

[5] Koch R. Die aetiologie der tuberculose, a translation by Berna Pinner and Max Pinner with an introduction by Allen K. Krause. Am Rev Tuberc 1932;25:285–323.

[6] Gouzy A, Nigou J, Gilleron M, et al. Tuberculosis 2012: biology, pathogenesis and intervention strategies; an update from the city of light. Res Microbiol 2013;164:270–80.

[7] Global tuberculosis report. Geneva (Switzerland): World Health Organization; 2014. Available at: http://www.who.int.

[8] Mandalakas AM, Starke JR. Current concepts of childhood tuberculosis. Semin Pediatr Infect Dis 2005;16:93–104.

[9] Perez-Velez CM, Marais BJ. Tuberculosis in children. N Engl J Med 2012;367:348–61.

[10] Lin S-Y, Desmond EP. Molecular diagnosis of tuberculosis and drug resistance. Clin Lab Med 2014;34:297–314.

[11] Bastos ML, Hussain H, Weyer K, et al. Treatment outcomes of patients with multidrug-resistant and extensively drug-resistant tuberculosis according to drug susceptibility testing to first- and second-line drugs: an individual patient data meta-analysis. Clin Infect Dis 2014;59:1364–74.

[12] Jackson-Sillah D, Hill PC, Fox A, et al. Screening for tuberculosis among 2381 household contacts of sputum-smear-positive cases in The Gambia. Trans R Soc Trop Med Hyg 2007;101:594–601.

[13] Morrison J, Pai M, Hopewell PC. Tuberculosis and latent tuberculosis infection in close contacts of people with pulmonary tuberculosis in low-income and middle-income countries: a systematic review and meta-analysis. Lancet Infect Dis 2008;8:359–68.

[14] Childhood TB. Tranining toolkit. Geneva (Switzerland): World Health Organization; 2014. Available at: http://www.who.int.

[15] Lawn SD, Mwaba P, Bates M, et al. Advances in tuberculosis diagnostics: the Xpert MTB/RIF assay and future prospects for a point-of-care test. Lancet Infect Dis 2013;13:349–61.

[16] Sandgren A, Cuevas LE, Dara M, et al. Childhood tuberculosis: progress requires an advocacy strategy now. Eur Respir J 2012;40:294–7.

[17] Marais BJ, Graham SM, Cotton MF, et al. Diagnostic and management challenges for childhood tuberculosis in the era of HIV. J Infect Dis 2007;196(Suppl 1):S76–85.

[18] Burki T. $ 1.4 billion funding shortfall for tuberculosis control. Lancet Infect Dis 2013;13: 1016–7.

[19] Flynn JL, Goldstein MM, Chan J, et al. Tumor necrosis factor-alpha is required in the protective immune response against Mycobacterium tuberculosis in mice. Immunity 1995;2: 561–72.

[20] Kaufmann SH, Dorhoi A. Inflammation in tuberculosis: interactions, imbalances and interventions. Curr Opin Immunol 2013;25:441–9.

[21] Philips JA, Ernst JD. Tuberculosis pathogenesis and immunity. Annu Rev Pathol 2012;7: 353–84.

[22] Kundu M, Basu J. Mycobacterium tuberculosis and the host macrophage: maintaining homeostasis or battling for survival? Curr Sci 2013;105:617–25.

[23] Cronan MR, Tobin DM. Fit for consumption: zebrafish as a model for tuberculosis. Dis Model Mech 2014;7:777–84.

[24] Hawn TR, Matheson AI, Maley SN, et al. Host-directed therapeutics for tuberculosis: can we harness the host? Microbiol Mol Biol Rev 2013;77:608–27.

[25] Divangahi M, Behar SM, Remold H. Dying to live: how the death modality of the infected macrophage affects immunity to tuberculosis. Adv Exp Med Biol 2013;783: 103–20.

[26] Pang JM, Layre E, Sweet L, et al. The polyketide Pks1 contributes to biofilm formation in Mycobacterium tuberculosis. J Bacteriol 2012;194:715–21.

[27] Abel L, El-Baghdadi J, Bousfiha AA, et al. Human genetics of tuberculosis: a long and winding road. Philos Trans R Soc Lond B Biol Sci 2014;369:20130428.

[28] Sabri A, Grant AV, Cosker K, et al. Association study of genes controlling IL-12-dependent IFN-gamma immunity: STAT4 alleles increase risk of pulmonary tuberculosis in Morocco. J Infect Dis 2014;210:611–8.

[29] Tobin DM, Roca FJ, Oh SF, et al. Host genotype-specific therapies can optimize the inflammatory response to mycobacterial infections. Cell 2012;148:434–46.

[30] Newton SM, Brent AJ, Anderson S, et al. Paediatric tuberculosis. Lancet Infect Dis 2008;8: 498–510.

[31] Tabarsi P, Marjani M, Mansouri N, et al. Lethal tuberculosis in a previously healthy adult with IL-12 receptor deficiency. J Clin Immunol 2011;31:537–9.

[32] Marais BJ, Gie RP, Schaaf HS, et al. The natural history of childhood intra-thoracic tuberculosis: a critical review of literature from the pre-chemotherapy era. Int J Tuberc Lung Dis 2004;8:392–402.

[33] Zumla A, Raviglione M, Hafner R, et al. Tuberculosis. N Engl J Med 2013;368:745–55.

[34] Marais BJ, Schaaf HS, Graham SM. Child health and tuberculosis. Lancet Respir Med 2014;2:254–6.

[35] Howley MM, Painter JA, Katz DJ, et al. Evaluation of QuantiFERON-TB Gold In-Tube and Tuberculin Skin Tests among Immigrant Children being Screened for Latent Tuberculosis Infection. Pediatr Infect Dis J 2015;34(1):35–9.

[36] Blumberg HM, Kempker RR. Interferon-gamma release assays for the evaluation of tuberculosis infection. JAMA 2014;312:1460–1.

[37] Mazurek GH, Jereb J, Vernon A, et al. Updated guidelines for using Interferon Gamma Release Assays to detect Mycobacterium tuberculosis infection - United States, 2010. MMWR Recomm Rep 2010;59:1–25.

[38] Machingaidze S, Wiysonge CS, Gonzalez-Angulo Y, et al. The utility of an interferon gamma release assay for diagnosis of latent tuberculosis infection and disease in children: a systematic review and meta-analysis. Pediatr Infect Dis J 2011;30:694–700.

[39] Debord C, De Lauzanne A, Gourgouillon N, et al. Interferon-gamma release assay performance for diagnosing tuberculosis disease in 0- to 5-year-old children. Pediatr Infect Dis J 2011;30:995–7.

[40] Garazzino S, Galli L, Chiappini E, et al. Performance of interferon-gamma release assay for the diagnosis of active or latent tuberculosis in children in the first 2 years of age: a multi-center study of the italian society of pediatric infectious diseases. Pediatr Infect Dis J 2014;33:e226–31.

[41] Pavic I, Topic RZ, Raos M, et al. Interferon-gamma release assay for the diagnosis of latent tuberculosis in children younger than 5 years of age. Pediatr Infect Dis J 2011;30:866–70.

[42] McMullen SE, Pegues DA, Shofer FS, et al. Performance of QuantiFERON-TB Gold and tuberculin skin test relative to subjects' risk of exposure to tuberculosis. Clin Infect Dis 2014;58:1260–6.

[43] Daley CL, Reves RR, Beard MA, et al. A summary of meeting proceedings on addressing variability around the cut point in serial interferon-gamma release assay testing. Infect Control Hosp Epidemiol 2013;34:625–30.

[44] Alexander TS, Miller MB, Gilligan P. Should interferon gamma release assays become the standard method for screening patients for Mycobacterium tuberculosis infections in the United States? J Clin Microbiol 2011;49:2086–92.

[45] Use of tuberculosis interferon-gamma release assays (IGRAs) in low–and middleincome countries: policy statement. Geneva (Switzerland): World Health Organization. Available at: http://www.who.int.

[46] Anderson ST, Kaforou M, Brent AJ, et al. Diagnosis of childhood tuberculosis and host RNA expression in Africa. N Engl J Med 2014;370:1712–23.

[47] Rangaka MX, Wilkinson KA, Glynn JR, et al. Predictive value of interferon-gamma release assays for incident active tuberculosis: a systematic review and meta-analysis. Lancet Infect Dis 2012;12:45–55.

[48] Cuevas LE, Petrucci R, Swaminathan S. Tuberculosis diagnostics for children in high-burden countries: what is available and what is needed. Paediatr Int Child Health 2012;32(Suppl 2):S30–7.

[49] Ghodbane R, Raoult D, Drancourt M. Dramatic reduction of culture time of Mycobacterium tuberculosis. Sci Rep 2014;4:4236.

[50] Van Rie A. Xpert MTB/RIF: a game changer for the diagnosis of pulmonary tuberculosis in children? Lancet Glob Health 2013;1:e60–1.

[51] Pang Y, Wang Y, Zhao S, et al. Evaluation of the Xpert MTB/RIF assay in gastric lavage aspirates for diagnosis of smear-negative childhood pulmonary tuberculosis. Pediatr Infect Dis J 2014;33:1047–51.

[52] Bates M, O'Grady J, Maeurer M, et al. Assessment of the Xpert MTB/RIF assay for diagnosis of tuberculosis with gastric lavage aspirates in children in sub-Saharan Africa: a prospective descriptive study. Lancet Infect Dis 2013;13:36–42.

[53] Sekadde MP, Wobudeya E, Joloba ML, et al. Evaluation of the Xpert MTB/RIF test for the diagnosis of childhood pulmonary tuberculosis in Uganda: a cross-sectional diagnostic study. BMC Infect Dis 2013;13:133.

[54] Nicol MP, Workman L, Isaacs W, et al. Accuracy of the Xpert MTB/RIF test for the diagnosis of pulmonary tuberculosis in children admitted to hospital in Cape Town, South Africa: a descriptive study. Lancet Infect Dis 2011;11:819–24.

[55] Reither K, Manyama C, Clowes P, et al. Xpert MTB/RIF assay for diagnosis of pulmonary tuberculosis in children: a prospective, multi-centre evaluation. J Infect 2015;70(4):392–9.

[56] Nhu NT, Ha DT, Anh ND, et al. Evaluation of Xpert MTB/RIF and MODS assay for the diagnosis of pediatric tuberculosis. BMC Infect Dis 2013;13:31.

[57] Rachow A, Clowes P, Saathoff E, et al. Increased and expedited case detection by Xpert MTB/RIF assay in childhood tuberculosis: a prospective cohort study. Clin Infect Dis 2012;54:1388–96.

[58] Raizada N, Sachdeva KS, Nair SA, et al. Enhancing TB case detection: experience in offering upfront Xpert MTB/RIF testing to pediatric presumptive TB and DR TB cases for early rapid diagnosis of drug sensitive and drug resistant TB. PLoS One 2014;9:e105346.

[59] Zar HJ, Workman L, Isaacs W, et al. Rapid diagnosis of pulmonary tuberculosis in African children in a primary care setting by use of Xpert MTB/RIF on respiratory specimens: a prospective study. Lancet Glob Health 2013;1:e97–104.

[60] Yin QQ, Jiao WW, Han R, et al. Rapid diagnosis of childhood pulmonary tuberculosis by Xpert MTB/RIF assay using bronchoalveolar lavage fluid. Biomed Res Int 2014;2014: 310194.

[61] Nicol MP, Spiers K, Workman L, et al. Xpert MTB/RIF testing of stool samples for the diagnosis of pulmonary tuberculosis in children. Clin Infect Dis 2013;57:e18–21.

[62] Companion handbook to the WHO guidelines for the programmatic management of drug-resistant tuberculosis. Geneva (Switzerland): World Health Organization; 2014. Available at: http://www.who.int.

[63] Lippincott CK, Miller MB, Popowitch EB, et al. Xpert MTB/RIF assay shortens airborne isolation for hospitalized patients with presumptive tuberculosis in the United States. Clin Infect Dis 2014;59:186–92.

[64] LaCourse SM, Chester FM, Preidis G, et al. Use of xpert for the diagnosis of pulmonary tuberculosis in severely malnourished hospitalized Malawian children. Pediatr Infect Dis J 2014;33:1200–2.

[65] Portevin D, Moukambi F, Clowes P, et al. Assessment of the novel T-cell activation marker-tuberculosis assay for diagnosis of active tuberculosis in children: a prospective proof-of-concept study. Lancet Infect Dis 2014;14:931–8.

[66] Blok N, Visser DH, Solomons R, et al. Lipoarabinomannan enzyme-linked immunosorbent assay for early diagnosis of childhood tuberculous meningitis. Int J Tuberc Lung Dis 2014;18:205–10.

[67] Nicol MP, Allen V, Workman L, et al. Urine lipoarabinomannan testing for diagnosis of pulmonary tuberculosis in children: a prospective study. Lancet Glob Health 2014;2: e278–84.

[68] Swingler GH, du Toit G, Andronikou S, et al. Diagnostic accuracy of chest radiography in detecting mediastinal lymphadenopathy in suspected pulmonary tuberculosis. Arch Dis Child 2005;90:1153–6.

[69] Bolursaz MR, Mehrian P, Aghahosseini F, et al. Evaluation of the relationship between smear positivity and high-resolution CT findings in children with pulmonary tuberculosis. Pol J Radiol 2014;79:120–5.

[70] Marais BJ, Schaaf HS. Tuberculosis in children. Cold Spring Harb Perspect Med 2014;4: a017855.

[71] Thwaites GE. Adjunctive corticosteroids for all forms of tuberculosis? Lancet Infect Dis 2013;13:186–8.

[72] Sterling TR, Villarino ME, Borisov AS, et al. Three months of rifapentine and isoniazid for latent tuberculosis infection. N Engl J Med 2011;365:2155–66.

[73] Weiner M, Savic R, Mac Kenzie W, et al. Rifapentine pharmacokinetics and tolerability in children and adults treated once weekly with rifapentine and isoniazid for latent tuberculosis infection. Journal of Pediatric infectious disease society 2014;3(2):132–45.

[74] Gillespie SH, Crook AM, McHugh TD, et al. Four-month moxifloxacin-based regimens for drug-sensitive tuberculosis. N Engl J Med 2014;371:1577–87.

[75] Madan K, Yadav SS, Wig N, et al. Corticosteroids for prevention of tuberculosis mortality. Lancet Infect Dis 2013;13:915.

[76] Schoeman JF, Van Zyl LE, Laubscher JA, et al. Effect of corticosteroids on intracranial pressure, computed tomographic findings, and clinical outcome in young children with tuberculous meningitis. Pediatrics 1997;99:226–31.

[77] Critchley JA, Young F, Orton L, et al. Corticosteroids for prevention of mortality in people with tuberculosis: a systematic review and meta-analysis. Lancet Infect Dis 2013;13: 223–37.

[78] Shaik J, Pillay M, Jeena P. The role of interferon gamma release assays in the monitoring of response to anti-tuberculosis treatment in children. Paediatr Respir Rev 2014;15:264–7.

[79] Hewitson JP, Von Oppell UO. Role of thoracic surgery for childhood tuberculosis. World J Surg 1997;21:468–74.

[80] Huish DW. The surgical treatment of pulmonary tuberculosis in childhood and adolescence. Thorax 1956;11:186–200.

[81] Vilaplana C, Marzo E, Tapia G, et al. Ibuprofen therapy resulted in significantly decreased tissue bacillary loads and increased survival in a new murine experimental model of active tuberculosis. J Infect Dis 2013;208:199–202.

[82] Bhattacharya D, Dwivedi VP, Maiga M, et al. Small molecule-directed immunotherapy against recurrent infection by Mycobacterium tuberculosis. J Biol Chem 2014;289: 16508–15.

[83] Mayer-Barber KD, Andrade BB, Oland SD, et al. Host-directed therapy of tuberculosis based on interleukin-1 and type I interferon crosstalk. Nature 2014;511:99–103.

[84] Al-Dabbagh M, Lapphra K, McGloin R, et al. Drug-resistant tuberculosis: pediatric guidelines. Pediatr Infect Dis J 2011;30:501–5.

[85] Zumla AI, Schito M, Maeurer M. Advancing the portfolio of tuberculosis diagnostics, drugs, biomarkers, and vaccines. Lancet Infect Dis 2014;14:267–9.

[86] Schaaf HS, Garcia-Prats AJ, Hesseling AC, et al. Managing multidrug-resistant tuberculosis in children: review of recent developments. Curr Opin Infect Dis 2014;27:211–9.

[87] Seddon JA, Perez-Velez CM, Schaaf HS, et al. Consensus statement on research definitions for drug-resistant tuberculosis in children. J Pediatric Infect Dis Soc 2013;2:100–9.

[88] Zignol M, Sismanidis C, Falzon D, et al. Multidrug-resistant tuberculosis in children: evidence from global surveillance. Eur Respir J 2013;42:701–7.

[89] Lange C, Abubakar I, Alffenaar JW, et al. Management of patients with multidrug-resistant/extensively drug-resistant tuberculosis in Europe: a TBNET consensus statement. Eur Respir J 2014;44:23–63.

[90] Kim SJ. Drug-susceptibility testing in tuberculosis: methods and reliability of results. Eur Respir J 2005;25:564–9.

[91] Ajbani K, Grace Lin SY, Rodrigues C, et al. Evaluation of pyrosequencing for detecting extensively drug-resistant tuberculosis (XDR-TB) in clinical isolates from four high-burden countries. Antimicrob Agents Chemother 2015;59(1):414–20.

[92] Zheng R, Zhu C, Guo Q, et al. Pyrosequencing for rapid detection of tuberculosis resistance in clinical isolates and sputum samples from re-treatment pulmonary tuberculosis patients. BMC Infect Dis 2014;14:200.

[93] Mignone F, Codecasa LR, Scolfaro C, et al. The spread of drug-resistant tuberculosis in children: an Italian case series. Epidemiol Infect 2014;142:2049–56.

[94] Franck C, Seddon JA, Hesseling AC, et al. Assessing the impact of multidrug-resistant tuberculosis in children: an exploratory qualitative study. BMC Infect Dis 2014;14:426.

Advances in Pediatrics 62 (2015) 91–103

ADVANCES IN PEDIATRICS

Child Advocacy in the Twenty-first Century

Lisa J. Chamberlain, MD, MPH[a,*], Nancy Kelly, MD, MPH[b]

[a]Department of Pediatrics, Stanford University School of Medicine, 1265 Welch Road, Stanford, CA 94305, USA; [b]Department of Pediatrics, University of Texas Southwestern Medical Center, 5323 Harry Hines Boulevard, 9063, Dallas, TX 75390, USA

Keywords
- Children • Advocacy • Pediatrician • Health

Key points
- The professional role of pediatricians should include advocacy.
- Children's physical, mental, and behavioral health are affected by social determinants of health.
- Several components of the Affordable Care Act are directed at improving the health of US children, but lack of health insurance for children, including those who are undocumented, remains a significant problem.
- There are numerous avenues that physicians may take in advocating for children, including patient-level, community-level, and legislative advocacy.
- Advocacy training is an important component of residency to ensure that the next generation of pediatricians has the skills necessary to address the growing challenges of health disparities.

ADVOCACY DEFINED

Advocacy has been defined by a consensus of leaders in pediatric advocacy training as follows: "To speak up, to plead, or to champion for a cause while applying professional expertise and leadership to support efforts on individual (patient or family), community, and legislative/policy levels, which result in the improved quality of life for individuals, families, or communities" [1].

WHY SHOULD PEDIATRICIANS ADVOCATE?

Children are a vulnerable population, unable to speak to their own needs. Their lives are dependent upon adults, and they are unable to vote or voice

*Corresponding author. E-mail address: lchamberlain@stanford.edu

0065-3101/15/$ – see front matter
http://dx.doi.org/10.1016/j.yapd.2015.04.010

their cause. Pediatricians are uniquely positioned to serve as advocates for children for several reasons [2]. They work with children on a daily basis and are able to directly observe the specific health issues afflicting their patients. Physicians have a trusting, personal relationship with their patients and families and are privy to details about their lives. Thus, they may be able to identify social, economic, or environmental problems that directly affect the health of their patients, such as hunger, which may affect a child's ability to perform well in school. They are able to identify issues affecting individual patients and simultaneously detect emerging trends impacting communities. When issues are identified that require action, pediatricians are well positioned to initiate efforts for change. In general, they are trusted and respected members of society and are viewed as experts in the care of children. Because of this status, pediatricians have the opportunity to access key local, state, and national leaders, and are not viewed as having an ulterior motive when championing a child health issue. For these reasons, the professional role of pediatricians should include child health advocacy.

Abraham Jacobi, MD, is considered the founder of pediatrics in the United States, and a trailblazer in child advocacy. His work to secure safe housing and safe milk for poor infants and children in the mid-1800s was an early example of physician advocacy, and serves as a model for current pediatricians [3]. Dr Jacobi illustrates his early recognition of the pediatrician's duty toward child advocacy. "… It is not enough, however, to work at the individual bedside at the hospital. In the near or dim future, the pediatrician is to sit in and control school boards, health departments, and legislatures. He is the legitimate advisor to the judge and the jury, and a seat for the physician in the councils of the republic is what the people have a right to demand."

THE STATE OF CHILDREN'S HEALTH

Advances over the past century have significantly improved child health. Infectious diseases that once claimed the lives of thousands of children pose far less of a threat thanks to vaccines and a better understanding of infection pathology. However, new threats face the children of the twenty-first century. Palfrey and colleagues [4] describe the health issues facing the children of today as the millennial morbidity. Examples of these are socioeconomic and technologic influences on health, obesity, mental health problems, and health disparities.

Health disparities are preventable differences in the burden of disease, injury, violence, or opportunities to achieve optimal health that are experienced by socially disadvantaged populations [5]. Racial and ethnic disparities noted in children's health and health care include, but are not limited to, mortality rates, access to care and use of services, prevention and population health, health status, and quality of care [6]. These disparities arise from differences in income, insurance status and area of residence. Despite federal efforts toward reduction, significant disparities remain based on race/ethnicity, income, and insurance status [7].

The sate of US child health leaves much room for improvement because numerous issues that affect the well-being of children remain paramount. Infant mortality (death before the age of 1 year) was 6.1 per 1000 live births in 2010, mostly attributed to preterm births. The most recent comparative international data find the United States to be 27th among industrialized nations for infant mortality [8]. Data from 2011 to 2012 from the Federal Interagency Forum on Child and Family Statistics shows concerning rates of childhood asthma (9%); obesity (19%); and emotional, concentration, and behavior problems (5%) [9]. In addition, data on social and environmental risks for children remain concerning. Nearly one-quarter of all children (22%) live in a household that the US Department of Agriculture defines as food insecure. Approximately 14.7 million children are living in poverty, nearly 1 in 5 children overall, with higher rates for Hispanic children (24%) and African American children (27%). Forty-six percent of children are experiencing inadequate or crowded housing or shelter cost burden, and two-thirds of children live in counties where the pollutant concentrations exceed the levels of current air quality standards.

It has become increasingly understood that children's physical, mental, and behavioral health is affected by social determinants. Healthy People 2020 defines the social determinants of health as "conditions in the environments in which people are born, live, learn, work, play, worship, and age that affect a wide range of health, functioning, and quality of life outcomes and risks" [10]. Lack of necessary resources, such as safe housing, availability of healthy food, transportation, quality education, social support, and literacy, can have significant impact on population health. Because primary care providers may be the only health professionals to interface with families on a regular basis, it imperative that they view advocacy as a part of their commitment to the medical profession.

THE AFFORDABLE CARE ACT AND IMPROVING POPULATION HEALTH

Health disparities widen when access to efficacious care is unequal. The last 5 years have seen significant shifts in the landscape of health coverage and the emerging realization of aligning reimbursement to incentivize prevention, which represent a fundamental shift in American medicine. The Patient Protection and Affordable Care Act (ACA) was passed by Congress and signed by President Obama in 2010. As with many advances in US health policy the ACA was driven to address the needs of adults, specifically cost containment, through the triple aim of improved health, streamlined health care, and reduced costs.

Despite the adult-oriented forces three advances for children are important to consider. First, a well liked aspect of the ACA is the extension of coverage for children under their parents' insurance policies from age 18 to 26 years. This extension has already had a measurable impact, reducing the number of this traditionally underinsured age group (young adults in their 20s) by 3 million. A second important component affects children with medical complexity. Previously insurance carriers could deny coverage for preexisting conditions and impose lifetime limits on coverage. Elimination of these components increases coverage for a vulnerable subset of our population: those with chronic illness resulting from a legacy of birth and/or childhood, who before the ACA were at high risk for being uninsured and thus unable to access necessary medical care, especially as they became adults. In addition, it is important to remember that expanding health insurance coverage through Medicaid expansion for low-income parents helps their children through increased engagement in the Medicaid system [11]. Medicaid expansion has not been evenly adopted: it was implemented in 29 states, is under discussion in 6 states, and has not been adopted by 16 states [12]. Unequal levels of adult coverage at the state level mirrors uneven coverage for children: undocumented children currently remain largely uninsured. Providing coverage for this particularly vulnerable population has been shown to reduce unmet health and dental needs, improve health status, and reduce child school absenteeism, so much remains to be done [13].

PATIENT-LEVEL ADVOCACY

Physicians advocate every day in their practices when they work to obtain services needed by their individual patients. Pediatricians may provide vaccines to low-income patients through the Vaccines for Children Program, ensuring their protection against several infectious agents. Questioning their patients and families about social determinants may identify food insecurity, leading to prompt referral to a local food pantry. In addition, pediatricians may communicate with a child's school to ensure that the child receives appropriate evaluation and services for learning difficulties. All of these actions qualify as individual patient-level advocacy.

COMMUNITY-LEVEL ADVOCACY

Advocacy should also extend beyond the individual level. The American Academy of Pediatrics (AAP) Council on Community Pediatrics calls for pediatricians to participate in "community activities to improve the health and welfare of all children" and further states that this should be considered "an integral part of the professional role and ethical obligation of all pediatricians" [14]. Some of these recommendations are as follows:

1. Use community data to better understand the effects of social determinants on child health
2. Work with community organizations to identify and decrease barriers to child health, and have access to information about local resources to improve the health and well-being of children in the community
3. Promote preventive strategies for common childhood issues on an individual level and on a population level within the community
4. Work with the community to improve all settings and organizations in which children spend time (eg, schools)

5. Advocate for universal access to health care in a medical home and for the social, economic, educational, and environmental resources essential for children's healthy development
6. Interface with the media and serve as trusted sources of information about public health issues

Effective physician engagement in advocacy that extends beyond the individual level can occur in numerous settings and to various degrees, as described by Earnest and colleagues [2]. Joining and supporting medical societies is a simple way to get started. Organizations such as the AAP, its local chapters, and the Academic Pediatric Association can benefit from physicians' financial support, and donation of their time, energy, and expertise. These organizations identify pertinent child health and wellness issues and work to effect change by drafting policy statements, forming coalitions to bring attention to issues, and working with legislatures to effect policy change.

Physicians working in hospital settings can lead or assist in efforts to make system-wide improvements or create programs that can benefit their patients and families. To date, 135 hospitals nationwide have joined forces with legal institutions to form medical-legal partnerships [15]. Providing legal services to patients and their families can lead to improved health and well-being. A medical-legal partnership can advocate for children who have been wrongly denied special education services or food assistance by helping the parents understand their rights, and facilitating the process of obtaining the services or benefits. Some children's hospitals have developed programs to provide influenza or pertussis vaccines at no cost to the household contacts of their pediatric patients in an effort to protect very young patients from these potentially deadly diseases [16,17]. Physicians are well positioned to advocate for implementation of programs such as these.

Earnest and colleagues [2] describe the following 2 scenarios that show how pediatricians can advocate within their communities to alleviate health issues pertinent to their own patient populations. Physicians may notice that obesity is a prominent health issue for school-aged patients in their practices. They question the families about contributing factors, and determine that lack of healthy food choices offered in the school may be a contributor. They raise the issue with the local school board and work to effect changes in the school's nutrition policy. This example shows the power of the pediatrician's voice and how collaborating and partnering with the community can effect change.

Injury prevention provides another example of physician advocacy. From car passenger safety to preventing falls from windows, physicians have had an active role in successfully advocating for change that has reduced unintended injuries and death. Other arenas of evolving injury prevention work include water safety and bike safety, the latter through increased adoption of laws requiring bike helmet use. As physicians care for children who are seriously injured their perspectives bearing witness to these preventable tragedies is very effective.

Physicians are also in an optimal position to bring pertinent health issues to public attention. Working with the media, pediatricians can share their stories to educate the public about disparities, safety dangers, disease risk, and benefits of prevention and treatment. Television and radio news interviews and letters to the editor are examples of avenues physicians use. Recent outbreaks of pertussis were brought to life in a personal manner by news pieces aired on television [18]. Infants with pertussis are featured in this news clip. One child is shown intubated and receiving treatment in the intensive care unit. His parents and a physician are interviewed and share information about the danger of the disease and the importance of vaccination. Physicians can share these real-life stories to bring health and safety concerns to the attention of the public. Not all physicians feel comfortable working with the media, but, for those who are, there are many accessible resources through the AAP's Council on Communications and Media that can provide valuable information and support services [19]. Furthermore, many hospitals have media relations departments and are able to assist physicians who wish to improve their skills in this area.

COMMUNITY PARTNERSHIPS

Another avenue for physicians is engagement in community-based advocacy. Pediatricians may wish to partner with a community group or organization to address a health issue within the population of the community rather than with patients in a hospital or clinic setting. This partnership requires a thoughtful and systematic approach to build a strong partnership that is effective and sustainable. Four basic concepts have been cited by Sanders and colleagues [20] as the necessary components to guide pediatricians if they wish to effect meaningful action with a community partner. The first is collaborating with the community to establish a specific, short-term, health-related goal. This step is paramount to building and sustaining a successful partnership. A physician may identify a presumed need in the community, but unless there is agreement on the ultimate goal, the partnership may not lead to change or, worse, it may deteriorate into a poor experience for both. It is imperative that the physician recognizes and acknowledges the community partner's assets and seeks input from the partner so the venture is mutually beneficial. Priorities of both the physician and community organization must be in alignment because both may have limited time and financial resources to dedicate to a project.

The second concept is identifying evidence-based best practices for achieving the shared goal. Substantial data on previously implemented community-based interventions are available to the public. Rather than starting from scratch, people can learn from and build on the prior experiences of other community-based advocates and researchers. The Community Guide is a publication of a scientific systematic review of health interventions by the Community Preventive Services Task Force [21]. Interventions are reviewed for effectiveness, populations and sites studied, cost, benefits or harm, and areas in need of further research. Based on this scientific review, interventions are rated as "recommended" if they have been found to be effective, "recommended against" if harmful or ineffective, and "insufficient evidence" if more research is needed to determine whether the intervention is effective or not.

The third concept is adapting a best practice to the specific community setting. Physicians may have ideas for how to implement an intervention within the community, but without knowing the community in depth, they may not anticipate barriers or understand the factors that may motivate individuals to participate in the program. For example, even the best program may be poorly attended if it is not held at a convenient location or at a time that works for the families it is meant to target. It is thus crucial to include community members in planning discussions so that physicians can better understand the population's needs and constraints. In addition, having buy-in from respected community leaders and organizations may help individuals gain trust in an otherwise unknown physician who is proposing a health intervention. Implementation of health promotion interventions in collaboration with faith-based organizations has been shown to be an effective strategy [22]. In addition, use of lay health workers can help in efforts to improve health outcomes of community members [23].

Program evaluation is also a critical component of community intervention. In today's cost-conscious society, demonstrating an intervention's effectiveness is usually necessary to secure funding to sustain it. In addition, much is learned from a well-designed program evaluation that can inform the development or revision of future successful health interventions.

LEGISLATIVE ADVOCACY

Many pediatricians seek to make a difference by working on policy change through legislative advocacy. There are a variety of ways to contribute to policy change depending on the amount of time and effort available. Organizations such as the AAP provide resources to help pediatricians become more adept at legislative advocacy. The AAP's Advocacy and Policy Web page provides information to keep busy pediatricians abreast of current legislation that is pertinent to children's health [24]. Letter templates in support of or against particular legislation are frequently available that can be edited, personalized, and sent to elected leaders. One medical center used the time before its pediatric departmental grand rounds to educate attendees about pertinent legislature and issues affecting children's health, and offered opportunities for interested persons to sign prewritten letters or to obtain information they could use to call or contact their legislator [25]. Efforts such as this can increase pediatricians' awareness of current issues and help them to actively advocate on a legislative level. Local chapters of the AAP and other organizations offer opportunities for medical students, residents, and practicing physicians to visit state or national legislatures as a group, and meet with law makers to discuss pertinent health issues. Physicians often provide testimony to members of Congress to support legislation deemed critical to child health. Groups such as the Academic Pediatric Association support its members by offering in-person educational workshops and on-line training to teach basic legislative advocacy tips to those who wish to learn these skills. Its Public Policy and Advocacy Web site provides valuable information for pediatricians and opportunities to get involved [26]. Palfrey and colleagues [27] summarize some of the efforts of pediatricians working with the Academic Pediatric Association in the passage of important legislation concerning vaccines, health insurance, lead toxicity, gun safety, and car and safety restraints.

ADVOCACY TRAINING FOR PEDIATRICIANS

It is well recognized that the future of pediatrics must include community engagement and collaboration, thus teaching the next generation of pediatricians must include curricula designed to this end. In 1996, the Pediatric Residency Review Committee of the Accreditation Committee for Graduate Medical Education (ACGME) required that residency programs provide the following for their trainees: "There must be a structured education experience that prepares residents for the role of advocate for the health of the children within the community" [1]. Effective July 2013, the ACGME specified that pediatric residency programs provide a specific number of "educational units" composed of ambulatory experiences including "elements of community pediatrics and child advocacy" [28]. Although the specifics of this training are not outlined, experts in pediatric advocacy have suggested that certain components of knowledge, attitudes, and skills should be taught to equip pediatricians for the role of child advocate [1]. In terms of knowledge, understanding the barriers that limit patient access to care, knowing local community characteristics and resources, and knowing how to access local and state government leaders were recognized as some of the most important concepts to be taught. Acquisition of advocacy skills was thought to be just as important as knowledge acquisition, if not more so. Skills such as assessing a patient's needs and assets; accessing community resources and collaborating with the community; and participating in advocacy efforts within a hospital, professional group, or on a grass-roots level were thought to be basic skills necessary for resident advocacy training. However, an advocacy curriculum that teaches knowledge and skills is inadequate if it does not ultimately instill in residents the attitude that advocating for children is part of the professional role of a pediatrician. Thus, advocacy training should be structured such that the ultimate goal is resident adoption of this attitude.

Programs such as the Anne E. Dyson Foundation Community Pediatrics Training Initiative have provided grant support to help pediatric residency programs develop their advocacy training [29]. This initiative provided 5 years of support to 10 pediatric residency programs beginning in 2000. Subsequent programs such as the AAP's Community Pediatrics Training Initiative (CPTI) supported by the Josiah Macy Jr. Foundation provided additional pediatric residency programs with financial support and mentorship from pediatric advocacy leaders to help them transform their community pediatrics and advocacy training. To date, the AAP's CPTI has supported more than 60 pediatric residency programs in strengthening their community pediatrics programming [30]. In a 2005 article, Shipley and colleagues [31] explore approaches and models for teaching community health and child advocacy to pediatric residents. They define 2 strategies considered crucial to this training: engaging residents and building strong community partnerships. Pediatric residency programs have implemented a variety of experiences in their curricula to instill knowledge, skills, and attitudes to promote child advocacy in their trainees and future pediatricians. Residency programs have worked to achieve these goals in various ways. Some incorporate this education into well-defined block rotations, whereas others use longitudinal experiences throughout the years of residency. Many programs include community organization site visits and tours, self-directed learning modules, community-based primary care opportunities, and longitudinal individual or group advocacy projects as curricular components. Each program's method of teaching advocacy should take advantage of the unique talents of the program's faculty, staff, and residents, and also those of the community in which it is located.

STATEWIDE COLLABORATIVES

Dissemination and uptake of educational innovation can occur at national meetings, in which best practices are presented, or it can spread through peer-to-peer or program-to-program engagement. These educational collaboratives offer a rapid approach to providing faculty development through train-the-trainer models, as well as sharing educational resources such as presentations, handouts, and readings to advance resident training. These approaches are important in novel areas of curricular development. Examples of statewide educational collaboratives include California [32], New Jersey [33] and Missouri, all of which have collaborated to share best practices around community pediatrics training. In California, 13 pediatric residency programs united in 2009 to improve advocacy training. The endeavor was evaluated and, following the collaboration, the programs showed an increase in advocacy activities and enhanced incorporation of curricular component. The impact of the collaboration extended beyond the impact of the learners. Qualitative evaluation showed that the collaboration (1) reduced faculty isolation and strengthened faculty academic development; (2) enhanced identification of curricular areas of weakness and provided curricular development from new resources; (3) helped to address barriers of limited resident time and program resources; and (4) sustained impact through curricular enhancement, the need for further resources, and a shared desire to expand the collaborative network [32]. Recently across the state of Missouri the 4 pediatric training programs formed an educational collaboration to strengthen training and, working in conjunction with their AAP chapter, a unified pediatric voice in the capital in Jefferson City. Similar initiatives are being considered in other states. Supporting the development and academic success of community pediatric faculty is a key component of sustaining community pediatrics and advocacy.

DOES TRAINING IN ADVOCACY CHANGE PEDIATRICIAN BEHAVIOR?

Evaluation of advocacy training has evolved as the field has grown. Assessment of the impact of such training required patience: evaluation of the impact had to wait until those residents who had been trained graduated and went into practice. Initial evaluations, gleaned from national survey data fielded by the AAP after examining pediatric practice patterns, revealed that although pediatricians found high interest in advocacy, there were declining rates of engagement in advocacy activity [34]. Respondents went on to note their inadequate skills in public speaking, poor understanding of health issues on a population level, and not being comfortable with their understanding of health policy issues as reasons for not participating. Simultaneously, most reported that they would participate if they had more training. This evaluation was followed by a more authoritative study of the graduates' community engaged behaviors from programs that had high levels of community pediatric training, and compared them with those with age-matched controls (43.6% vs 31.1%; $p < .01$) [35]. These findings were particularly important in the context of waning community engagement for child health by pediatricians nationally. It seems that education in community pediatric training "immunized" graduates, moving the field forward in terms of meeting both the required training mandates and the timely mandate of training the next generation of pediatricians to work to address the growing challenges of health disparities.

NEXT STEPS

Although debate about the role of physicians engaging beyond the clinic walls continues for some fields of medicine [2,36,37], pediatrics has committed to move community engagement forward. This commitment is fortuitous as recent health reform begins to align this prescient work with sustainable mechanisms for reimbursement. This fundamental shift will move community engagement from a volunteer activity, at risk of being eclipsed by busy pediatricians' many competing priorities (young families and high levels of educational debt), to a central, reimbursable part of practice. As mentioned previously, the ACA has shifted the health care landscape. This massive piece of health legislation established Accountable Care Organizations, which use novel payment models that shift physician responsibility from the health of the individual patient to the health of the community. This paradigm shift seamlessly aligns with community pediatrics and its emphasis on population level health. This model moves academic medical centers and clinical pediatric practice into the spheres of community nonprofit organizations and departments of public health; an area of expertise for the community pediatrician. A system of care in which prevention drives revenue by allowing practitioners to capture the savings will ensure a greater collaboration between public health, medicine, and community pediatrics. As always, critical evaluation will be needed of how pediatricians are practicing in local communities in which these models are already underway.

The confluence of an increasing number of US children confronting the millennial morbidities with the next generation of pediatricians being trained to effectively address them, all practicing within an environment in which the financial incentives align with prevention, all come together to create a significant shift in the way pediatrics is practiced. For the first time, the opportunity to take to scale physicians engaged in community exists. This change moves toward the day when physician advocacy grows from professional aspiration to a defined obligation [38].

References

[1] Wright CJ, Katcher ML, Blatt SD, et al. Toward the development of advocacy training curricula for pediatric residents: a national Delphi study. Ambul Pediatr 2005;5(3): 165–71.

[2] Earnest M, Wong S, Federico S. Professional behaviors of physicians and pursuing social justice. JAMA 2009;302(12):1269 [author reply: 1269–70].

[3] Burke EC. Abraham Jacobi, MD: the man and his legacy. Pediatrics 1998;101(2):309–12.

[4] Palfrey JS, Tonniges TF, Green M, et al. Addressing the millennial morbidity–the context of community pediatrics. Pediatrics 2005;115(4 Suppl):1121–3.

[5] Centers for Disease Control and Prevention. Community health and program services (CHAPS): health disparities among racial/ethnic populations. Atlanta (GA): US Department of Health and Human Services; 2008.

[6] Flores G, Committee on Pediatric Research. Technical report—racial and ethnic disparities in the health and health care of children. Pediatrics 2010;125(4):e979–1020.

[7] Dougherty D, Chen X, Gray DT, et al. Child and adolescent health care quality and disparities: are we making progress? Acad Pediatr 2014;14(2):137–48.

[8] US Department of Health and Human Services. Maternal Child Health Bureau. 2015. Available at: http://mchb.hrsa.gov/infantmortality/index.html. Accessed September 1, 2015.

[9] Federal Interagency Forum on Child and Family Statistics. America's children in brief: key national indicators of well-being, 2014. 2014. Available at: http://www.childstats.gov/americaschildren/glance.asp. Accessed September 1, 2015.

[10] Office of Disease Prevention and Health Promotion. Social determinants of health. 2015. Available at: http://www.healthypeople.gov/2020/topics-objectives/topic/social-determinants-health. Accessed August 2, 2015.

[11] Dubay L, Kenney G. Expanding public health insurance to parents: effects on children's coverage under Medicaid. Health Serv Res 2003;38(5):1283–301.

[12] The Henry J. Kaiser Family Foundation. Status of state action on the Medicaid expansion decision. State health facts Available at: http://kff.org/health-reform/state-indicator/state-activity-around-expanding-medicaid-under-the-affordable-care-act/. Accessed March 27, 2015.

[13] Howell E, Trenholm C, Dubay L, et al. The impact of new health insurance coverage on undocumented and other low-income children: lessons from three California counties. J Health Care Poor Underserved 2010;21(2 Suppl):109–24.

[14] American Academy of Pediatrics Council on Community Pediatrics. Community pediatrics: navigating the intersection of medicine, public health, and social determinants of children's health. Pediatrics 2013;131:623–8.

[15] National Center for Medical-Legal Partnership. Partnerships across the U.S. 2015. Available at: http://medical-legalpartnership.org/partnerships/. Accessed January 23, 2015.

[16] Kelly NR, Kromelis MR, Jordan D, et al. Feasibility of delivering influenza vaccine to household contacts of pediatric patients in a residents' continuity clinic. Am J Infect Control 2012;40(7):627–31.

[17] Dylag AM, Shah SI. Administration of tetanus, diphtheria, and acellular pertussis vaccine to parents of high-risk infants in the neonatal intensive care unit. Pediatrics 2008;122(3): e550–5.

[18] CBS News. Two infants dead in Texas whooping cough epidemic. Available at: http://www.youtube.com/watch?v=l_e57WaKLzw. Accessed February 8, 2015.

[19] American Academy of Pediatrics. Council on Communications and Media. 2015. Available at: http://www.aap.org/en-us/about-the-aap/Committees-Councils-Sections/Council-on-Communications-Media/Pages/default.aspx. Accessed May 11, 2015.

[20] Sanders LM, Robinson TN, Forster LQ, et al. Evidence-based community pediatrics: building a bridge from bedside to neighborhood. Pediatrics 2005;115(4 Suppl):1142–7.

[21] The Guide to Community Preventive Services. What is the community guide? 2015. Available at: http://www.thecommunityguide.org/about/index.html. Accessed February 8, 2015.

[22] DeHaven MJ, Hunter IB, Wilder L, et al. Health programs in faith-based organizations: are they effective? Am J Public Health 2004;94(6):1030–6.

[23] Raphael JL, Rueda A, Lion KC, et al. The role of lay health workers in pediatric chronic disease: a systematic review. Acad Pediatr 2013;13(5):408–20.

[24] American Academy of Pediatrics. Advocacy and policy. 2015. Available at: http://www.aap.org/en-us/advocacy-and-policy/Pages/Advocacy-and-Policy.aspx. Accessed February 8, 2015.

[25] Bensen R, Roman H, Bersamin M, et al. Legislative advocacy: evaluation of a grand rounds intervention for pediatricians. Acad Pediatr 2014;14(2):181–5.

[26] Academic Pediatric Association. Public Policy and Advocacy Committee. 2015. Available at: http://www.academicpeds.org/public_policy/public_policy_index.cfm. Accessed February 8, 2015.

[27] Palfrey JS, Cheng TL, Schuster MA. A history of the Academic Pediatric Association's Public Policy and Advocacy initiatives. Acad Pediatr 2011;11(3):205–10.

[28] Accreditation Council for Graduate Medical Education. Program Requirements for Graduate Medical Education in Pediatrics. 2011. Available at: http://www.acgme.org/acWebsite/downloads/RRC_progReq/320_pediatrics_07012007.pdf. Accessed June 5, 2011.

[29] Palfrey JS, Hametz P, Grason H, et al. Educating the next generation of pediatricians in urban health care: the Anne E. Dyson Community Pediatrics Training Initiative. Acad Med 2004;79(12):1184–91.

[30] Community Pediatrics Training Initiative. Current grantees. Available at: http://www2.aap.org/commpeds/cpti/grantees.htm. Accessed April 10, 2014.

[31] Shipley LJ, Stelzner SM, Zenni EA, et al. Teaching community pediatrics to pediatric residents: strategic approaches and successful models for education in community health and child advocacy. Pediatrics 2005;115(4 Suppl):1150–7.

[32] Chamberlain LJ, Wu S, Lewis G, et al. A multi-institutional medical educational collaborative: advocacy training in California pediatric residency programs. Acad Med 2013;88(3):314–21.

[33] Schwartzberg P. Catch Corner: New Jersey Residency Advocacy Program. The New Jersey Pediatrician. 2010;Summer:12.

[34] Minkovitz CS, O'Connor KG, Grason H, et al. Pediatricians' involvement in community child health from 1989 to 2004. Arch Pediatr Adolesc Med 2008;162(7):658–64.

[35] Minkovitz CS, Goldshore M, Solomon BS, et al. Five-year follow-up of Community Pediatrics Training Initiative. Pediatrics 2014;134(1):83–90.

[36] Huddle TS. Perspective: medical professionalism and medical education should not involve commitments to political advocacy. Acad Med 2011;86(3):378–83.

[37] Palfrey JS, Chamberlain LJ. Do medical professionalism and medical education involve commitments to political advocacy? Acad Med 2011;86(9):1062–3 [author reply: 1065].

[38] Gruen RL, Pearson SD, Brennan TA. Physician-citizens–public roles and professional obligations. JAMA 2004;291(1):94–8.

Advances in Pediatrics 62 (2015) 105–136

ADVANCES IN PEDIATRICS

ELSEVIER
MOSBY

Children in Immigrant Families
The Foundation for America's Future

Joyce R. Javier, MD, MPH[a], Natalia Festa, BA[b],
Ellynore Florendo, MS[a], Fernando S. Mendoza, MD, MPH[b],*

[a]Division of General Pediatrics, Department of Pediatrics, Children's Hospital Los Angeles, University of Southern California Keck School of Medicine, 4650 Sunset Boulevard MS#76, Los Angeles, CA 90027, USA; [b]Division of General Pediatrics, Department of Pediatrics, Lucile Packard Children's Hospital, Stanford University School of Medicine, Stanford, 1265 Welch Road, MSOB 238, Stanford, CA 94305-5459, USA

Keywords
• Latino • Immigrant • Health care

Key points

- The consequences of the 1965 Immigration and Naturalization Act Amendments (INAA) resulted in a dramatic shift in those who immigrated to the United States.
- Children in immigrant families (CIF) are changing the demographics of the United States.
- As one examines the health and well-being of CIF, one needs to not just start from the present but also understand their past.
- There are differences in the health status that first-generation immigrant children experience as opposed to second- or third-generation US children.
- Overall, low-income immigrants are likely to be more uninsured than low-income United States–born citizens because of decreased access to public and private health insurance.

INTRODUCTION

The United States is one of the few countries of the world where immigrants are considered core to the country's foundation. It has been the children of those immigrants who have made the nation successful and a leader in the global community. One of our national symbols, the Statue of Liberty, proclaims, "Give me your tired, your poor, your huddled masses yearning to breathe free." This message has been heard around the world by those seeking freedom and an improved economic status. They have come not only seeking

*Corresponding author. E-mail address: fmendoza@stanford.edu

0065-3101/15/$ – see front matter
http://dx.doi.org/10.1016/j.yapd.2015.04.013

freedom and economic opportunities for themselves but also hoping to create a new and rewarding life for their children and subsequent generations. Over the years, the push-pull of the immigration process has basically remained the same. The push from the country of origin has been created by persecution, violence, lack of freedom, and limited economic opportunities. The pull to the United States has centered on the freedoms of our society and the economic opportunities of our country. Yet, the value that we philosophically place on immigrants is clouded by the reality of the history of the immigrant experience and the legislative efforts to shape it. This article on children in immigrant families (CIF) addresses the health and well-being of CIF; it starts with background information on the history of immigration to the United States including recent changes and the demographic impact it has had on the US population, particularly its children.

FROM THE PAST TO THE PRESENT: IMMIGRATION POLICY

The first immigration law of the country was the Naturalization Act of 1790, which establishes that only "white persons of good moral character" could become citizens in the newly formed United States [1]. Early in our country's history, most of the immigration came from Northern Europe, primarily England, Germany, and Ireland. Immigrants from Ireland came after the social disruption caused by the potato famine of the mid-nineteenth century, whereas others came for religious freedom and economic opportunity. Citizenship became more of a racial issue with the 1882 Chinese Exclusion Act that prohibited naturalization of Chinese individuals, and an ethnic issue with the 1921 Emergency Quota Act and Immigration Act of 1924, which put quotas on individuals from Southern and Eastern Europe [1]. Among these immigrants were Jews, Italians, and Slavs. These legislative actions were intended to maintain the racial makeup of the United States stable. Post World War II in 1952, racial restrictions were abolished, but a quota system with ethnic preference was maintained in the Immigration and Nationality Act that sought aliens with skills needed in the United States to spur economic growth. The eventual elimination of racial/ethnic-based immigration legislation was accomplished with the 1965 Immigration and Nationality Act (INAA) which eliminated national origin quotas and developed immigration regulations based on family reunification and employment skills. It also set, for the first time, a quota for Western Hemisphere immigration and a 20,000 immigrant limit for countries from the Eastern Hemisphere.

The consequences of the 1965 INAA resulted in a dramatic shift in those who immigrated to the United States. In 1960, 75% of foreign-born individuals living in the United States were from Western and Northern Europe. Since 1965, there has been a persistent drop in the proportion of foreign-born individuals in the United States from Western and Northern Europe, down to 12.1% in 2010, and concurrently, there has been a significant increase in the proportion of foreign-born individuals from Latin America and Asia, 53.1% and 28.2%, respectively [2]. Furthermore, higher birth rates of immigrants from Latin America and Asia have led to a significant increase in the proportion of newborns from these groups. Consequently, since 1990 to the present, 75% of the population growth of children has come from the Latin American and Asian American populations [3,4] This growth has changed the demographics of US children, with growing Latino and Asian American proportions. In states such as California, Latinos are becoming the majority; 50% of all newborns in California are Latino. This demographic change has two components: immigrant children (children born outside of the United States) and children born in the United States to immigrant mothers. As such, the construct of CIF has become a useful term to identify families with both types of children born to immigrant mothers. Approximately 86% of the CIF are US citizens, with another 8% documented and only 6% identified as undocumented [3].

Since the passage of the INAA in 1965, other laws have been passed that have modified the immigration process and have affected CIF. In 1990, the Congress passed the Immigration Act of 1990 with the Temporary Protection Status (TPS) that allowed the US Attorney General to designate a foreign country unsafe and allow individuals from those countries TPS, which meant that they could have work permits, but not permanent residence, a green card [5]. The Homeland Security Act of 2002 moved the processing of the TPS into Homeland Security. The countries currently covered by this act are Haiti, Somalia, Sudan, Syria, El Salvador, Honduras, and Nicaragua. (The recent influx of unaccompanied minors was from El Salvador and Honduras). In 2000, the Trafficking Victims Protection Act was passed, which required undocumented immigrant children from noncontiguous states to be transferred to the Office of Refugee and Resettlement within 72 hours while starting the process for removal by the Executive Office for Immigration Review. These 2 acts involving TPS and human trafficking victims emphasize the importance of defining an individual as a migrant or refugee. The United Nation's High Commission on Refugees considers a migrant as an individual who chooses to move to improve the economic status of themselves and their families. In contrast, refugees have to move if they are to save their lives or preserve their freedom. The US Immigration service states that, "Refugee status or asylum may be granted to people who have been persecuted or fear they will be persecuted on account of race, religion, nationality, and/or membership in a particular social group or political opinion" [6]. Thus, the immigration experience of Latino immigrants from Mexico, El Salvador, Honduras, and Nicaragua can be different because all Mexicans are considered migrants, whereas refugee status is possible for individuals from El Salvador, Honduras, and Nicaragua. Cubans have been considered refugees since the 1960s because of the Cuban communist regime. Consequently, immigrants are considered migrants or refugees depending on the political and social dysfunction status of their country of origin. Determining whether an immigrant family has migrant or refugee status is important in assisting them in adapting to their new communities.

Lastly, in addition to Congressional laws, the Supreme Court and the Executive branch of the government also have affected the lives of CIF. In 1982, the Supreme Court in *Plyler v Doe* established that illegal immigrant children had a right to public education, from K to 12th grade, allowing undocumented immigrant children to be educated. In June 2012, President Obama established the Deferred Action for Childhood Arrivals (DACA), which instructed the US Department of Homeland Security to not deport certain undocumented youth who had come to the United States as children and were in school and had not committed any crime. Undocumented youth can apply for DACA and receive 2 years of deferred action.

The complications of immigration policy were exemplified during the past years (2011–2014) when there was a 10-fold increase in unaccompanied children and youth from El Salvador, Honduras, and Guatemala [7]. Although this flow of children and youth has lessened along the US southern border, there was still an increase in apprehension of immigrant children and youth by the Immigration Service in fiscal year 2013–14 compared with prior baseline years: 177% increase in children 5 years and younger, 111% increase in children 6 to 12 years, and 12% increase in adolescents 13 to 17 years. The driving force behind this increased migration was the increased violence and social disruption in those sending countries. Because of these children's age and the fact that they were from countries not contiguous to the United States, these children were placed with the Office of Refugee and Resettlement until their immigration status could be determined. This created significant confusion and overload of the immigration services dealing with children. However, through cooperation between federal agencies, communities, and professional groups, these children were managed, being seen as victims caught between their country's violence and our immigration laws. Nonetheless, in a recent report on the outcomes of these children and youth, most were deported. Those from Mexico where immediately deported, whereas those not from Mexico (noncontiguous country) were sent to an immigration court, where less than half (48%) had a lawyer [8]. Among those children and youth with lawyers, 53% were deported, whereas among those without lawyers, 90% were deported. Perhaps more so than any other event, the recent influx of unaccompanied children along the southern border has brought greater attention to the issue of immigrations and children. This event has given the country an opportunity to consider the effects of immigration law on the well-being of CIF, including when the lives of children are changed when parents are deported.

DEMOGRAPHICS AND SOCIAL DETERMINANTS OF CHILDREN IN IMMIGRANT FAMILIES

CIF are changing the demographics of the United States. In 2014, 1 of every 4 child lives in an immigrant family, a family having at least 1 parent born outside of the United States. It is estimated that by 2050, this will increase to 1 of every 3 children [4]. At present, approximately 60% of Latino children and 85% of Asian American children live in an immigrant family. During the past decade, the immigrant population has come principally from Latin America/Caribbean and Asia, 54% and 25.9%, respectively [9]. Mexico has provided the most immigrants of any country, 29.2% of immigrants during the past 10 years. Other regions of the world have contributed significantly lower proportions: Europe 8.7%, Africa 5.0%, Middle East 4.2%, Canada 1.5%, and Australia/others 0.6%.

Yet, the growth of the population of CIF is primarily because these families have higher birth rates compared with native families. The US Census Bureau estimates that by 2050 there will be equal proportions of Latino and non-Latino white children in the United States [10]. In the face of a growing elderly population estimated to achieve 18.6% of the total US population by 2050 and a falling proportion of children in the population, currently 24%, the proportion of children to elderly will be approaching 1:1. This ratio implies that the economic success of CIF is critical to the future support of the nation's elderly population [11]. Without children becoming productive adults and supporting the tax-supported services for the elderly, the nation will be in economic difficulty.

The primary social determinates of CIF are established by their parents' educational level, their income, family structure, and their immigration status. The Urban Institute's review of family and parental characteristics shows this variability [12]. For example, 47% of immigrant parents from Mexico have less than a high school education, whereas 70% of parents from the Middle East and South Asia have college degrees. This variation is closely linked with the levels of poverty that are seen in these families; 69% of Mexican immigrant families are less than 200% of poverty, compared with 23% of immigrant families from the Middle East and South Asia and 35% of native families. In contrast, the family structure of immigrant families is similar. Most have 2-parent families at the same proportion as native non-Latino white families at 76% and have a similar rate of working fathers, 80%. Yet, the educational levels of these fathers determine their hourly wage and work benefits, such as health insurance. Thus, although there is significant variability among immigrant families, when one examines the situation for the most populous group, those from Mexico and Central America, their profile is one of low education and higher poverty but still with robust family structure.

The immigration status of the parents is an important social determent of immigrant families. It is estimated that 5.5 million children live with 1 unauthorized parent, and 4.5 million are born in the United States [13]. These values mean that children with unauthorized parents are one-third of all CIF and make up 8% of US children. A review of this area by Yoshikawa and Kholopseva [13] suggest that these parents are at risk for removal, are less likely to use public services for the families, and are more likely to have poorer working conditions with increased stress and persistent economic hardship. The impact on their children's development as a result of this chronic stress can lead to lower cognitive skill in early childhood, lower levels of general positive development in middle school years, higher levels of anxiety and depressive symptoms in adolescent years, and overall less school years. Consequently, among the social determinants for CIF, one of the most influential may be their parents' residential status [13].

THE IMMIGRANT EXPERIENCE AND HEALTH

As one examines the health and well-being of CIF, one needs to not just start from the present but also understand their past. Having knowledge about why the family (or individual child) migrated to the United States and the experiences of that process can inform the understanding of current and future health problems, which can be key in understanding the emotional stress causing health problems in children and their parents. In 2014, the media highlighted the experiences of unaccompanied minors from Latin America involving violence and physical and emotional stress. Yet, these experiences have been reported among immigrant children more than a decade ago, with one-third having clinically significant posttraumatic stress [14]. Thus, this emphasizes the need for pediatricians to explore the family social history to achieve a comprehensive understanding of the health and well-being of CIF.

The Academy of Pediatrics through the Council on Community Pediatrics made a policy statement on providing care for immigrant, migrant, and border children [15]. They divided children into immigrants (children with 1 immigrant parent), migrants (children of families who migrate to the United States for work opportunities), and border children (children who live within 100 km of the Mexican border), with most migrant and border children being immigrants as well. Although some migrant and border children have 2 parents who are US citizens and therefore the immigration issues noted earlier do not apply to them, they share the common environment of poverty, lower educational levels, barriers to access of quality health care, and detachment from social institutions. Moreover, the issue of the border environment of lower resources is something that is not uncommon in other areas of the country where these children reside. Therefore, this article focuses on immigrant children, with the caveat that some migrant and border children are in nonimmigrant families but have similar health profiles.

In this article, the term CIF is used rather than immigrant children to emphasize that predominantly these children are US citizens, even though they have an immigrant parent.

Lastly, the health issues of CIF direct the focus to the model of health proposed by Tarlov [16] and adopted by the Centers for Disease Control, which has integrated social determinants into the predictors of population health outcome (Fig. 1). In this model, the ecology of a population plays a major part in determining health, even more so than other factors usually thought of as significant health determinants: genetic, health care access, and health behaviors. Yet, as one examines CIF, the one issue that needs to be kept in mind is that within these families, the ecology and medical care may be different from one child to another based on their citizenship status, which is the dilemma for the parents and health providers of these children.

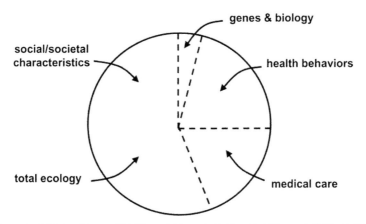

Fig. 1. Relative influence of the five major determinant categories of population health: rough approximations. (*From* Tarlov AR. Public policy frameworks for improving population health. Socioeconomic status and health and industrial nations: social, psychological, & biologic pathways. Ann N Y Acad Sci 1999;896:283; with permission.)

THE FIRST 5 YEARS: OPPORTUNITIES TO DEVELOP HUMAN CAPITAL IN EARLY CHILDHOOD

As noted earlier, CIF represent the most diverse and rapidly growing segment of the US child population, yet they are disproportionately represented among the poor, with their poverty likely to persist into adulthood. Within the population of CIF, Latino children, especially those of Mexican origin, are the most likely to live in poverty and are at highest risk of poor academic outcomes with subsequent limited occupational opportunities [17]. As this already sizable demographic population achieves increasing representation in our schools and subsequently in our workforce in a time of growing social expenditures to support an aging population, it is imperative that CIF are afforded the opportunity to become productive citizens by way of healthy growth and development. Pediatricians are often the first professionals to encounter these children. As such, they are presented with the unique opportunity to facilitate healthful development as these children go on to face the challenges and opportunities of the educational system and their community.

Opportunities to develop the human capital of immigrant children during early childhood can be broadly divided into the infancy period, ages 1 to 3 years, and ages 3 to 5 years. In each of these periods, as per Bright Futures, pediatricians are charged with supporting the child's physical and developmental health and also supporting the parenting skills of mothers and fathers to provide a nurturing environment for the child. Traditionally, this has included ensuring proper growth and nutrition, treatment of acute diseases, educating parents about child development and parenting, providing preventive health care through the provision of immunizations, and, more recently, obesity prevention advice. For some children, there is also the specter of chronic disease developed either in the neonatal period or later in childhood that complicates the health care of these children. CIF bring additional factors, both positive and negative, that can affect their health care. The following sections cover health and development issues during the first 5 years of life aside from chronic illness, which is discussed in subsequent sections.

NEONATAL HEALTH

The US infant mortality rate of approximately 6 per 1000 live births [18] is higher than that of most industrialized nations. Although these rates are likely reflective of differences in the measurement and reporting of infant mortality globally, further analysis has shown that higher rates in the United States as compared with its industrialized counterparts are attributable to prematurity [19]. A persistent finding of infants born to immigrant mothers is that infants born to these mothers tend to have better outcomes (lower prevalence of low birth weight and lower infant mortality) than do children born to nonimmigrant mothers, even though immigrant mothers have less education, higher poverty, and less access to health care. This phenomenon has been termed the immigrant paradox, because it would be expected that those mothers with the mentioned risk factors would have poor infant outcomes. Unfortunately, the immigrant paradox dissipates with time in the United States, resulting in these mothers approaching the levels of low birth weight, prematurity, and infant mortality of nonimmigrant mothers with the same risk factors. This trend of worsening health outcomes with the length of stay in the United States is of importance, as immigrants and their descendants are projected to account for approximately 80% of the national population growth by 2050 [20]. Given that the initial immigrant advantage in birth outcomes regresses with duration in the United States, it is pressing that the drivers of poorer birth outcomes in this population are more accurately characterized and addressed [20]. Markides and Coreil [21] established the concept of the epidemiologic or immigrant paradox in 1986 in their review of the literature on the health status of Latino immigrants in the Southwestern United States. In analyzing patterns of infant mortality, overall mortality, subjective reports of physical and mental health, and trends in chronic disease, Latino immigrants were found to have health status more similar to that of white Americans despite sociodemographic characteristics that resemble those of black Americans [21,22]. It was suggested that these findings were likely to be linked with cultural health behaviors, particularly as the acculturation process seems to lessen the immigrant paradox effect.

More recent scholarship has favored intraethnic assessments of health status, so as to allow for comparison to immigrants with longer duration of stay within the United States and to those individuals who have remained in their countries of origin. The concept of in-group comparisons has also precipitated questions as to former analyses of rates of low birth weight as an indicator of neonatal health, given that birth weight is most appropriately assessed within racial and ethnic groups rather than by conventional birth with curves, based on a population of neonates primarily of European descent [23]. Such intraethnic assessments of birth outcomes have found that immigrants to the United States tend to have improved health outcomes and longevity as compared with both individuals who remain in their countries of origin and United States–born individuals of the same race or ethnicity, although these advantages dissipate with time. Such findings have demonstrated a curvilinear association by which rates of prematurity and low birth weight decline during the first few years in the United States and increase thereafter. Although applicable to all immigrant groups, this relationship is especially strong in the case of Latino immigrants [22].

This relationship between increased rates of low birth weight within immigrant families and time in the United States has become a matter of concern as CIF, a predominately Latino population, account for one-quarter of the national child population and are predicted to drive nearly all of the growth in the national workforce during the next several decades [4]. With the rapid growth of this population prefiguring the ways in which the face of schools and the workforce are to change [24], increased risk of premature birth and low birth weight with time in the United States are tantamount to greater incidence of suboptimal childhood growth and developmental outcomes and chronic health conditions such as asthma in later childhood [25,26]. With the increasing number of survivors of prematurity and the increased health care and educational costs that are required by these children, it is important to better understand the curvilinear association between adverse birth outcomes and time in the United States for the most rapidly growing demographic, nationally. Can the worsening neonatal outcomes of CIF be avoided?

EARLY PREVENTION

The early childhood years serve as a critical window for the implementation of preventive health measures for CIF, particularly for those born outside of the United States. Immunizing children against communicable diseases is one core element of preventive care for children. Although CIF born outside of the United States depend on the public health resources of their country of origin, these have historically been limited, leading to immunized rates lower than their native-born peers [27]. However, more recently, children in sending nations such as Mexico and China have rates of immunization comparable or higher than those of US children for all infectious diseases [28]. Yet, despite improved rates of immunization in sending nations, once in the United States, CIF depend on our health service system for completion and continued adherence to the immunization schedule. A 2002 analysis of the National Immunization Survey demonstrates comparable rates of the diphtheria, pertussis, and tetanus/polio/measles, mumps, and rubella immunization series coverage between United States– and foreign-born children between 19 to 35 months of age. However, this same analysis raises concern for lower rates of vaccination coverage against Hib and hepatitis B among foreign-born children, with foreign-born Asian children least likely to be protected. Another study using data from the National Health Interview Survey 2000–03 demonstrated that immigrant mothers who had resided in the United States for less than 5 years were most likely to have their children fully immunized, but this decreased after 10 years in the country [29]. Nonetheless, the United Nations Children's Fund 2011 estimates of immunization rates internationally show that children in many sending nations are vaccinated at either comparable or higher rates than children within the United States, overall. As compared with 94% of children in the United States, children from Guatemala, Mexico, and China are vaccinated against polio at rates of 97%, 86%, and 99% respectively. Although the prevalence of hepatitis B is greater in the US foreign-born population, disparities in prevalence between immigrant and native-born children have narrowed over time [30]. Overall, the task of the pediatrician with respect to immunizations of this population is to identify the completeness of the immunization series and encourage immigrant mothers to continue to adhere to the recommended vaccination schedule.

In addition to ensuring that foreign-born children are appropriately immunized, screening for other disease conditions should also be part of the initial evaluation of these children. The American Academy of Pediatrics (AAP), through the Council of Community Pediatrics, has developed a tool kit to assist in the assessment of foreign-born children [31]. This tool kit recommends screening for infectious diseases, such as tuberculosis and patristic diseases, based on the prevalence in their country of origin. Although the rates of tuberculosis are declining in the United States, they are 13 times higher among foreign-born individuals than among native born individuals and the highest among foreign-born non-Hispanic Asians, 26 times higher [32]. Concurrently, an assessment of the overall nutritional status should also be done, including testing for iron deficiency anemia. Malnutrition in both calories and nutrients can lead to poorer immune response and in some cases anergy, which may affect the screen for tuberculosis. Screening for possible toxins, such as lead, also should be considered.

Although in the past, malnutrition implied lower weight and stature, in the present world of high-caloric low-nutrient foods, malnutrition is also linked with obesity. The years immediately after birth are a critical time frame during which significant racial and ethnic differences in rates of obesity emerge, with United States–born CIF at greatest risk within their respective racial and ethnic groups [33]. As CIF have been found to have lower levels of physical activity than their native-born peers [34], they remain at significantly greater risk for overweight, obesity, and concomitant comorbidities [35]. In an analysis of rates of overweight and obesity within a population of disadvantaged households, Latino children were nearly twice as likely to be overweight or obese as white children [34]. In this same analysis, Latino children were also twice as likely to be overweight or obese as black children despite similar socioeconomic status (SES). This difference may be partly attributable to cultural differences in parental feeding practices [34], as well as reported lower levels of physical activity within immigrant families that are not attenuated by accounting for socioeconomic or neighborhood characteristics [33]. Analysis by panethnic group and generation has identified second-generation Latino children to be at greatest risk of obesity, with a 55% greater likelihood than their native-born white peers. Contrastingly, Asian CIF were found to be at lesser risk, with first-generation children 63% less likely to be obese than native-born white children. As patterns of obesity among CIF vary greatly by generational status and ethnicity, pediatricians should consider the cultural factors that may be influencing the dietary and exercise habits of children in diverse families [36].

PROMOTION OF SCHOOL READINESS IN THE HOUSEHOLD SETTING: AGES 0 TO 3 YEARS

Although much of the national discussion on the topic of school readiness has focused on access to early childhood programming, such as Head Start, there has been a shift toward characterizing the types of parental behaviors and involvement that promote school readiness and academic success within the home. In support of this concept are analyses indicating that the academic and behavioral benefits offered to children vary between interventions that are directed toward cultivating parental engagement versus those that are institutionally based, such as Head Start [37]. In a comparison of the benefits of Early Head Start (partially home-based intervention for children ages 0–3 years) with traditional Head Start (center-based programming for children ages 3–5 years), benefits in language acquisition, behavior, and parental involvement were associated with Early Head Start. In longitudinal analyses, children younger than 3 years whose families participated in home-based interventions have been found to have higher receptive vocabulary scores, arithmetical achievement test scores, and fewer behavioral problems than peers at the conclusion of kindergarten [38], with benefits continuing through adolescence [39]. The enduring effects of home-based intervention on parental engagement and child functioning lend support to growing interest in how parental engagement can best be promoted in the home from birth.

The effects of verbal engagement in early infancy are directly reflected in emergent language skills and the ability to direct attention in social interaction as early as 24 months [40]. With mounting evidence to support the importance of early cognitive engagement for later language acquisition, literacy, and school readiness, there is concern that CIF are more likely to be at risk for delayed development of these skills as a result of residing in poverty in linguistically isolated non-English-speaking households compared with children in native-born families [41–43], It was thought that such demographic factors entirely explained the lower likelihood of immigrant parents to verbally engage and share books with children. However, a recent study determined that in controlling for factors formerly thought to explain decreased frequency of parental book sharing with children (a proliteracy behavior), residing in an immigrant household itself is highly predictive of decreased parental book sharing behavior within the home for children of Asian and Latino descent [44]. Thus, it is now hypothesized that targeting immigrant mothers as early as possible to engage in book sharing with their children may promise significant impact in the early cognitive development and school readiness of this population.

Interventions such as Reach Out and Read (ROR), which capitalize on the anticipatory guidance offered in the pediatric primary care setting, have proved to be an effective means of engaging parents to best facilitate the early cognitive development and school readiness of their children [45]. A substantial evidence base has shown that parents whose children receive primary care at ROR participating sites are likelier to share books, to have reading materials at home, and to describe reading aloud as a regular activity [46]. A longitudinal analysis of Latino CIF whose parents were engaged with ROR from the time of the first well-child visit were found to have greater phonemic awareness and familiarity with print at the time of kindergarten entry [47]. Despite risk factors for poor academic achievement, most of these children were determined to be average or above average in reading proficiency by the completion of kindergarten.

As early cognitive development, emergent literacy and school readiness have become increasingly established as predictors of educational and occupational outcomes [48–50]. both the AAP and the Bright Futures guidelines have stressed the importance that pediatricians promote parental engagement through behaviors that support early literacy and language acquisition [51,52]. Promoting ROR is a means of promoting early literacy and language development through the medical encounter [45], but it remains unclear why CIF are sharing books with parents at rates much lower than that of their native-born counterparts despite comparable rates of health care access [44]. Although it has been suggested that immigrant families are more likely to read to children if provided with books during the well-child visit [53,54], engaging parents in immigrant families with early literacy and language and cognitive development is important to achieve rates akin to their native-born counterparts.

PROMOTION OF SCHOOL READINESS IN THE EDUCATIONAL SETTING: AGES 3 TO 5 YEARS

As noted earlier, in the past decade, births have outpaced immigration as the main driver of growth in the Latino and Asian population, with these groups projected to account for most of the US population growth in the coming decades [20]. As a result, this exceedingly young cohort will soon represent most of the students in public schools nationally [17,55]. The established disadvantage in school readiness of CIF underscores the importance of early childhood intervention in allowing these children, particularly those of Latino origin, to overcome their relative disadvantage and enter kindergarten with foundational skills comparable to that of their peers in native-born families.

With increased evidence that the years between birth and school entry represent a time frame during which school readiness disparities in disadvantaged CIF emerge, modifiable factors such as access to preschool have been identified as possible ways to augment early cognitive development and childhood learning trajectory [56,57]. As early as kindergarten, CIF perform worse on several indicators of school readiness, and such disparities not only persist but also tend to worsen during the educational course [58]. An analysis of the US Department of Education's Early Childhood Longitudinal Study, Kindergarten (ECLS-K) cohort data set reveals that, even before kindergarten, the average cognitive score of children in the highest SES group are 60% more than the scores of the lowest SES group, conferring relative disadvantage to CIF given their disproportionate representation among the poor [58].

An analysis of the ECLS-K data by race and ethnicity indicates considerable diversity in school readiness among CIF, as demonstrated by performance on standardized math examination at the conclusion of third grade. Of first-generation CIF, Asian children are found to greatly outperform their Latino peers [59]. In assessing for differences in school performance by national origin within broader ethnic groups, significant differences in academic performance by nationality have emerged; for example, children of Vietnamese and Chinese immigrants surpass their peers of Laotian or Cambodian and Filipino descent in early math competency [60]. Beyond differences by national origin, time and generations in the United States have been associated with poorer academic outcomes of Latino immigrants, a trend that remains to be more clearly understood [60].

Disparities at the time of kindergarten entry for CIF are problematic as academic performance at this juncture is found to be predictive of later educational outcomes. For example, disparities in foundational literacy and language skills are known to widen rather than narrow over the course of the educational trajectory [59,61]. In addition to promoting parental facilitation of children's early literacy and language development, research has demonstrated improvements in school readiness among CIF enrolled in center-based early childhood care and educational programming [41]. Despite the advantages of such programming to early cognitive development, immigrant families are less likely to enroll their children (31%) than native-born families (37%), overall [3,62]. In subsequent generations within immigrant families, Filipino- and Mexican American children in particular have been much less likely to enroll in center-based care than their Asian-American, white, and black counterparts [63].

Of CIF, those in linguistically isolated households, defined as homes in which little or no English is spoken, are at the greatest risk of disadvantage on entering kindergarten and often the least likely to have exposure to formal educational programming before this time [62]. These predominately Latino children are most likely to be classified as English learners on kindergarten entry and have been shown to make gains in early literacy and language skills as a result of preschool enrollment [62]. Lower rates of enrollment among Latino children have been shown to be associated with demographic characteristics, particularly low parental education, increased household size, and undocumented status [62].

The advantages conferred to CIF by participation in center-based child care and their relative underutilization of this resource have provided impetus to better characterize the demographics of children less likely to use this resource. Common to all children with socioeconomic disadvantage are barriers of financial and geographic access, as well as the limited enrollment capacity of programs in their communities, such as Head Start [3]. More specific to immigrant families are gaps in knowledge regarding eligibility and documentation status of household members as well as language and potential cultural barriers [64]. Although 86% of CIF are born in the United States, families often do not take advantage of means-tested services and benefits, citing lack of knowledge about the programs, confusion about eligibility requirements, language barriers, and fear of adverse immigration consequences for other family members who are undocumented [65]. This situation can be partially attributed to limitations in their eligibility and to reluctance among these families to disclose information in seeking out such social supports. An understanding of the characteristics of families least likely to enroll their children in formal early childhood programming will allow pediatricians to more readily identify families in need of anticipatory guidance focused on the promotion of school readiness.

Before entering school, well-child visits present a unique and perhaps singular opportunity to educate immigrant parents as to early care and education programs in helping children to achieve school readiness. Because the pediatric primary care setting is often the first institutional encounter for many CIF, providers in this setting have the opportunity to actively engage with immigrant families in addressing the barriers to the early cognitive development and school readiness of their children. Just as CIF stand to benefit greatly in their early literacy and language development by increased book sharing from birth to 3 years of age, these children are poised to gain further developmental benefit by connection to the early formal educational system through the health care setting. Because pediatricians have access to CIF from the time of birth, they are in a unique position to combat these substantial disparities in school readiness and subsequent academic outcomes through the medical encounter.

CHILDREN IN IMMIGRANT FAMILIES: HEALTH ISSUES FOR SCHOOL-AGED CHILDREN AND ADOLESCENT YOUTH

There are differences in the health status that first-generation immigrant children experience as opposed to second- or third-generation immigrants, including differences in the manifestations of asthma, teen births, obesity, physical activity, nutrition, and behavioral disorders. These health conditions can have a significant impact on the well-being of an individual. As mentioned previously, a phenomenon known as the immigrant paradox has been used to describe the differences in the birth outcomes of foreign-born versus native-born mothers and between the health statuses of first-generation and later-generation children. Among Hispanic immigrants, this paradox has been particularly consistent during the infancy period. The immigrant paradox describes that despite the fact that recent immigrant families are among the poorest, least educated, and often uninsured resulting in less access to health care, they have better than expected health outcomes in some measures of health status. Further, those who acculturate have poorer health behaviors (increased rates of smoking, drinking, and drug use) [21]. Although this phenomenon is seen in some health conditions and in risky adolescent behaviors for CIF, it does not apply to all of their health outcomes, especially for children with asthma and special health care needs. This section reviews some of these complex relationships between health and outcomes among CIF for common illnesses and risk behaviors.

ASTHMA

Rates of asthma are higher in United States–born than in foreign-born children [66]. Likewise, rates of allergic diseases that are triggered by a similar biological mechanism of action as asthma, such eczema, hay fever, and food allergies, are lower for children born outside of the United States but increase after residing in the United States for one decade [67]. Consequently, like their mothers' perinatal outcomes, the length of stay in the United States worsens health outcomes for immigrant children and therefore requires us to consider the immigrant paradox as a temporary phenomenon that may be reversed with exposure to the American environment.

The immigrant paradox has been implied when examining the relationship of immigrant status with childhood asthma. Compared with children with asthma in nonimmigrant families, children with asthma in immigrant families are more likely to report access barriers, such as lacking a usual source of care or reporting delays in medical care. They are also less likely to report asthma symptoms and utilization of an emergency room in the past year, yet more likely to report fair or poor perceived health status [68]. Although these data support the immigrant paradox, because they are based on parental reports, like many self-reported surveys, the results might be significantly influenced by the lack of health care access to identify the child's condition. However, there may be other factors in play for a lower rate of asthma in immigrant children, among them genetic factors. For example, in Latino children, there is a 3-fold difference in prevalence between Mexican American first-generation and island Puerto Rican children (7% vs 20%, respectively; NCHS 2005) [69]. This difference seems to be a result of greater genetic propensity for asthma among Puerto Ricans. Genetic studies have revealed that Latino's risk for asthma is determined by the degree of Native American and African genes related to asthma. These findings correlate with the observed lower prevalence of asthma among Mexican American children (immigrant and nonimmigrant) who have a higher proportion of Native American genes and lower proportion of African genes than Puerto Ricans [70]. The prevalence of asthma has been reported the lowest for Mexican Americans (4.8%), followed by European Americans (8.2%), African Americans (14.6%), and Puerto Ricans (18.4%) [71]. Thus, Latino subgroups may have different epigenetic risk for asthma, and the risk may change as they are exposed to their US environment.

Overall, immigrants need to be assessed by their genetic propensity for asthma by their family histories and the risk they incur from their population of origin. As genomic studies continue to expand our understanding of different populations, greater attention needs to be given to targeting the most at-risk group of children. Once identified, children with asthma need 2 things: access to health care and quality care for asthma. The former is driven by access to health insurance and availability of health services. The latter is driven by the cultural and linguistic competency of the medical services to maximize the therapeutic outcomes of these children.

In 2014, The Pew Research Center reported that, overall, foreign-born Hispanics were twice as likely to be uninsured (39% vs 17%), whereas among those Hispanics 18 years or younger, the difference was almost 3 times greater (34% vs 12%). Although as noted previously the great majority of CIF are US citizens (86%), these children still have a higher rate of being uninsured (12.8% vs 5.4%) than non-Hispanic white US children [72]. Moreover, even with Children's Health Insurance Program (CHIP) and the Affordable Care Act (ACA), CIF still have access issues because of regulation requirements, problems in understanding the application processes, and fear of affecting future immigration opportunities for parents, many of whom are undocumented (approximately 30%). Noncitizen but documented children in some states have to wait 5 years for access to CHIP benefits. Although the Immigrant Children's Health Improvement Act (ICHIA) allows states to remove this requirement, not all states have done so, resulting in differences between states in accessing care by immigrant children. Furthermore, although the ACA improves access to care for all lawfully present, it will not affect undocumented individuals or those who have been given temporary stays (DACA and TPS). Still, even for those CIF who are US citizens, significant barriers exist in accessing ACA benefits because of their family's income and documented status. For example, the Urban Institute analysis in 2014 noted that 19% of those Medicaid/CHIP eligible children were uninsured if they had an undocumented parent versus 8.8% for those who were documented [73]. Major barriers for undocumented parents are their reluctance to participate in governmental programs and problems in understanding the application processes. Thus, pediatricians treating all CIF, and more so those with a chronic illness such as asthma, need to engage the parents of these children in discussion about health coverage and link them with groups or agencies that can assist them in insuring their children.

Culturally and linguistically competent care is one of the goals of Bright Future and has been well documented to improve the outcomes of care including in children with asthma. In a study of Medicaid quality monitoring of children with asthma, those clinical sites that had the highest cultural competency scores had mothers who were less likely to report underusing preventive asthma medication, (odds ratio [OR], 0.15; 95% confidence interval, 0.06–0.41) after controlling for practice variables [74]. With most immigrant parents being limited English proficient (LEP) (50%–80%) and having a culture different from that of the provider, providing cultural and linguistic competent care for CIF with asthma and other chronic diseases is vital to provide high-quality care.

Lastly, although cultural and linguistic competent care can be provided, assessing the parents' health literacy is also critical in developing a therapeutic plan for their child with asthma. Parents with low health literacy are more likely to report that their children with asthma have had emergency room visits (OR, 1.4), hospitalizations (OR, 4.6), and missed school days (OR, 2.8) [75]. Given that among the largest immigrant group, Latinos, there is a high level of limited English proficiency and low levels of education, health literacy needs to be assessed when working with these parents. In a study of Latino caregivers of young children, there was a strong relationship between low acculturation and low health literacy, with both affecting health-related skills [64]. Therefore, in managing a child with asthma in an immigrant family, the best practice is to provide evidence-based care in a culturally and linguistically appropriate manner that is conscious of the health literacy of the parents.

CHILDREN WITH SPECIAL HEALTH CARE NEEDS

Concurrent with the earlier discussion about CIF who have asthma, children in special health care need have similar issues. Compared with children with special health care needs (CSHCN) in nonimmigrant families, CSHCN in immigrant families are more likely to report health care access barriers such as lack of insurance, lack of a usual source of care, and delays in medical care. Similar to CIF with asthma, they are less likely to report utilization of an emergency room visit in the past year, yet more likely to report fair or poor perceived health status [76]. Concurrent with children with asthma who are part of an immigrant family, CSHCN in undocumented families are at greater risk for decreased access, utilization, and poorer health status. As the medical condition becomes more complicated, these children may be seen by more pediatric subspecialists and are more likely to be referred to a subspecialty child center for care, which can add to difficulty in coordinating care and the coverage of such care by public insurance, which may be state dependent. For example, in California, CIF can be insured by private insurance (if parents either pay for insurance or have employer insurance), by Medicaid or CHIP if eligible, or if not by local programs for children ineligible for Medicaid/CHIP (Healthy Kids in Santa Clara County, CA, USA). If the child has a specific chronic condition covered by California Children Services (a state insurance program for specific chronic conditions), it provides both payment for services and a coordinating care system that is available independent of residential status. Therefore, there are communities where care for all children is available, with and without special health care needs. However, this is currently not the case throughout the nation. Consequently, pediatricians need to strongly advocate for health care to all children in their communities, and as shown in California, with the support of state and local government this is possible.

OBESITY IN CHILDREN IN IMMIGRANT FAMILIES

In a study examining the health status of 91,532 children of immigrant and United States–born parents from the 2007 National Survey of Children's Health (parental reporting), obesity prevalence was assessed and ranged from the lowest of 7.7% for children for native-born Asian parents to approximately 25% for children of immigrant Hispanic and native-born non-Hispanic black parents [77]. Hispanic children in immigrant and nonimmigrant families were approximately 1.5 times as likely to be obese compared with native non-Hispanic whites. In contrast, immigrant and native Asian families had children who were 50% less likely to be obese. Although immigrant children generally reported lower physical activity levels than native-born children, only Hispanic CIF had a significant OR of 2.5 for inactivity compared with non-Hispanic native white children [77]. Thus, CIF vary in the risk of obesity and sedentary behaviors, and these ethnic-nativity differentials with non-Hispanic native white children remained marked after covariate adjustment [77]. For example, after adjusting for social determinants, Asian adolescents' health remained better than that of whites with respect to their obesity risk. In contrast, Latino adolescents have poorer preventive health behaviors and nutritional status with respect to white adolescents, and in the case of nutrition, their diets worsened with acculturation [26,78].

More research is needed to examine risk factors for development of diabetes and cardiovascular disease other than obesity. For example, although Asian populations are less obese than other minority populations, the American Diabetes Association recently lowered the body mass index (BMI) cut point at which it recommends screening Asian Americans for type 2 diabetes. According to the Joslin Diabetes Center, Asians, the nation's fastest growing ethnic group, under recognized as a group at risk for diabetes because they develop diabetes at lower BMI levels compared to other ethnic groups. This has been attributed to differences in their body composition (ie, Asians have more central adiposity around the waist, an area that is more harmful from a disease standpoint, rather than in other parts of the body) [79]. Latinos, African Americans, and Native Americans still remain the populations with the greatest risk for diabetes [80]. With two-thirds of Latino children living in an immigrant family, the risk for obesity and future diabetes is a significant issue for these children.

TEEN PREGNANCY IN IMMIGRANT YOUTH

Teenage pregnancy is another significant health concern among all adolescents but particularly among the immigrant population. Compared with European American adolescents, Hispanic adolescents have a higher prevalence of having sex before age 13 years (8.3% vs 4.2%) and having 4 or more sexual partners (15.7% vs 10.8%) [81]. In addition, Hispanic adolescents reported a lower rate of condom use at last intercourse in comparison with European American adolescents (ie, 57.4 vs 62.5%) [81]. In a study of 2016 first- and second-generation Hispanic immigrant adolescents from the National Longitudinal Study of Adolescent Health (Waves I and II), maternal support and communication about sex were significantly associated with risky sexual behaviors over time (ie, positive parenting among Hispanic families were associated with less risky sexual behaviors among youth) [82].

Among Asians, Filipinos have higher rates of adolescent pregnancy and human immunodeficiency virus infection than other Asian subgroups [83]. In a study of 120 pairs of Filipino American parents and adolescents, few adolescents (22%) reported regularly discussing sex with parents [84]. Community-academic collaborations aimed at engaging particular aspects of Filipino culture (ie, religion and intergenerational differences) have been implemented to promote parent-adolescent communication about sex to prevent adolescent pregnancy in this population [85]. Thus, the role of the pediatrician is to provide an open environment in which sexual health can be address between CIF teens and their parents.

MENTAL HEALTH AND BEHAVIORAL CONDITIONS

Data from the 2007 National Survey of Children's Health shows that immigrant children in each racial/ethnic group (ie, black, Asian, and Hispanic) had a lower prevalence of depression and behavioral problems: autism; attention-deficit/hyperactivity disorder; developmental delay and learning disability; speech, hearing, and sleep problems; and school absence than native-born children, with prevalence increasing markedly in relation to parents' duration of residence in the United States [77]. However, as noted for asthma and obesity, the patterns in child health and health-risk behaviors differ by ethnicity, generational status, and length of time since immigration. For example, Huang and colleagues [86] examined mental health disparities among young children of Asian immigrants and found that children of foreign-born Asian families from east (eg, Korea), southeast (eg, Philippines and Vietnam), and south Asia (eg, India and Pakistan) were at greater risk for internalizing problems (eg, sadness, loneliness, anxiety, and self-esteem) and inadequate interpersonal relationships compared with children of United States–born white families. Thus, generalization of immigrant children's health should be done cautiously, with attention being paid to the variability among different ethnic and generational groups.

Physical and emotional trauma can have significant impact on the health and well-being of children. CIF who are foreign born may have experienced physical and psychological trauma in their country of origin or in the process of migration. Events such as endured separation from family, forced labor and starvation, physical or sexual assault, or exposure to violence can lead to an impact on the health of children and youth [15]. For example, children of Mexican immigrants in the United States are at risk for developing posttraumatic stress disorder (PTSD) due to increased levels of violence related to drug wars in Mexico [87]. Refugee children also have a greater risk of developing PTSD, with reports as high as 50% among Cambodian youth [88]. Unaccompanied children at the Southern border of the United States have gained national attention, and the need to address physical, mental, and emotional trauma that these youth have faced through mental health and primary care linkages has been recommended [89].

EDUCATIONAL OUTCOMES OF IMMIGRANT YOUTH

Consistent with the immigrant paradox in health, most CIF seem to fare well in their educational performance compared to native born children. The educational immigrant paradox, however, is more evident among children from Asian and African immigrant families. However, some immigrant children, including those of Mexican origin are more likely to be below grade level, and less likely to graduate [17].

Immigrant teens in certain ethnic groups have a higher dropout rate than the national average. According to Morse, the use of a "status dropout rate" that includes all youth whether or not they enrolled in school in the US, and not just whose who are enrolled, may better estimate the problem of poor educational performance among immigrant youth. Hispanics, aged 16 to 24, have a status dropout rate of 27% compared with 11% for black non-Hispanic, 7% for white non-Hispanic, and 4% for Asian/Pacific Islander youth. The high dropout rate seen among Hispanics overall is due in part to the high dropout rates among Hispanic immigrants. Greater than half of Hispanic immigrant youth never enrolled in a US school and are counted as dropouts if they did not complete high school in their country of origin [90].

According to Fry at the Pew Hispanic Center, Hispanic youth in US schools have a dropout rate twice that of non-Hispanic whites, 15%. Fry suggests that in developing educational programs for immigrants, it is important to determine whether they have been in US schools and for how long, since greater time in US schools increases their likelihood of having better English fluency [91].

For example, among Hispanic youth, those with limited English proficiency have higher rates of school drop-out compared to those who speak English [90].

POLICY RECOMMENDATIONS FOR CHILDREN IN IMMIGRANT FAMILIES

Given that immigrant children are a large and growing population in the United States, it is of utmost importance that our health, education, immigration, and economic policies address the wellness and potential of these children and their families. This section provides policy recommendations based on our current understands about CIF in 6 key areas: (1) immigration (2) access to health care, (3) quality of health care, (4) maintaining family structure, (5) early education and promotion of childhood development, and (6) economic development.

IMMIGRATION REFORM AND HEALTH CARE COVERAGE

Overall, low-income immigrants are likely to be more uninsured than low-income United States–born citizens because of decreased access to public and private health insurance. Immigrants have less access to insurance because of 3 reasons: (1) the 1996 welfare reform law restricted access for recent lawful permanent residents (LPRs) for public insurance; (2) undocumented immigrants remain ineligible for health insurance through any federal program, including the ACA; and (3) immigrants are more likely to work in sectors such as agriculture, food service, and construction, which are less likely to offer job-based insurance [92].

In 2009, the CHIP Reauthorization Act was signed and included a provision called the Immigrant Children's Health Improvement Act (ICHIA). ICHIA removed the five-year waiting period for Medicaid coverage for LPR children and pregnant women. ICHIA is optional for states, and as of 2012, only 24 states adopted the option to extend Medicaid coverage to LPR children, whereas 16 states opted to extend coverage to LPR pregnant women [93]. Unfortunately, immigrant children and pregnant mothers living in those states that did not take this option are not receiving the benefits of the CHIP Reauthorization Act, which has limited the impact of the CHIP Reauthorization Act to improve the health of children and mothers living in our country.

The ACA helps many legal immigrants by expanding Medicaid coverage and offering better opportunities to purchase private health insurance in new health insurance exchanges, with income-related tax subsidies to help make them more affordable. If lawfully present immigrants with incomes less than 100% of the federal poverty line are ineligible for Medicaid, because they have fewer than 5 years of permanent residency, they are eligible for these exchanges and tax credits. However, the current controversy over immigration reform suggests that ACA subsidies will not be provided to immigrants who have only a provisional and not a permanent resident status [92]. Likewise, undocumented immigrants will not have access to ACA benefits.

In June 2012, the Obama administration announced a new DACA Policy, which grants temporary permission to remain in the United States legally for certain unauthorized young people who arrived in the country before age 16 years and who have graduated from high school, are still in school, or have served in the military and do not have a criminal record. However, DACA youth remain ineligible for insurance coverage under Medicaid, CHIP, and the ACA's subsidies and health exchanges [94]. It is premature to assess how comprehensive immigration reform bills may affect health care access for immigrants, including those who may be on a path toward citizenship. Initial legislative proposals have shown reluctance to provide access to health insurance coverage to undocumented immigrants who gain provisional status on the path toward citizenship. Regardless of the controversies surrounding health care and immigration policies, a large number of states have improved coverage for immigrant children based on the 2009 law that eliminated the 5-year waiting period for LPR children and pregnant women and the ACA [92]. Nonetheless, comprehensive immigration reform would markedly clarify the status of immigrant families and thereby improve their health status.

Policy recommendation

1. Comprehensive immigration reform with a pathway to citizenship for current undocumented immigrants
2. Separation of health policies from immigration policies to allow for health insurance coverage for all CIF

ACCESS TO HEALTH CARE

Although progress has been made, there is much that remains to be done to help improve health access for immigrant children, particularly those who have entered the country legally, including encouraging states to expand Medicaid coverage and adopt options to eliminate waiting periods for legal immigrant children and pregnant women. Supporting the health care safety net by expanding community health centers will also help improve access, particularly to whose remain uninsured. Some states with large immigrant populations, such as California, New York, and Massachusetts, are adopting the ICHIA option to provide Medicaid to cover all LPRs regardless of their length of US residency. Even with these changes, outreach to and education of immigrant communities regarding health insurance exchanges need to occur to improve understanding of these programs among immigrants and, thereby, increase the health insurance coverage of legal immigrants.

Beyond the federal and state governments' efforts to provide health care to immigrants children, innovative local initiatives have taken the next step in providing health care coverage for all immigrant children, whether documented or undocumented. For example, in California, the Santa Clara Family Health Plan established Healthy Kids, a comprehensive health insurance for children not covered by Medicaid or Healthy Families. The primary targets of this initiative were undocumented immigrant children. This additional health care coverage meant that all children up to 19 years of age in Santa Clara County had coverage by health insurance. The initiative is funded by local support, and its success has lead to other regional counties undertaking similar initiatives. Moreover, Healthy Kids has made a difference. In a study comparing children continuously insured by Health Kids for 1 year and a group of newly insured children, the study group was significantly less likely to be in fair/poor health and to have functional impairments than the comparison group of newly insured children (15.9% vs 28.5% and 4.5% vs 8.4%, respectively). Impacts were largest among children who enrolled for a specific medical reason [95]. Overall, the fundamental principal of these local initiatives is that children should not be without health insurance because it is a societal responsibility to keep all children healthy and well.

Policy recommendation

1. All children and youth should have access to health care.
2. All pregnant mothers should have access to health care.

ADDRESSING BARRIERS TO IMPROVING QUALITY OF HEALTH CARE

Having insurance coverage is not equivalent to receiving access to quality care [92]. There must be providers who are willing to serve vulnerable populations and the elimination of provider-patient (literacy, linguistic, and cultural differences) and health care system barriers (geographic availability and cultural competency of staff) to quality health care. In addition, social determinants of health must be addressed for CIF in the form of addressing the consequences of poverty and societal disenfranchisement resulting from the immigrant experience.

Key to addressing these barriers are federally qualified health centers (FQHC), designed to provide health care to medically unserved populations and supported by federal grants under Section 330 of the Public Health Service Act. A measure of their service to immigrant communities is that one-quarter of health center patients need language assistance, and this number has risen from 4.3 million in 2007 to 4.7 million in 2011 [92]. The innovation in health care for immigrant communities by FQHC is exemplified by AltaMed in Los Angeles, the largest independent FQHC in the country, which has spearheaded efforts with safety-net hospitals to take advantage of care coordination activities under the ACA for underserved populations. Similar to other FQHCs, AltaMed serves multicultural communities and makes special efforts to provide language assistance by employing interpreters and using language lines and other multilingual staff to help meet language needs. AltaMed has also obtained grant funding to conduct community-level obesity prevention activities, such as body mass index screenings [96]. Overall, connecting closely with the immigrant community is an effective way to address barriers to health care for these communities; this is especially true for mental health. For example, the Filipino Family Initiative, a community engagement program to promote mental health among immigrant Filipino youth, involved a pediatrician partnered with churches, schools, and community-based organizations to offer an evidence-based parenting intervention to Filipino parents of school-aged children [97]. This program demonstrated positive effects for youth and parents.

Integrating behavioral health with primary care is viewed as an especially important building block for safety-net providers serving immigrant children given the high rates of mental health disorders, such as PTSD among refugee populations. Offering mental health screening and services in a primary care setting may help overcome stigma associated with going to a mental health clinic [97]. For instance, at an AltaMed site located in Children's Hospital Los Angeles, evidence-based parenting interventions have been implemented in a pilot project with Spanish-speaking parents of preschool children, and developmental-behavioral pediatricians [98,99] and child psychiatrists see children in their primary care settings. In addition, AltaMed Health Services has earned The Joint Commission's Gold Seal of Approval in compliance with The Joint Commission's standards for Primary Care Medical Home (PCMH). Under the PCMH model, AltaMed primary care doctors work closely with an interdisciplinary team to support the patient and ensure comprehensive and coordinated care, treatment, and services.

Other barriers to improving health outcomes sometimes require services outside the health care system; among those are legal services to address factors that affect health such as unhealthy housing and immigration issues. The development of medical-legal partnerships across the country has been critical to overcome these barriers to care for immigrant families. An excellent example of a medical-legal partnership exists at the Boston Medical Center (Boston, Massachusetts, USA). Its three core undertakings are education of health care professionals in how the legal system can be used to advocate for children's basic needs, provision of direct legal assistance to patients, and systems-based advocacy [100]. Thus, improving the quality of care to CIF requires a comprehensive, multisystem, community-centered approached that adapts to the needs of the particular immigrant group and their community.

Recommendation

1. Primary health care services should be culturally competent and accessible for the population being served.
2. Community-based health care needs to be part of the health services delivered to immigrant communities.
3. Mental health services should be part of the comprehensive care to immigrant children and youth.
4. Medical homes for immigrant children and youth need to be culturally competent and have access a medical-legal partnership to address issues involving the family's social determinants of health.

FAMILY CENTER POLICIES

The AAP's Task Force on the Family in 2003 reported on the importance of family structure and function on the health, development, and emotional well-being of children [101] and youth. They noted that from 1970 to 2000, the proportion of 2-parent families decreased from 85% to 69%. This decrease raised concern with the Task Force because family income among female-headed household was 47% of that of married couples, and children raised in female-headed household are 5 times more likely to live in poverty. Moreover, the research found that family income is strongly related to children's health and well-being and that children need strong families to provide social support, socialization, and coping and life skills. They conclude by stating, "Unequivocally, children do best when they are living with 2 mutually committed and loving parents who respect and support one another, who have adequate social and financial resources, and who are actively engaged in the upbringing of their children." The Task Force terms the practice of pediatrics in support of families Family Pediatrics and encouraged pediatric practices to support their families, of all kinds, in their function and development.

In the area of education, research on single parents, particularly divorced parents, show that children in 2-parent families do better in academic performance and other developmental processes [102]. Review of the literature from the 1960s through the 1990s by Amato and Keith showed [103] the consistent finding that children from 2-parent families do better than those from single-parent families in academic performance, conduct, psychological well-being, self-esteem, and peer relationships. Thus, 2-parent families on the average are better for the outcomes of children's health, emotional development, academic performance, and social integration.

Although immigrant families tend to have a higher proportion of 2-parent families [104], 24% of parents are undocumented but only 6% of children are such; this puts approximately 1 in 4 families at risk for parental loss, even though the children in these families are 94% US citizens or have legal status. Therefore, immigration policy can potentially leave these US children in a single-parent environment, with its subsequent family disruption and poorer child outcomes. In 2013, the Immigration and Customs Enforcement Agency reported that 72,000 undocumented immigrant parents of United States–born children were deported [105]. This action has resulted in an increase in single-parent household among American children. With the loss of income from these parents and their support of family's stability, emotionally and socially, these families are more likely to become dysfunctional and stressed. If research has shown for the past 4 decades that this scenario leads to poor children and subsequent adult outcomes, then one needs to consider this as critical collateral damage from our immigration policies and work to mitigate it.

Recommendation

1. Pediatricians should follow the Family Pediatrics model established by the AAP Task Force on the Family particularly when it comes to immigrant families.
2. Advance and maintain a family supportive immigration policy and assess this policy and its effects on the well-being of the US citizen children of immigrant parents.
3. Research should be conducted to inform pediatricians about the impact of immigrant policies on the children of immigrant families and develop interventions to mitigate them.

EDUCATIONAL POLICY FOR CHILDREN IN IMMIGRANT FAMILIES

Educational research has shown that preschool and early intervention for educational problems is the most effective in producing successful students [106]. Recent research has shown that immigrant children younger than 5 years have less book sharing with their parents compared with other children [44]. CIF participate in preschool less than children in native families [63]. The implication of these findings is that more effort should be taken to improve the early educational environment of CIF. In addition, as these families are linguistically and culturally different from the later generations of these groups, educational transitions must be offered to avoid making these differences barriers to academic success. Bilingual education has been part of the effort to provide effective transition, and overall, bilingual education seems to have positive influence in the transition [107]. Given the right educational environment, educators report an immigrant paradox in education, that is, poor CIF performing better than poor native children [17]. Unfortunately, those undocumented immigrant youth who do achieve academic success can be stymied by their risk of deportation and inability to proceed to the next step, college. The proposed

Development, Relief, and Education for Alien Minors (DREAM) Act, would defer action on deportation for two years for qualified youth, thereby providing the opportunity to proceed with their education. These youth are called "Dreamers". Overall, if one considers the issue of educational achievement as an important health outcome, that is, achieving a productive citizen, then one needs to consider the effects of educational policy on the well-being of CIF.

Recommendations

1. Support early book sharing between immigrant parents and their children through improved support for the ROR program.
2. Increase the proportion of CIF who attend preschool by providing universal preschool.
3. Support the best practices of bilingual education for immigrant children to have an effective transition into schools.
4. Support policies that allow DREAMERS to move on with their education and add value to our national workforce.

ECONOMIC POLICY AND CHILDREN IN IMMIGRANT FAMILIES

Economic policy is usually not a pediatric topic, yet if our nation's future workforce will come from our children, then we have to be concerned about the path from childhood to adulthood and the workforce. Moreover, the change in the demographics of our country predicts 2 important facts that should influence policies affecting immigrant children. First, the proportion of children to elderly is significantly decreasing, so that in 2020, the estimated percentage of the population younger than 18 years compared with that older than 65 years will be in a ratio of approximately 2 to 1, the lowest it has ever been in the United States [4]. This value comes in the context of Latinos and Asian Americans being responsible for 75% of the growth of the child population since 1990, a trend that will continue into the future. That future as estimated by the US Census Bureau will have children in immigrant family representing 1 of every 3 children in the United States and the Latino child population equaling the non-Hispanic white population by 2050. Thus, the future human capital of the United States lies with immigrants and those populations that have been traditionally thought of as minority. Recent estimates of the economic loss from children living in poverty and their subsequent outcomes as adult shows that the nation loses 4% of gross domestic product or approximately $500 billion a year. That is, for every poor child in the country, we will lose $38,000 annually in cost or losses in reduced economic output, increased crime, and increased health expenditures [108]. Thus, the well-being of CIF as well as all children becomes an important economic factor in the well-being of our nation's economic future.

Recommendations

1. Economic policies need to examine their effects on children, particularly on CIF, poor children, and children in economically disadvantaged families.

2. The economic community needs to work with the health and educational communities to advance the development of children in our country, the nation's human capital.
3. Economic development of immigrant and minority communities to improve family incomes and opportunities needs to be advanced by government and business.

In the final analysis, the history of our country has taught us that strength comes from using the human talent of our immigrant populations. Yet, unlike the past when tapping into that talent has taken generations, the competitive global economy and rapidly changing technology of the work place means that we must tap the talent of all our children now rather than later; this will help build a stronger nation.

References

[1] Starkweather S. U.S. immigration legislation online. Available at: http://library.uwb.edu/guides/USimmigration/USimmigrationlegislation.html. Accessed December 1, 2014.
[2] The foreign-born population in the United States: 2010. American Community Survey Reports. United States Census Bureau, May 2012.
[3] Hernandez D, Cervantez W. Children in immigrant families: ensuring opportunity for every child in America. New York: First Focus and Foundation for Child Development; 2011.
[4] Passel JS. Demography of immigrant youth: past, present and future. Future Child 2011;21(1):19–42.
[5] Messick M, Bergeron C. Temporary protected status in the United States: a grant of humanitarian relief that is less than permanent. Washington, DC: Migration Policy Institute; 2014.
[6] U.S. Citizenship and Immigration Services. 2011. Available at: http://www.uscis.gov/humanitarian/refugees-asylum.
[7] Southwest Border Unaccompanied Alien Children. U.S. Customs and Border Protection. 2014. Available at: http://www.cbp.gov/newsroom/stats/southwest-border-unaccompanied-children.
[8] New data on unaccompanied children in immigrant court. Syracuse University's Transactional Records Access Clearinghouse (TRAC) Immigration. 2014. Available at: http://trac.syr.edu/immigration/reports/359/. Accessed February 13, 2015.
[9] Camarota S. Immigrant in the United States, 2010: a profile of America's foreign-born populations. Washington, DC: Center for Immigration Studies; 2012.
[10] Federal Interagency Forum on Child and Family Statistics. America's children: key national indicators of well-being. Washington, DC: Government Printing Office; 2013.
[11] Pew Research Center. Attitudes about aging: a global perspective in a rapidly graying world, Japanese are worried, American aren't. 2014. Available at: http://www.pewglobal.org/2014/01/30/chapter-2-aging-in-the-u-s-and-other-countries-2010-to-2050/. Accessed February 13, 2015.
[12] Chaudry A, Fortuny K. Children of immigrants: family and parental characteristics. Washington, DC: Urban Institute; 2010. Brief No. 2.
[13] Yoshikawa H, Kholoptseva J. Unauthorized immigrant parents and their children's development: a summary of the evidence. Migration Policy Institute; 2013. p. 1.
[14] Jaycox LH, Stein B, Kataoka SH, et al. Violence exposure, posttraumatic stress disorder, and depressive symptoms among recent immigrant schoolchildren. J Am Acad Child Adolesc Psychiatry 2002;41(9):1104–10.
[15] Council on Community Pediatrics. Providing care for immigrant, migrant, and border children. Pediatrics 2013;131(6):e2028–34.
[16] Tarlov AR. Public policy frameworks for improving population health. Socioeconomic status and health and industrial nations: social, psychological, & biologic pathways. Ann N Y Acad Sci 1999;896:281–93.

[17] Crosnoe R, Lopez-Turley RN. K-12 educational outcomes of immigrant youth. Future Child 2011;21(1):129–52.

[18] United Nations Inter-agency Group for Child Mortality Estimation. World development indicators: mortality rate, infant. 2014. Available at: http://www.childmortality.org.

[19] MacDorman MF. Behind international rankings of infant mortality: how the United States compares with Europe. Available at: http://www.cdc.gov/nchs/data/databriefs/db23.pdf. Accessed February 1, 2015. 2009.

[20] Passel JS, Cohn D. United States population projections: 2005–2050. Washington, DC: Pew Hispanic Center; 2008. Available at: http://www.pewhispanic.org/files/reports/85.pdf. Accessed February 2, 2015.

[21] Markides KS, Coreil J. The health of Hispanics in the southwestern United States: an epidemiologic paradox. Public Health Rep 1986;101(3):253–65.

[22] Ray JG, Sgro M, Muhammed M, et al. Birth weight curves tailored to maternal world region. J Obstet Gynaecol Can 2012;34(2):159–71.

[23] Teitler JO, Hutto N, Reichman NE. Birthweight of children of immigrants by maternal duration of residence in the United States. Soc Sci Med 2012;75(3):459–68.

[24] Hernandez DJ, Charney E. Executive summary. In: Hernandez DJ, Charney E, editors. From generation to generation: the health and well-being of children in immigrant families. Washington, DC: Committee on the Health and Adjustment of Immigrant Children and Families; Board on Children, Youth, and Families; National Research Council; Institute of Medicine; National Academy Press; 1998. p. 1–16.

[25] Hack M, Klein NK, Taylor GH. Long-term developmental outcomes of low birth weight children. Future Child 1995;5(1):176–96.

[26] Singh GK, Yu SM, Siahpush M, et al. High levels of physical inactivity and sedentary behaviors among US immigrant children and adolescents. Arch Pediatr Adolesc Med 2008;162(8):756–63.

[27] Strine TW, Barker LE, Mokdad AH, et al. Vaccination coverage of foreign-born children 19 to 35 months of age: findings from the National Immunization Survey, 1999–2000. Pediatrics 2002;110(2):e15.

[28] UNICEF. Immunization summary: a statistical reference containing data through 2011. New York: World Health Organization; 2013. Available at: http://www.childinfo.org/files/32775_UNICEF.pdf. Accessed February 1, 2015.

[29] Buelow VH, Van Hook J. Timely immunization series completion among children of immigrants. J Immigr Minor Health 2008;10(1):37–44.

[30] Wasley A, Kruszon-Moran D, Kuhnert W, et al. The prevalence of hepatitis B virus infection in the United States in the era of vaccination. J Infect Dis 2010;202(2):192–201.

[31] Immigrant Child Health Toolkit. Available at: http://www.aap.org/en-us/about-the-aap/Committees-Councils-Sections/Council-on-Community-Pediatrics/Pages/Immigrant-Child-Health-Toolkit.aspx. Accessed February 1, 2015.

[32] Alami N, Yen C, Miramontes R, et al. Trends in tuberculosis - United States 2013. MMWR Morb Mortal Wkly Rep 2014;63(11):229–33.

[33] Kimbro RT, Brooks-Gunn J, McLanahan S. Racial and ethnic differentials in overweight and obesity among 3-year-old children. Am J Public Health 2007;97(2):298–305.

[34] Sherry B, McDivitt J, Birch LL, et al. Attitudes, practices, and concerns about child feeding and child weight status among socioeconomically diverse white, Hispanic, and African-American mothers. J Am Diet Assoc 2004;104(2):215–21.

[35] Brewer N, Kimbro RT. Neighborhood context and immigrant children's physical activity. Soc Sci Med 2014;116:1–9.

[36] Power TG, Sleddens EF, Berge J, et al. Contemporary research on parenting: conceptual, methodological, and translational issues. Child Obes 2013;9(s1):S87–94.

[37] Love JM, Kisker EE, Ross C, et al. The effectiveness of early head start for 3-year-old children and their parents: lessons for policy and programs. Dev Psychol 2005;41(6):885–901.

[38] Olds DL, Kitzman H, Cole R, et al. Effects of nurse home-visiting on maternal life course and child development: age 6 follow-up results of a randomized trial. Pediatrics 2004;114(6): 1550–9.

[39] Olds DL, Kitzman HJ, Cole RE, et al. Enduring effects of prenatal and infancy home visiting by nurses on maternal life course and government spending: follow-up of a randomized trial among children at age 12 years. Arch Pediatr Adolesc Med 2010;164(5):419–24.

[40] Cates CB, Dreyer BP, Berkule SB, et al. Infant communication and subsequent language development in children from low income families: the role of early cognitive stimulation. J Dev Behav Pediatr 2012;33(7):577–85.

[41] Fortuny K, Hernandez D, Chaundry A. Young children of immigrants: the leading edge of America's future. Washington, DC: Urban Institute; 2010.

[42] Tienda M, Haskins R. Immigrant children: introducing the issue. Future Child 2011;21(1): 3–18.

[43] Borjas G. Poverty and program participation among immigrant children. Future Child 2011;21(1):247–66.

[44] Festa N, Loftus-Gagli P, Cullen M, et al. Disparities in early exposure to book sharing within immigrant families. Pediatrics 2014;134:e162–8.

[45] Zuckerman B. Promoting early literacy in pediatric practice: twenty years of Reach Out and Read. Pediatrics 2009;124(6):1660–5.

[46] Klass P, Dreyer BP, Mendelsohn AL. Reach Out and Read: literacy promotion in pediatric primary care. Adv Pediatr 2009;56:11–27.

[47] Diener ML, Hobson-Rohrer W, Byington CL. Kindergarten readiness and performance of Latino children participating in Reach Out and Read. J Community Med Health Edu 2012;2(133).

[48] Shonkoff JP. From neurons to neighborhoods: the science of early childhood development. Washington, DC: National Academy Press; 2000.

[49] Regalado M, Halfon N. Primary care services promoting optimal child development from birth to age 3 years: review of the literature. Arch Pediatr Adolesc Med 2001;155(12): 1311–22.

[50] Halfon N, Regalado M, McLearn KT, et al. Building a bridge from birth to school: improving developmental and behavioral health services for young children. New York: The Commonwealth Fund; 2003.

[51] American Academy of Pediatrics Committee on Psychosocial Aspects of Child and Family Health. Guidelines for health supervision III. Elk Grove Village (IL): American Academy of Pediatrics; 2002.

[52] Green M, Palfrey JS. Bright futures: guidelines for health supervision of infants, children, and adolescents. Arlington (VA): National Center for Education in Maternal and Child Health; 2002.

[53] Sanders LM, Gershon TD, Huffman LC, et al. Prescribing books for immigrant children: a pilot study to promote emergent literacy among the children of Hispanic immigrants. Arch Pediatr Adolesc Med 2000;154(8):771–7.

[54] Needlman R, Toker KH, Dreyer BP, et al. Effectiveness of a primary care intervention to support reading aloud: a multicenter evaluation. Ambul Pediatr 2005;5(4):209–15.

[55] Frey WH. Census projects new "majority minority" tipping points. Washington, DC: The Brookings Institution; 2012. Available at: http://www.brookings.edu/research/opinions/2012/12/13-census-race-projections-frey. Accessed February 1, 2015.

[56] Cascio EH, Whitmore-Schanzenbach D. The impacts of expanding access to high-quality preschool education. Washington, DC: Brookings Institute; 2013.

[57] High PC. School readiness. Pediatrics 2008;121(4):e1008–15.

[58] Lee S, Juon HS, Martinez G, et al. Model minority at risk: expressed needs of mental health by Asian American young adults. J Community Health 2009;34(2):144–52.

[59] Takinishi R. Leveling the playing field: supporting immigrant children from birth to eight. Future Child 2004;14(2):61–79.

[60] Glick JE, Hohmann-Marriott B. Academic performance of young children in immigrant families: the significance of race, ethnicity, and national origins. Int Migr Rev 2007;41(2): 371–402.

[61] Crosnoe R. Preparing the children of immigrants for early academic success. Migration Policy Institute Report. 2013. Available at: http://www.google.com/url?sa=t&rct= j&q=&esrc=s&frm=1&source=web&cd=1&ved=0CCAQFjAA&url=http%3A%2F%2F www.migrationpolicy.org%2Fsites%2Fdefault%2Ffiles%2Fpublications%2FCrosnoeFINAL. pdf&;ei=mnvmVMq9DYKXgwSdhoGYBQ&usg=AFQjCNHmwfwytxSU4bY9fgmFuvXf0ai WAg&bvm=bv.86475890,d.eXY. Accessed January 15, 2015.

[62] Zambrana RE, Morant T. Latino immigrant children and inequality in access to early schooling programs. Zero to Three 2009;29:46–53.

[63] Karoly LA, Gonzalez GC. Early care and education for children in immigrant families. Future Child 2011;21(1):71–101.

[64] Ciampa PJ, White PO, Perrin EM, et al. The association of acculturation and health literacy, numeracy, and health-related skills in Spanish-speaking caregivers of young children. J Immigr Minor Health 2013;15(3):492–8.

[65] Shields M, Behrman R. Children of immigrant families: analysis and recommendations. Future Child 2004;14(1):4–29.

[66] Iqbal S, Oraka E, Chew GL, et al. Association between birthplace and current asthma: the role of environment and acculturation. Am J Public Health 2014;104(Suppl 1):S175–82.

[67] Silverberg JI, Simpson EL, Durkin HG, et al. Prevalence of allergic disease in foreign-born American children. JAMA Pediatr 2013;167(6):554–60.

[68] Javier JR, Wise PH, Mendoza FS. The relationship of immigrant status with access, utilization, and health status for children with asthma. Ambul Pediatr 2007;7(6):421–30.

[69] Children's environmental health disparities: Hispanic and Latino American children and asthma. United States Environmental Protection Agency. 2014. Available at: http:// www2.epa.gov/sites/production/files/2014-05/documents/hd_hispanic_asthma.pdf. Accessed February 1, 2015.

[70] Pino-Yanes M, Thakur N, Gignoux CR, et al. Genetic ancestry influences asthma susceptibility and lung function among Latinos. J Allergy Clin Immunol 2014;135(1):228–35.

[71] Moorman JE, Zahran H, Truman BI, et al. Current asthma prevalence - United States, 2006-2008. MMWR Surveill Summ 2011;60(Suppl):84–6.

[72] Krogstad JM, Lopez MH. Hispanic nativity shift: U.S. births drive population growth as immigration stalls. Washington, DC. 2014. Available at: http://www.pewhispanic.org/2014/ 04/29/hispanic-nativity-shift/. Accessed February 1, 2015.

[73] McMorrow G, Kenney G, Coyer C. Addressing barriers to health insurance coverage among children: new estimates for the Nation, California, New York, and Texas. Washington, DC: Health Policy Center, Urban Institute; 2012.

[74] Lieu TA, Finlelstein JA, Lozano P, et al. Cultural competency policies and other predictors of asthma care quality for Medicaid-insured children. Pediatrics 2004;114: e102–10.

[75] Dewalt DA, Dilling MH, Rosenthal MS, et al. Low parental literacy is associated with worse asthma care measures in children. Ambul Pediatr 2007;7:25–31.

[76] Javier JR, Huffman LC, Mendoza FS, et al. Children with special health care needs: how immigrant status is related to health care access, health care utilization, and health status. Matern Child Health J 2010;14(4):567–79.

[77] Singh GK, Yu SM, Kogan MD. Health, chronic conditions, and behavioral risk disparities among U.S. immigrant children and adolescents. Public Health Rep 2013;128(6): 463–79.

[78] Buttenheim AM, Pebley AR, Hsih K, et al. The shape of things to come? Obesity prevalence among foreign-born vs. US-born Mexican youth in California. Soc Sci Med 2013;78:1–8.

[79] Hsu WC, Araneta MR, Kanaya AM, et al. BMI cut points to identify at-risk Asian Americans for type 2 diabetes screening. Diabetes Care 2015;38(1):150–8.

[80] Centers for Disease Control and Prevention. National Diabetes Statistics Report: estimates of diabetes and its burden in the United States, 2014. Atlanta (GA): US Department of Health and Human Services; 2014.

[81] Youth Risk Behavior Surveillance. Morbidity and Mortality Weekly Report 53/No. SS-2. 2004. Available at: http://www.cdc.gov/mmwr. Accessed February 2, 2015.

[82] Trejos-Castillo E, Vazsonyi AT. Risky sexual behaviors in first and second generation Hispanic immigrant youth. J Youth Adolesc 2009;38(5):719–31.

[83] Javier JR, Huffman LC, Mendoza FS. Filipino child health in the United States: do health and health care disparities exist? Prev Chronic Dis 2007;4(2):A36.

[84] Chung PJ, Borneo H, Kilpatrick SD, et al. Parent-adolescent communication about sex in Filipino American families: a demonstration of community-based participatory research. Ambul Pediatr 2005;5(1):50–5.

[85] Javier JR, Chamberlain LJ, Rivera KK, et al. Lessons learned from a community-academic partnership addressing adolescent pregnancy prevention in Filipino American families. Prog Community Health Partnersh 2010;4(4):305–13.

[86] Huang K, Calzada E, Cheng S, et al. Physical and mental health disparities among young children of Asian immigrants. J Pediatr 2012;160(2):331–6.e1.

[87] Unruh S. Mexico's violence and posttraumatic stress disorder in immigrant children: a call for collaboration among educators. The Journal of Multiculturalism in Education 2011;7(1):1–18.

[88] Kinzie J, Sack W, Angell R, et al. The psychiatric effects of massive trauma on Cambodian children. J Am Acad Child Adolesc Psychiatry 1986;25:370–6.

[89] Robinson LK. Arrived: the crisis of unaccompanied children at our southern border. Pediatrics 2015;135(2):205–7.

[90] Morse A. A look at immigrant youth: prospects and promising practices. National Conference on State Legislatures Children's Policy Initiative: A Collaborative Project on Children and Family Issues. Washington, DC: 2005.

[91] Fry R. Hispanic youth dropping out of U.S. schools: measuring the challenge. Pew Hispanic Center; 2003.

[92] Leighton Ku, Jewers M. Health care for immigrant families: current policies and issues. Washington, DC: Migration Policy Institute; 2013.

[93] Georgetown University Health Policy Institute Center for Children and Families. Coverage of lawfully residing immigrant children and pregnant women without a 5-year waiting period. 2012. Available at: http://ccf.georgetown.edu/wp-content/uploads/2012/04/ICHIA.pdf. Accessed January 12, 2015.

[94] National Immigration Law Center. Frequently Asked Questions: Exclusion of people granted 'Deferred Action for Childhood Arrivals' from affordable health care. 2012. Available at: http://www.nilc.org/acadacafaq.html.

[95] Howell EM, Trenholm C. The effect of new insurance coverage on the health status of low-income children in Santa Clara County. Health Serv Res 2007;42(2):867–89.

[96] Maxwell J, Bailit M, Tobey R, et al. Early observations show safety-net ACOs hold promise to achieve the triple aim and promote health equity. Health Aff 2014;2014.

[97] Javier JR, Supan J, Lansang A, et al. Preventing Filipino mental health disparities: perspectives from adolescents, caregivers, providers, and advocates. Asian Am J Psychol 2014;5(4):316–24.

[98] Javier JR, Coffey DM. Promoting the importance of play using evidence-based parenting interventions. Pediatrics eLetter. March 12, 2012.

[99] Bauer N, Webster-Stratton C. Prevention of behavioral disorders in primary care. Curr Opin Pediatr 2006;18:654–60.

[100] Zuckerman B, Lawton E, Morton S. From principle to practice: moving from human rights to legal rights to ensure child health. Arch Dis Child 2007;92(2):100–1.

[101] Family Pediatrics. Report on the Task Force on the Family. Pediatrics 2003;111(6): 1541–71.

[102] Amato PR. The impact of family formation change on the cognitive, social and emotional well-being of the next generation. Future Child 2005;15(2):75–96.

[103] Amato PR, Keith B. Consequences of Parental Divorce for Children's Well-Being: A Meta-Analysis. Psychological Bulletin 10(1991):26–46.

[104] Landale NS, Thomas KJ, Van Hook J. The living arrangement of children of immigrants. Future Child 2011;21(1):42–70.

[105] Foley E. Deportation separated thousands of U.S. born children from parents in 2013. Hunnington Post 2014.

[106] Barnett WS. Preschool education and its lasting effects: research and policy implications. Boulder (CO): National Education Policy Center; 2008.

[107] Rolstad K, Mahoney K, Glass G. The big picture: a meta-analysis of program effectiveness research on English language learners. Educ Pol 2005;19(4):572–94.

[108] Holzer HJ, Schanzenbach DW, Duncan GJ, et al. The economic cost of poverty in the United States: subsequent effects of children growing up poor. Washington, DC: Center for American Progress; 2007.

Advances in Pediatrics 62 (2015) 137–164

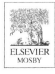

ADVANCES IN PEDIATRICS

ELSEVIER
MOSBY

Preparing for Transition from Pediatric to Adult Care
Evaluation of a Physician Training Program

Janet S. Hess, DrPH, MPH[a],*, Diane M. Straub, MD, MPH[a], Jazmine S. Mateus, MPH[b], Cristina Pelaez-Velez, MD[a]

[a]Department of Pediatrics, University of South Florida Morsani College of Medicine, 2 Tampa General Circle, Tampa, FL 33606, USA; [b]All Children's Hospital Johns Hopkins Medicine, 501 Sixth Avenue South, St. Petersburg, FL 33701, USA

Keywords

• Physician training program • Education • Health care transition • Young adults
• Youth with special health care needs • Adolescents • Self-management
• Experiential learning

Key points

- Clinical guidelines published by the American Academy of Pediatrics, the American Academy of Family Physicians, and the American College of Physicians recommend systematic processes for transition from pediatric to adult health care as a standard of care for all adolescent and young adult patients (A/YA), with and without special health care needs.

- To address a knowledge gap in physician education, University of South Florida Health used a behavior change planning framework to develop and evaluate a transition training model for pediatrics and combined internal medicine and pediatrics residents that emphasizes the use of the electronic health records (EHR) as an experiential learning tool.

- Examination of program reach, effectiveness, adoption, and implementation indicates a positive intervention effect on selected dimensions of resident knowledge, confidence, and experience in health care transition as well as areas for program improvement.

Continued

The authors affirm they have no financial relationships relevant to this article or conflicts of interest to disclose.

This study was part of a dissertation project supported by the USF College of Public Health Student Research Scholarship Project and the USF Community and Family Health Graduate Student Research Award.

*Corresponding author. Department of Pediatrics, University of South Florida, 2 Tampa General Circle, 5th Floor, Tampa, FL 33606. E-mail address: jhess@health.usf.edu

0065-3101/15/$ – see front matter
http://dx.doi.org/10.1016/j.yapd.2015.04.003

Continued

- The model is distinctive in addressing health care self-management skills with all A/YA, consistent with an increasing recognition of the importance of patient engagement in every aspect of health care, including health literacy and shared decision making.
- Study findings show that a programmed transition tool in the EHR provides a convenient, forced reminder of essential patient discussion items; provides a mechanism for both physician education and practice improvement; reduces the time needed for didactic instruction; and can be replicated across EHR systems, residency programs, and clinical practices.

INTRODUCTION

The Maternal and Child Health Bureau (MCHB), the federal agency tasked with improving the health, safety and well-being of mothers and children, defines children and youth with special health care needs (C/YSHCN) as those "who have or are at increased risk for a chronic physical, developmental, behavioral, or emotional condition and who also require health and related services of a type or amount beyond that required by children generally" [1].[pp137] It is estimated that 10.2 million C/YSHCN from birth to 17 years of age currently reside in the United States [2]. The proportion of C/YSHCN increases dramatically with age: Approximately 9% of children younger than 6 years have special health needs, but the proportion almost doubles to about 17% for those aged 12 to 17 years [2]. The large and growing number of adolescents and young adults (A/YA) with chronic health conditions and disabilities is a result of advances in treatment (eg, pharmacology, surgical techniques, medical technology) that have been made over the last 3 decades. Today, about 90% of children with conditions that were previously fatal in childhood are surviving into adulthood [3].

Although many of these young people will move smoothly into adulthood, others will have difficulty transitioning to independence and autonomy without assistance [4]. Transitions may include movement from a family home to living alone or with peers, from high school to postsecondary education or work, and from pediatric to adult health services [5]. Blum and colleagues [6][pp570] are credited with defining health care transition (HCT) in 1993 as "the purposeful, planned movement of adolescents and young adults with chronic physical and medical conditions from child-centered to adult-oriented health care systems." Despite a general understanding among health care professionals about the value of providing an uninterrupted hand-off from pediatric to adult care, national data show that only about 40% of YSHCN aged 12 to 17 years are adequately prepared for transition to adult systems of care [2].

By current estimates, 15% to 20% of 20 million A/YA with SHCN aged 14 to 26 years living in the United States have needs that necessitate utilization of health care services across the lifespan at much higher rates than the general population [7,8]. For this population, access to appropriate, affordable adult care is critical yet problematic. Factors that interfere with smooth HCT are numerous and well documented [9–14]: A/YA with SHCN often find it difficult to secure adequate and affordable insurance coverage after they age out of childhood plans; they have problems finding adult providers who receive training in childhood-onset diseases or who take Medicaid or Medicare; they are not adequately prepared to assume responsibility for managing their own health care; there is no systematic linkage between pediatric and adult medical systems to guide them. Without ongoing care, A/YA with SHCN are likely to experience disease complications, increased emergency department visits and hospitalizations, and development of secondary disabling conditions.

Over the last 20 years, numerous professional organizations have responded to this emerging health care system problem by issuing policy and position statements about the need for transition services [15,16]. In 2001, the MCHB identified HCT as one of 6 core outcomes for improving care for C/YSHCN: all YSHCN will receive the services necessary to make transitions to adult life [17]. In 2010, MCHB's operational measure, transition preparation, was used to develop a new Healthy People 2020 (HP 2020) objective "to increase the proportion of youth with special health care needs whose health care provider has discussed transition planning from pediatric to adult health care" [8]. Further, a clinical report jointly published in 2011 by the American Academy of Pediatrics (AAP), the American Academy of Family Physicians (AAFP), and the American College of Physicians (ACP) outlined guidelines to transition *all* A/YA to an adult model of care, not just those with chronic health conditions [18]. These events highlight the need to develop a competent, knowledgeable health care workforce that is trained to facilitate HCT, particularly in light of data showing that most YSHCN are unprepared to move to adult health care systems [2].

HEALTH CARE TRANSITION GUIDELINES
The introduction of the HP 2020 HCT objective [8] and the new clinical report [18] reflect increasing public recognition of the importance of HCT as well as a shift in its conceptualization among health care professionals. The report, entitled "Supporting the Health Care Transition from Adolescence to Adulthood in the Medical Home," provides detailed guidance for transition preparation, planning, and implementation within a medical home. A cornerstone of the new algorithm is that A/YA, as developmentally able, should be introduced to an adult model of care beginning in early adolescence (eg, encouraging self-management skills, involvement in health care decision making, speaking to physician alone), regardless of provider type (eg, pediatrician, combined internal medicine and pediatrics [Med-Peds], family practitioner, subspecialist). By 18 years of age, the adolescent should be fully transitioned to the adult care model; transfer to an adult provider, if needed, ideally occurs between 18 to 21 years of age.

The report lays out clear steps for HCT timing and interventions for both pediatric and adult medical homes. Use of electronic health records (EHR) and other information technology is a critical component of the new guidelines. Got Transition [19], the federally funded Center for Health Care Transition Improvement, developed a corresponding set of tools to document and support transitional care processes. Important HCT process components include use of EHR and information technology. Using a Plan-Do-Study-Act (PDSA) quality improvement (QI) approach, Got Transition has introduced practice-based HCT learning collaboratives for pediatric and adult practices and health systems [20–22]. Primary care and subspecialty providers are encouraged to adapt the instruments to fit the unique needs and requirements of their own practices.

RESIDENCY EDUCATION

HCT curricula have also been introduced in several residency programs in recent years [23,24]. In a study of primary care residents in South Carolina, Mennito [25] found that residents preferred for HCT curricula to include a combination of teaching modalities, with clinical experience ranked as the most preferred means for information presentation. They also preferred a continuous HCT training experience throughout the residency rather than a short-term, month-long experience. However, few studies have examined the effectiveness of HCT teaching models; to the authors' knowledge, no residency programs have incorporated guidelines to systematically address transition with *all* patients.

To address this knowledge gap, the authors developed and piloted a training model among University of South Florida Health (USF Health) pediatrics and Med-Peds residents. Using a quasi-experimental, mixed methods research design, the authors explored the effect, acceptability, and feasibility of the intervention; factors that influenced adoption of intervention elements; and ways to improve the program. The authors describe here the framework used to design and evaluate the intervention, report quantitative and qualitative findings from the study, and discuss implications for ongoing implementation and replication in other training programs and clinical practice.

METHODS
Planning and evaluation framework
Drawing from adult learning [26] and behavior change theory [27,28], the authors developed a conceptual model for residency education program planning and evaluation that illustrates the integration of individual, interpersonal, and organizational factors in influencing behavior change (Fig. 1). The RE-AIM evaluation framework [29,30] is useful in assessing theory-based multilevel interventions, with the goal of translating health behavior research into practice. A central tenet of RE-AIM is that the ultimate impact of an intervention is caused by its combined effects on 5 dimensions: reach (proportion of target audience participating in the intervention); efficacy/effectiveness (impact of intervention on important outcomes), adoption (proportion of practitioners or settings that adopt the intervention), implementation (extent to which the

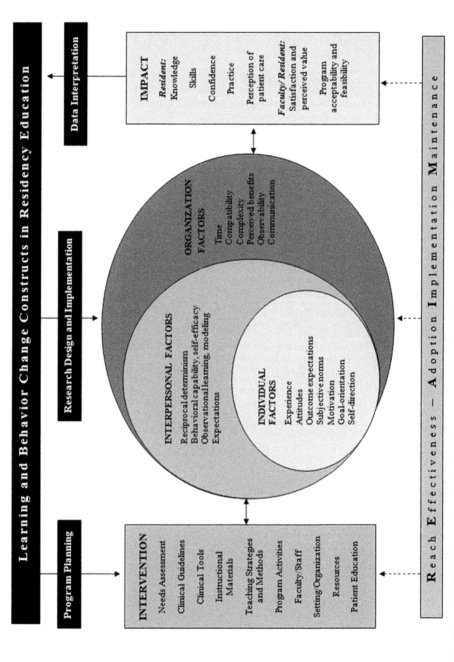

Fig. 1. Conceptual model for residency education program planning and evaluation.

intervention is implemented as intended), and maintenance (extent to which the intervention is sustained over time).

Although many evaluation models emphasize strong internal validity in controlled, homogeneous environments, RE-AIM gives equal importance to external validity, that is, its generalizability across settings. Recognizing the complexity and various levels of behavioral determinants, the model pays close attention to the elements of a program that can most easily be translated into other programs or practices [29]. Using a combination of quantitative and quantitative methods, the authors' evaluation focused on the first 4 dimensions of the RE-AIM framework; the last dimension, maintenance, requires long-term follow-up assessment [17] and was not within the scope of the pilot. The USF Institutional Review Board approved the study.

Intervention elements

Introduction of the HCT intervention was coordinated with the authors' departmental Medical Home Demonstration Project, which participates in a statewide AAP-sponsored learning collaborative for practice improvement. Using a QI approach of introducing small changes, then recalibrating as needed in subsequent PDSA implementation cycles (similar to QI methods used by Got Transition [19]), the authors introduced residents to important processes in *preparing* adolescents for an adult care model, with future cycles to focus on transition planning and transfer-of-care processes.

The intervention was launched in 2012 among 50 pediatrics and 17 Med-Peds residents who were at various stages in their residency programs. Physician preceptors and chief residents were informed about the intervention before its launch and were asked to encourage residents to use the new transition protocol. Key components are described next.

Didactic presentation

A 45-minute lecture about HCT clinical guidelines and the pilot program was presented twice during the intervention at weekly resident conferences. The presentation was taped and posted on the authors' course material Web site. E-mail communication informed all residents of the new protocol and availability of the taped presentation and other educational materials.

Electronic health records transition tool

The core component of the authors' model is using EHR as an experiential learning tool. In a literature review, the authors identified several existing transition readiness tools and age-specific checklists [31,32] that could be implemented within the EHR platforms (Allscripts [Chicago, IL] and Epic [Verona, WI]) used in their 3 pediatrics and Med-Peds continuity clinics. Additional considerations in the development of the tool were that it be thorough but not overly time consuming as well as relevant for A/YA with and without SHCN. A panel of USF Health faculty and HCT experts reviewed the authors' adapted transition checklist (Box 1) for content validity.

Box 1: EHR transition checklist for well visits among patients aged 12 to 21 years

Health Care Self-Management: 12 to 14 years

Patient can name his/her chronic conditions, if any *(yes/needs help/no)*

Patient can name his/her allergies, if any *(yes/needs help/no)*

Patient can name his/her medications, if any *(yes/needs help/no)*

Patient answers questions asked by provider *(yes/needs help/no)*

Patient asks questions of provider *(yes/needs help/no)*

Discussed importance of keeping a personal health care record *(yes/no)*

For YSHCN

Family is working with patient to help him/her be independent *(yes/no/NA)*

Patient has attended an IEP meeting *(yes/no/NA)*

IEP includes HCT goals/activities, such as health care self-management *(yes/no/NA)*

Patient has applied for APD/Medicaid Home and Community-Based Waiver *(yes/no/NA)*

Subspecialty provider contacts *[type text here]*

Health Care Self-Management/Transition: 15 to 17 years

Patient can describe how his/her chronic conditions (if any) impact their health *(yes/needs help/no)*

Patient can describe how his/her medications (if any) impact their health *(yes/needs help/no)*

Patient can take his/her medications (if any) without supervision *(yes/needs help/no)*

Patient has tried to refill a medication *(yes/needs help/no)*

Patient has scheduled a doctor's appointment on his/her own *(yes/needs help/no)*

Patient meets with provider without parents/caregivers present (for part of visit) *(yes/no)*

Patient is keeping his/her own health care summary *(yes/needs help/no)*

Patient knows source of own medical insurance *(yes/needs help/no)*

Patient/family are investigating adult doctors for both primary and specialty care *(yes/needs help/no)*

Patient/family are investigating secondary education or vocational opportunities *(yes/no)*

Patient has received "10 Steps to Successful Health Care Transition" handout *(yes/no)*

For YSHCN

Family has begun vocational rehabilitation application *(yes/no/NA)*

Family has begun guardianship applications (by 17 years of age) *(yes/no/NA)*

Transition IEP includes HCT goals/activities, such as health care self-management (yes/no/NA)

Patient has applied for APD/Medicaid Home and Community-Based Waiver (yes/no/NA)

Subspecialty Provider Contacts: [type text here]

Transition/Transfer: 18 to 21 years

Patient has selected adult doctors for primary and specialty care (yes/no)

   Include name/address

Patient can refill own medication (yes/needs help/no)

Patient has insurance/Supplemental Security Income benefits (yes/no)

Patient has received "Just the Facts" insurance guide (yes/no)

Transfer summary has been/will be forwarded to new providers (yes/no)

For YSHCN

There is a formal plan in place for postsecondary education/adult living/vocation (yes/no/NA)

Have/will verbally communicate with new providers (yes/no/NA)

Family has completed vocational rehabilitation application (yes/no/NA)

Family has addressed guardianship (yes/no/NA)

Transition IEP includes HCT goals/activities, such as health care self-management (yes/no/NA)

Patient has applied for APD/Medicaid Home and Community-Based Waiver (yes/no/NA)

Subspecialty provider contacts: (type text here)

Abbreviation: APD, agency for persons with disabilities; IEP, individualized education program; NA, not applicable.

After several months of testing positions within the EHR to maximize utilization, the checklist was programmed in the adolescent well-visit template for new and established patients aged 12 to 21 years. It prompts residents to engage patients and families in age-appropriate HCT discussion and activities at every well visit, with additional items specifically for YSHCN. For patients aged 18 years and older, a transfer summary of relevant diagnostic, treatment, and social-behavioral information can be forwarded to new adult providers.

Guidelines for Adolescent Preventive Services questionnaire

A/YA patients at the 3 clinics are routinely asked to complete the American Medical Association's *Guidelines for Adolescent Preventive Services* (GAPS) questionnaire in the waiting area before their visit. The physician then reviews the questionnaire and addresses any items of concern with patients and their families. The authors added 5 HCT self-management questions to the form, providing another prompt for physicians to engage in transition discussions.

Patient materials and resources
EHR tasks include providing patients with print and Web-based HCT educational materials. Materials developed by the authors' state HCT initiative, Florida Health and Transition Services (FloridaHATS) [33], were distributed to each clinic. In addition, each patient receives a summary at the conclusion of the visit that includes age-appropriate anticipatory guidance recommended by the AAP Bright Futures program, transition-specific recommendations, and the FloridaHATS Web address.

Survey

A pretest/post-test survey design with a comparison group was used to assess the degree to which the intervention changed resident knowledge, confidence, and experience in HCT. The authors invited all 67 residents (50 pediatrics and 17 Med-Peds residents) who received the intervention to complete an online self-report survey as well as a control group of 52 graduated USF Health pediatrics and Med-Peds residents from the previous 5 years for whom the authors had an e-mail address (obtained from the authors' Department of Pediatrics program office).

Survey instrument
The 35-item survey was composed of close-ended questions with a Likert-type response scale along with general demographic information (pediatrics vs Med-Peds program, year of residency) and the last 4 digits of the respondent's social security number to match pretest and post-test data. It was adapted from an instrument originally developed at the University of Kansas School of Medicine, modified to include key HCT activities outlined in the clinical report. Survey questions were reviewed by a panel of USF faculty and field tested before administration. It was administered through Qualtrics (Provo, UT), a secure online survey software program. All residents and controls were invited via e-mail to participate in the 10-minute preintervention and postintervention survey; reminder e-mails were sent once weekly over 4 weeks to ensure that everyone saw the communication and had an opportunity to complete the questionnaire.

Analytical procedures
Ten knowledge questions were combined to create 2 composite measures for knowledge: exposure to HCT learning activities (eg, heard or read about HCT, attended lecture or training on HCT, assisted with HCT in clinic) and familiarity with HCT tools and processes (familiar with standardized HCT tools and resources, patient self-management skills, adult health care providers, insurance coverage options for patients, health/social/legal services for YSHCN). Confidence was assessed by asking residents about their confidence level in providing primary care for YSHCN and in developing a transition plan for YSHCN. Eight experience items (frequency of discussing HCT issues with patients, encouraging self-management skills, discussing insurance options, developing individualized HCT plans, using standardized tools and resources,

communicating with adult providers, and spending time alone with adolescent patients) were combined to create one composite measure for experience: implementation of HCT processes and activities.

Analytical tests were conducted to compare pretest and post-test mean scores for the intervention and control groups, using statistical analysis system (SAS) 9.3 and statistical package for software sciences (SPSS) Statistics 21. Analysis of covariance (ANCOVA) was used to determine whether differences between the two groups from pretest to post-test were statistically significant. Effect size was estimated using Cohen's d. Calculated Cronbach's alpha coefficients suggested that knowledge (0.51) and experience (0.38) questions had a low consistency of responses within the authors' construct, with confidence (0.73) items found to be consistent. However, the authors chose to include all of the questions in the analysis because each one represented a unique yet important attribute within their composite measures.

Chart review

The authors retrospectively reviewed charts of patients seen by residents in the 3 continuity clinics over a period of 60 days. Inclusion criteria for the reviews included all well-care visits for new and established patients aged 12 to 21 years, conducted by pediatrics and Med-Peds residents at the 3 clinics. Patient data extracted included age, sex, and presence of an SHCN (at least one chronic condition or disability). Residency data extracted from the EHR and department records included sex, residency program, residency year, clinic location, and EHR system. For each qualified encounter, the authors noted resident documentation of HCT tasks that were performed (yes/no) during the visit. The number of items to be addressed ranged from 5 to 16, based on patient age and presence of an SHCN.

Descriptive statistics and correlation procedures using SAS 9.3 were conducted to calculate EHR utilization rates and associations between utilization (dependent variable) and patient or resident factors (independent variables). Fisher's Exact and Chi-squared tests of significance were conducted for patient and resident variables. Comparison of tool utilization for each independent variable was conducted using General Linear Mixed Effect Modeling.

Interviews

Qualitative methods, which are often able to capture issues that cannot be captured by statistics alone, were used to explore and better understand resident and faculty perceptions about the intervention [34,35]. The authors used semistructured telephone interviews to collect the data. The research team was composed of the primary researcher, residency program associate director, and 2 colleagues from public health and social work.

Sampling and recruitment

Using a stratified probability sample of pediatrics and Med-Peds residents enrolled at USF Health 9 months after intervention launch, the authors invited 25 pediatrics and 5 Med-Peds residents to participate in the study. A purposive sample of 6 faculty preceptors was selected based on experience and availability. The authors' sampling estimate was guided by theory of saturation, understanding that adjustment might be required during data collection. Potential subjects were contacted via e-mail by the primary researcher, and residents were offered a $50 gift card to thank them for their participation.

Instrument

A semistructured interview guide was developed based on the authors' study objectives and the RE-AIM framework. Table 1 illustrates how multilevel learning and behavior constructs guided its development. The interview consisted of opened-ended questions about HCT experiences and perceptions, generally, and about intervention elements, specifically. Effectiveness rating scales for various aspects of the program were embedded within the interview protocol.

Procedures

Telephone interviews were conducted by the primary researcher and lasted an average of 25 minutes each. They were digitally recorded, and audiotaped interviews were transcribed verbatim. Deidentified transcripts and field notes were analyzed with the assistance of MAXQDA 11 (VERBI Software, Berlin, Germany), a qualitative data management program. Transcripts were coded by the primary researcher using an a priori and emergent coding system in a constant comparative, iterative process. Two other team members independently coded a portion of the interviews; coded data were discussed, and coding strategies were revised until intercoder agreement scores were acceptable and consistent. The data were grouped by common themes, organized within the RE-AIM framework, and reviewed for commonalities, differences, frequency, extensiveness (degree of detail), and co-occurrence of codes. Two team members then conducted a final review of all coded transcripts, coding strategies, and narrative analysis to improve accuracy of the information.

RESULTS

Participants

Survey

Among 67 residents who completed the intervention and were invited to participate in the survey, 40 completed the pretest and 34 completed the post-test, resulting in 11 useable, matched pretests and post-tests. Among 52 graduated residents in the control group, 29 completed the pretest and 28 completed the post-test, with 13 useable, matched tests. Table 2 shows the composition of intervention and comparison group respondents with matched surveys. Although the intervention sample was composed of pediatrics residents only, the authors have no reason to think there would be significant differences in responses between pediatrics and Med-Peds residents.

Chart review

The authors reviewed patient charts for 108 well-care visits conducted by 51 residents (76.1% of all residents) at 3 continuity clinics over a 60-day period.

Table 1
RE-AIM evaluation matrix, interview questions for residents and faculty preceptors

RE-AIM dimension	Ecological level	Learning and behavior constructs/variables	Interview questions and probes
Reach	Individual	Awareness (of intervention)	Are you familiar with each of the HCT training program components?
Efficacy/ effectiveness	Individual, interpersonal	Knowledge	What was your preresidency level of experience in HCT?
		Attitudes	What is your current level of experience in HCT?
		Skills	Is transition preparation a valid, relevant need?
		Satisfaction	How important is it for physicians to prepare adolescents for transition to adult health care?
		Outcome expectations	How important is HCT for all patients vs YSHCN?
		Motivation	Are there particular patient groups that are more difficult to transition?
		Reciprocal determinism	To what extent do you think HCT activities will lead to better health outcomes in adulthood?
		Behavioral capability	
		Self-efficacy	
		Observation/modeling	What is the most useful activity in teaching residents about HCT?
		Expectations	Do you like or dislike particular intervention components?
		Reinforcement	How frequently do you use the HCT checklist in the EHR?
		Learning should be	To what extent do you address all of the checklist tasks in the EHR?
		Relevant	What are motivating factors for you to use the HCT protocol and materials?
		Based on valid needs	Are there consequences for not adhering to the protocol?
		Self-directed	To what extent do attending physicians encourage you to discuss transition with your patients and to use the new HCT transition tools?
		Experiential	
		Beneficial to the learner	Overall, how effective are the training components in preparing pediatrics and Med-Peds providers to transition their patients?
		Participatory	

	Level	Constructs	Questions
Adoption	Individual, organizational	Communication channels Time Compatibility Complexity Perceived benefits Observability	What factors influence how often you use each intervention task and activity? What is the degree of ease or difficulty in implementing the new HCT protocol? Do you think any HCT tasks are unclear or unnecessary? Are there intervention tasks that you think are more important than other items? Were training activities explained adequately? Are time requirements adequate to implement the new HCT protocol? Which training materials and educational resources are the most useful and practical? What are the most effective ways for you to receive information on transition materials?
Implementation	Individual, organizational	Integrity of delivery Consistency in utilization	To what extent are intervention activities consistent or in conflict with USF Health policies? Are there any organizational barriers to implementation? Do you have suggestions to improve the training?
[a]Maintenance	Individual, organizational	—	—

[a]Maintenance was not addressed in pilot study.

Table 2
Composition of resident and control group survey respondents

Independent variables	Resident (N = 11)		Control (N = 13)	
	n	%	n	%
Residency Program				
Pediatrics	11	100.0	10	76.9
Med-Peds	0	0.0%	3	23.1
Year of Residency				
Year 1	4	36.4	—	—
Year 2	5	45.5	—	—
Year 3	2	18.2	—	—
Year 4	0	0.0	—	—
Graduation Year				
2006	—	—	1	7.7
2007	—	—	3	23.1
2008	—	—	5	38.5
2009	—	—	1	7.7
2010	—	—	3	23.1
Postresidency Specialty				
Primary Care	3	27.3	5	38.5
Hospitalist	1	9.1	3	23.1
Subspecialist	6	54.5	4	30.8
Undecided	0	0.0	1	7.7
Other	1	9.1	0	0.0

Note: For residents, anticipated postresidency specialty.

The remaining 23.9% of residents did not see any patients aged 12 to 21 years during the review time frame.

Interviews

A total of 22 telephone interviews were conducted with 16 residents and 6 faculty preceptors. Among residents, 12 (75%) were female; 12 (75%) were in the pediatrics program (vs Med-Peds); one (6%) was a first-year resident, 6 (37.5%) were second year, 6 (37.5%) were third year, and 3 (19%) were fourth-year residents. Among faculty, 4 (68%) were female and 4 (68%) were in the pediatrics department.

Quantitative and qualitative findings are reported next, organized within the first 4 dimensions of RE-AIM: reach, effectiveness, adoption, and implementation.

Reach

All 67 residents and 12 faculty members in the general pediatrics and Med-Peds continuity clinics were provided with intervention materials, delivered through one or a combination of communication channels (lecture, e-mail, course Web site, printed handouts, and the EHR). However, most residents and several faculty interviewed reported they were unfamiliar with some program components. Only one-third of residents said they attended the didactic presentation during a noon conference, and none reported viewing the recorded session on the course Web site. Similarly, another third did not see printed patient materials that were provided to each clinic or knew that the GAPS questionnaire had been modified to include HCT questions. The transition tool in the EHR was the only program element that all interview subjects reported using.

Residents
- "Noon conferences are a great way to spread information but there's a huge percentage of residents that miss it."
- "There are 6 million pamphlets in that clinic so they just become another pamphlet."
- "I've heard of all of them [patient materials] but I don't personally know where they're located in the clinic."

Faculty
- "I've seen the emails but have not had time to read through them."

Effectiveness

Effectiveness was assessed in surveys, chart reviews, and interviews with respect to resident knowledge, confidence, and experience in preparing A/YA for HCT. After controlling for corresponding pretest values in the survey, residents scored significantly higher than controls on the post-test in 2 of 5 outcome variables: exposure to learning activities ($P = .0005$) and confidence in providing primary care for YSHCN ($P = .0377$). Table 3 provides summary data along with pretest to post-test change statistics. It is noteworthy that resident mean scores increased from pretest to post-test in all 5 outcome variables, whereas controls showed little gain, and even loss, in some post-test scores. The magnitude of differences between resident and control mean scores from pretest to post-test were especially large for implementation activities ($d = 2.74$), familiarity with HCT processes ($d = 1.91$), and exposure to learning activities ($d = 1.58$).

Chart review data showed the EHR checklist was used by 34 residents (66.7%) to address at least one HCT task in 57 of 108 visits, representing a 52.8% overall utilization rate. Most residents (56.9%) saw more than one patient, with almost one-third seeing 3 to 7 patients. When the tool was used, the average number of tasks addressed was 9.3 (out of 5 to 16 tasks, based on age and presence of an SHCN). Almost all residents (96.1%) addressed at least 5 HCT tasks, and more than 50% addressed 9 to 16 tasks. However, tool usage was somewhat inconsistent. Among 29 residents with 2 or more patient visits, 44.8% ($n = 13$) used the tool in some visits and not in others. Utilization rates were highest in visits with female patients (66.7%), non-SHCN patients (59.4%), and 12 to 14 year olds (55.6%). In comparing HCT tool utilization by both patient and resident variables, only patient sex was significantly associated with utilization ($P = .0395$). Table 4 shows the demographic breakdown of patient visits and the effect of patient and resident factors on utilization.

Table 3
Comparison of resident versus control group survey composite scores for HCT knowledge, confidence, and experience

Composite outcome variables	Maximum score	Resident (N = 11)			Control (N = 13)				Cohen's d	ANCOVA coefficient	Change P value
		Mean				Mean					
		Pre	SD	Post	SD	Pre	SD	Post	SD			
Knowledge (10 items)												
Exposure to HCT learning activities (4 items)	4	1.64	1.03	3.18	0.87	3.08	0.86	3.08	0.95	1.58	0.65	.0005
Familiarity with HCT processes and tools (6 items)	30	11.45	3.98	16.73	3.38	17.46	4.45	18.15	4.45	1.91	1.77	.3164
Confidence (2 items)												
Confidence in providing primary care for YSHCN	4	2.82	0.40	3.27	0.47	3.08	0.76	2.83	0.72	0.90	0.52	.0377
Confidence in developing a transition plan for YSHCN	4	2.27	0.47	2.55	0.52	2.92	0.64	2.85	0.55	0.60	0.08	.6855
Experience (8 items)												
Implementation of HCT processes and activities	40	15.18	3.43	21.27	3.29	25.31	7.3	24.85	5.46	2.74	2.42	.1689

Note: Response scales for knowledge/exposure items are no = 0, yes = 1; knowledge/familiarity items are 1 = low to 5 = high; confidence items are 1 = low to 4 = high; experience items are 1 = low to 5 = high. P values less than .05 (P <.05).

Table 4
Chart review demographic composition of patients, effect of factors in HCT tool utilization

Variables	Composition of patient visits		Effect of patient and resident variables on utilization			
	N	%	Estimate	SE	t value	P value
Patient Visits	108	100.0	—	—	—	—
Patients						
Total	108	100.0	—	—	—	—
Age	—	—	0.10	0.34	0.28	.7778
12–14 y	54	50.0	—	—	—	—
15–17 y	44	40.7	—	—	—	—
18–21 y	10	9.3	—	—	—	—
Sex	—	—	−0.98	0.46	−2.11	.0395
Male	54	50.0	—	—	—	—
Female	54	50.0	—	—	—	—
Presence of SHCN	—	—	0.59	0.48	1.22	.2258
With SHCN	44	40.7	—	—	—	—
Without SHCN	64	59.3	—	—	—	—
Residents						
Total	51	100.0	—	—	—	—
Sex	—	—	−1.23	0.70	−1.75	.0857
Male	10	19.6	—	—	—	—
Female	41	80.4	—	—	—	—
Program	—	—	1.11	0.70	1.58	.121
Pediatrics	39	76.5	—	—	—	—
Med-Peds	12	23.5	—	—	—	—
Year of residency	—	—	−0.04	0.39	−0.10	.9201
1 y	11	21.6	—	—	—	—
2 y	20	39.2	—	—	—	—
3–4 y	20	39.2	—	—	—	—

Notes: (1) Number of items in the HCT tool to be addressed per visit ranged from 5 to 16, based on patient age and presence of SHCN (Box 1). (2) General linear mixed effect modeling used for independent variables. P values less than .05 (P <.05).

In interviews, residents and faculty uniformly said that preparing A/YA for adult health care is an important physician responsibility and that HCT training is a valid, relevant need (Table 5). They stated that it is particularly important to assist patients with complex medical conditions and other vulnerable groups, such as those with mental illness, in low socioeconomic environments, or without a strong social support system. Faculty members stipulated that, although it is a physician's role to provide HCT services, there should be additional clinical support to assist patients with access to adult-oriented social service and public benefits programs.

Almost all residents interviewed (94%) said they had minimal or no experience in HCT before starting their residency, but all reported moderate or extensive HCT experience at the time of the interview. Several faculty members expressed concern that, though residents could attend to the HCT preparation questions listed in the EHR tool, they were not necessarily more

Table 5
Resident and faculty perceptions of program effectiveness, embedded interview scales

Effectiveness scales	Residents (n = 16) Mean	Faculty (n = 6) Mean
Importance of physician-driven HCT services for all A/YA 1 (unimportant) to 5 (very important)	4.44	4.50
Provider *utilization* of HCT tool in the EHR 1 (never) to 4 (always)	3.47	2.75
^aResidents' current level of *experience* in HCT 1 (very minimal) to 5 (very extensive)	3.78	—
Overall *effectiveness* of the HCT training program 1 (not effective) to 5 (very effective)	3.81	3.08

^aMean score for residents' current level of experience in HCT compares with a mean score of 1.31 for pre-residency experience in HCT.

knowledgeable about the complexities of HCT or how to help A/YA access adult services. Some faculty conveyed their personal frustration in adequately addressing the barriers that many YSHCN encounter in transition and guiding them to appropriate adult care.

When asked about the most useful intervention element, most residents (81%) and providers (67%) interviewed cited the EHR tool, followed by the noon conference presentation. More than half of residents (56%) reported that they *always* use the EHR tool during A/YA well visits; 25% *usually* use it and 19% *sometimes* use it. No residents said they *never* use the tool. Faculty perceptions of EHR tool utilization were somewhat lower, with most faculty participants (83%) reporting that the HCT tool is used *usually* or *sometimes*. Although many residents were not familiar with patient educational materials, some (31%) said they had used the materials or the FloridaHATS Web site and found them useful; others said they intended to explore the materials following the interview. In assessing overall intervention effectiveness, faculty was again more conservative than residents, with an average of rating of *somewhat effective* compared with residents' *mostly effective.*

Residents
- "I'm definitely more comfortable than I was before I started."
- "I've gotten more aggressive with it in the last 6 months...I would say my experience is pretty good."
- "It's brought our attention to it [HCT]; I don't think it's something that a lot of residents really thought about much."

- "I thought it [noon conference] was really helpful. It brought up some issues I hadn't really thought about... like teenagers having a voice in what their medical solutions are."

Faculty
- "I've heard from various attendings... and everybody feels like they need to be more knowledgeable and take the time to really better study and understand what the questions are [in the EHR template]".

Adoption
Interview subjects described a confluence of factors that influenced the degree to which intervention activities were adopted. Frequently cited barriers and facilitators were accessibility of program materials, ease of use, time constraints, patient age or maturity level, complexity of patients' health condition, and involvement of attending physicians in enforcing the protocol. Table 6 provides a more comprehensive description of factors associated with use of the EHR tool.

Limitations with communication channels also impacted adoption. In addition to the relatively small number of residents who were able to attend a noon conference presentation, several residents and faculty said they do not regularly use the course Web site. Others acknowledged that they missed or did not remember reading program e-mails, though most still identified e-mail as a preferred method of receiving program information. Many emphasized the importance of easy access to information; that is, if participants had to search for an item, they were less likely to find and use it. Respondents universally cited the visibility, convenience, and ease of the EHR tool as important utilization factors.

Residents
- "I think all of the pieces are there. I just think it's so hard to get everybody in the same place at one time to do the teaching."
- "Email is probably the best way [to communicate], as long as it's to the point and not a 30-page email!"

Faculty
- "People will miss it if they can't do it super conveniently."

Implementation
Interview participants reported several individual and organizational factors that impacted uniformity of intervention implementation. First, residents assigned to a particular continuity clinic that primarily serves young children (more than 50% are less than 5 years of age) had fewer opportunities to interact with A/YA, a fact noted by several residents and faculty. Another clinic did not have computers in every examination room, so residents used laptops, as available, to log into the EHR during patient visits. When a laptop was not available, residents did not have the programmed HCT checklist to prompt discussion. One resident remarked that nurses occasionally forget to give the GAPS questionnaire to patients.

Table 6
Factors associated with utilization of the EHR transition tool, reported in interviews

Factors	Description	Resident quotes	Faculty quotes
Convenience/ accessibility	Participants consistently identified convenience as an important factor in utilization. Most said the EHR tool was the most useful element in the intervention because it served as a forced reminder to address HCT during the visit.	• "That's been the most helpful because it reminds us every single time." • "It's so easy to use. Why not use it?" • "You don't always remember to do it if you don't see it on the template."	• "Anything new…almost has to be 'in your face' for a little while to make it part of your routine."
Time	Both residents and faculty said that time constraints can be a barrier to addressing questions in the HCT tool. Several residents estimated the checklist took 5 minutes to administer, but it depended on factors such as the patient's medical condition and developmental stage.	• "If I have X number of things to cover, is this going to be one of them with the time I have allotted?" • "If there are a lot of issues going on, I can't always use it because of time constraints."	• "There is barely enough time to just do the actual medical stuff." • "I don't think it's a physician's role to act as a social worker all the time. There's no time for stuff like that."
Patient medical condition	Most participants said they think HCT preparation is particularly important for YSHCN, and some said they were more likely to use the tool with those patients. Several faculty members said they are more likely to remind residents about HCT if the patient has complex needs.	• "If I'm sure the patient doesn't have anything chronic…that's when I may skip them [HCT questions]." • "If they have a lot of medical conditions, it's something I spend a little more time with."	• "I'm much better at it when kids have a chronic condition or special health care need."

Patient age	Several residents said they were more likely to skip questions in the HCT tool with younger patients than with older ones who were close to transferring to adult care.	• "For some of the youngest kids, I felt that maybe it was not yet appropriate to be spending the limited time I had discussing that kind of stuff." • "I assess whether they have the intellectual capability as well as their age." • "I think the older they get, the more likely the resident will ask those questions."
Reinforcement from attending physicians and chief residents	Both residents and faculty emphasized the importance of attending physician enforcement of the HCT protocol. Reminders from chief residents were also perceived by residents as an effective way to increase tool utilization.	• "If the attending wants you to do it, everyone does it without question." • "Whatever my attending says, I definitely take notice of that." • "If I were to push it... it would then become habit." • "We just have to keep reminding them... to have it become the template in their head as well."

There was also considerable variation in the degree to which attending physicians reinforced the HCT protocol with residents. When asked to what extent faculty encouraged transition discussions, resident responses ranged from *none to minimal* (from a pediatrics resident) to *a lot* (from a Med-Peds resident). As with residents interviewed, faculty frequently alluded to the challenge of time constraints and prioritizing tasks during adolescent well visits, particularly for patients with complex conditions. Some also expressed discomfort in their knowledge of adult programs and ability to direct patients to appropriate services. All pediatrics faculty members said they (as attending physicians) needed additional guidance in effective modeling of HCT interactions with A/YA and families.

Finally, several participants offered suggestions on ways to improve adoption and implementation of the training program. In addition to adding faculty development activities, recommendations were to conduct noon conferences that focus on patient educational materials and resources, place HCT reminders and materials in clinic resident rooms, integrate HCT updates in chief resident communications, and enhance the EHR with HCT pop-up banners on A/YA patient charts.

Residents
- "I think some of the attendings might not totally understand [about HCT]. So they may have trouble telling us what to do."

Faculty
- "You just run out of hours in the day to do every single thing that's good and necessary, and you just have to prioritize what things you actually have time to do."
- "I'm not sure if I know all the answers to the questions I'm asking."
- "We, the individual attendings, need to stress to the residents why it's so important."

DISCUSSION

The authors' study aimed to address a knowledge gap about effective models of physician training in preparing A/YA for transition to adult health care. Using a multilevel program planning framework for behavior change, this pilot intervention integrates AAP/AAFP/ACP guidelines to systematically provide HCT services for all A/YA and emphasizes the use of the EHR as an experiential learning tool. The authors assessed intervention impact by examining program reach, effectiveness, adoption, and implementation—the first 4 dimensions of the RE-AIM evaluation model.

Study data show both strengths and areas for program improvement. Both residents and faculty perceived residency education in HCT as a highly relevant need. The data indicate that residents had little knowledge or experience in HCT before the intervention but felt more confident in their abilities to assist A/YA after participating in HCT training activities. However, some faculty questioned whether residents were truly more knowledgeable and could appropriately refer patients to adult services or whether they were simply attentive to the HCT preparation questions in the EHR. These data support survey findings that showed significant change in some aspects of knowledge (exposure to learning activities) and confidence (in providing primary care for YSHCN) but not in others (familiarity with HCT processes and tools, confidence in developing a transition plan for YSHCN). Because the pilot intervention focused on HCT preparation rather than plan development or transfer of care, it is not surprising that the latter outcome variables did not increase significantly. Experience, as measured in the survey (implementation of HCT processes), showed no significant change compared with controls, though residents interviewed reported considerable gains in experience. Certainly, differences between survey constructs and interview subjects' notions of knowledge, confidence, and experience are important considerations in data interpretation and triangulation.

Utilization of the EHR checklist provided stronger evidence of change in experience and practice, that is, the degree to which residents engaged patients in HCT discussions. Largely because of the forced reminder of HCT prompts in the EHR, the residents interviewed reported fairly high utilization of the tool (81% said they used it *usually* or *always*), despite the time constraints they often encountered. In comparison, chart review data indicated only 41.2% of residents used the tool in every patient visit. The overall utilization rate of 52.8% from chart review data was well below the authors' long-range QI goal of 90%, but it was not surprising for the introduction of an entirely new protocol. A consideration for optimal usage is specific location of the checklist within the EHR. The authors think that integrating it as part of the adolescent well visit template (vs creating a separate transition section, which was tested early in the intervention) provides greater visibility and accessibility for providers. Given utilization among two-thirds of residents during the 9-month intervention period, the authors expect usage to increase over time with continued exposure.

The authors noted a few interesting findings in EHR utilization patterns and associations from chart review data. Several residents used the HCT tool inconsistently (used it in one patient visit and not the next), which may be explained, in part, by time constraints or failure to document task completion. When the tool was used, most or all of the HCT tasks were addressed (vs 1 or 2 completed tasks). Residents were significantly more likely to use the tool in visits with female patients, though reasons for the association are not clear. Although the presence of SHCN was not a significant factor, the authors were surprised that utilization was higher for patients *without* SHCN than for those with SHCN. Perhaps this was, again, a reflection of time constraints rather than the resident's perception of patient need for transition preparation. Chart review data showed no other significant differences in intervention effect among subgroups of residents based on residency program (pediatrics vs

Med-Peds), year of residency, and sex. Interview data seem to support this finding, but survey sample sizes were too small to examine associations between resident characteristics and program effectiveness.

Both residents and faculty described several barriers to consistent use of the new protocol, such as time constraints, reminders from attending physicians, availability of laptops in examination rooms, and patient age and medical condition. A critically important aspect of the program, one that the authors underestimated, is to ensure that faculty preceptors are comfortable in their knowledge and ability to implement HCT clinical guidelines within the context of an adolescent well visit. Several faculty members said they are not familiar with local resources available to young adults with disabilities or chronic health conditions or where to refer patients for assistance in accessing adult programs. Further, most feel challenged in integrating HCT preparation tasks when office visit time is limited, particularly for patients with complex needs. Targeted training for both physicians and support staff about community resources and how to easily access patient materials should reduce patient visit time.

In addition, most faculty said they typically associate HCT with YSHCN who are close to transfer-of-care age (eg, 18 years). They are not accustomed to engaging healthy, young adolescents in discussion about self-care management skills and preparing for an adult model of care. However, the guidelines outline a transition process that occurs over time for all A/YA, not just for YSHCN. The authors' findings underscore the necessity of integrating faculty education activities into the intervention model and engaging faculty in enforcing the clinical protocol with residents.

Other barriers to program adoption and implementation may be attributed, in part, to logistical difficulties in reaching the full cohort of residents with all intervention elements, including the didactic lecture and patient educational materials. Background information covered in the didactic presentation provides context for the new protocol, allowing for a deeper understanding of the issues; the educational materials provide a plethora of resources to help guide patients to needed services. Increased attention to alternative teaching venues and communication channels, as well as continued implementation of program elements, may improve reach, effectiveness, and adoption of the intervention over time. Given residents' busy schedules, providing uniform training is a struggle generally shared by residency programs.

Limitations

Using a mixed methods research approach in this study allowed the authors to compare and triangulate data to better understand modifying factors, barriers, and facilitators that influenced intervention impact, thus providing a more comprehensive and credible view of results. However, there were several study limitations. The small sample size limits the degree to which results can be generalized or transferred to other residency programs as well as the authors' ability to measure associations between resident factors and outcome variables. The survey instrument was adapted from one used previously at another institution. Although the use of this tool allows for comparison across residency programs, survey questions addressed all aspects of the transition process rather than preparation only (the focus of the authors' intervention). Reliability and validity of findings could be improved with a larger study sample and a redesigned survey instrument that focused primarily on knowledge, confidence, and experience in HCT preparation.

Structural factors that were identified as barriers to consistent use of the HCT protocol also influenced the validity of overall findings (eg, awareness among residents about educational materials, number of A/YA patients seen in continuity clinics, availability of laptops in examination rooms, and faculty knowledge of transition). Further, chart reviews depended on truthful documentation of activities by residents, and self-report measures raise questions of accuracy. Threats to credibility and validity of qualitative findings include recall and response bias among interview subjects as well as researcher bias. Although the authors' research team had the dual role of developing and evaluating the intervention and one team member is a residency program administrator, they attempted to take appropriate methodological steps to minimize bias and maintain objectivity.

Implications

The authors think the USF Health pilot program has important implications for physician education in HCT. First, it is distinctive in its emphasis on training residents to systematically address health care self-management skills with all A/YA, which is consistent with an increasing recognition of the importance of patient engagement in all aspects of health care, including health literacy and shared decision making [36]. Second, the program is unique in its use of the EHR as a primary teaching tool. This point is noteworthy because all physicians are expected to start using an EHR system over the next few years; it provides a mechanism for both physician education and practice improvement; it can reduce the time needed for didactic instruction; and materials can be replicated across EHR systems, residency programs, and clinical practices. Despite time constraints often experienced during adolescent visits, the EHR tool provides a convenient, forced reminder of essential HCT discussion items and uniformly reaches all residents. It may be more easily sustained over time than other types of educational programs, addressing the last dimension of the RE-AIM model: maintenance.

Importantly, an EHR teaching tool should be accompanied by other teaching strategies, that is, there should be instructional methods that can provide background and context about the importance of physician-driven HCT services as well as education about local adult services and resources. Faculty engagement and commitment to reinforcing the HCT guidelines with residents are critical, as is comfort in providing HCT services to A/YA with and without chronic health conditions or disabilities.

Viewed through the lens of a QI approach, the pilot training program reflects an ongoing, dynamic process that has allowed the authors to assess whether proposed changes actually work in practice. The authors' next steps are to incorporate improvement strategies for HCT preparation and introduce new activities for transition plan development and transfer of care. The authors also hope to address new research questions that emerged from the study, which include examining intervention effect over time (Do tool utilization rates change with continued exposure?), assessing the impact of program enhancements (Can faculty training improve intervention adoption rates?), and exploring the sustainability of resident skills in postresidency practice (Do residents who engage in HCT preparation discussions with their patients continue to provide HCT services in community practice?)

Acknowledgments

The authors wish to thank the following dissertation committee members for their guidance and review: Russell Kirby, PhD; Martha Coulter, DrPH; Elizabeth Perkins, PhD; and Steve Freedman, PhD.

References

[1] McPherson M, Arango P, Fox H, et al. A new definition of children with special health care needs. Pediatrics 1998;102(1):137–40.

[2] Child and Adolescent Health Management Initiative. National survey of children with special health care needs. Available at: http://cshcndata.org. Accessed November 1, 2014.

[3] Gortmaker SL, Sappenfield W. Chronic childhood disorders: prevalence and impact. Pediatr Clin North Am 1984;21:3–18.

[4] Gortmaker SL, Perrin JM, Weitzman M, et al. An unexpected success story: transition to adulthood in youth with chronic physical health conditions. J Res Adolesc 1993;3: 317–36.

[5] Scal P, Evans T, Blozis S, et al. Trends in transition from pediatric to adult health care services for young adults with chronic conditions. J Adolesc Health 1999;24(4):259–64.

[6] Blum RW, Garrell D, Hodgman CH, et al. Transition from child-centered to adult health-care systems for adolescents with chronic conditions: a position paper of the Society of Adolescent Medicine. J Adolesc Health 1993;14(7):570–6.

[7] U.S. Census Bureau. 2010 U.S. demographic profile data. Available at: http://factfinder2. census.gov/faces/tableservices/jsf/pages/productview.xhtml?pid=DEC_10_DP_DPDP1. Accessed November 8, 2014.

[8] U.S. Department of Health and Human Services. Healthy people 2020. Available at: http://healthypeople.gov/2020/topicsobjectives2020/objectiveslist.aspx?topicId=9. Accessed October 25, 2014.

[9] Reiss J, Gibson R. Health care transition: destinations unknown. Pediatrics 2002;110: 1307–14.

[10] Cooper WO. Continuity of health insurance coverage among young adults with disabilities. Pediatrics 2007;119:1175–80.

[11] Greenen SJ, Powers LE, Sells W. Understanding the role of health care providers during the transition of adolescents with disabilities and special health care needs. J Adolesc Health 2003;32:225–33.

[12] Rosen DS, Blum RW, Britto M, et al. Transition to adult health care for adolescents and young adults with chronic conditions: position paper of the Society for Adolescent Medicine. J Adolesc Health 2003;33:309–11.

[13] Scal P, Ireland M. Addressing transition to adult health care for adolescents with special health care needs. Pediatrics 2005;115:1607–12.

[14] McManus M, Fox HB, O'Connor K, et al. Pediatric perspectives and practices transitioning adolescents with special needs to adult health care Fact sheet No 6. Washington, DC: National Alliance to Advance Adolescent Health; 2008. Available at: www.thenational alliance.org/pdfs/FS6.%20Pediatric%20Perspectives%20and%20Practices%20on% 20Transitioning.pdf. Accessed November 1, 2014.

[15] American Academy of Pediatrics, American Academy of Family Physicians, the American College of Physicians – American Society of Internal Medicine. A consensus statement on health care transitions for young adults with special health care needs. Pediatrics 2002;110:1304–6.

[16] Society for Adolescent Medicine. Transition to adult health care for adolescents and young adults with chronic conditions. J Adolesc Health 2003;33:309–11.

[17] U.S. Department of Health and Human Services, Maternal and Child Health Bureau. All aboard the 2010 express: a 10-year action plan to achieve community-based services systems for children and youth with special health care needs and their families. Washington, DC: Maternal and Child Health Bureau; 2001.

[18] Cooley WC, Sagerman PJ. American Academy of Pediatrics, American Academy of Family Physicians, American College of Physicians, Transitions Clinical Report Authoring Group. Clinical report: supporting the health care transition from adolescence to adulthood in the medical home. Pediatrics 2011;128:182–200. Available at: http://pediatrics.aap publications.org/content/128/1/182.full.html. Accessed October 25, 2014.

[19] Got transition, National Health Care Transition Center. Available at: www.gottransition.org/ UploadedFiles/Files/Six_core_Elements_PDF_Package1.pdf. Accessed October 27, 2014.

[20] McAllister JW. The medical home and the health care transition of youth: a perfect fit. Med Home News 2011;3(9).

[21] White PH, McManus MA, McAllister JW, et al. A primary care quality improvement approach to health care transition. Pediatr Ann 2012;41(5):e1–7.

[22] Lemly DC, Weitzman ER, O'Hare K. Advancing healthcare transitions in the medical home: tools for providers, families and adolescents with special healthcare needs. Curr Opin Pediatr 2013;25(4):439–46.

[23] Patel MS, O'Hare K. Resident training in transition of youth with childhood-onset chronic disease. Pediatrics 2010;123:S190–3. Available at: http://pediatrics.aappublications.org/content/126/Supplement_3/S190.full.pdf+html. Accessed October 27, 2014.

[24] Sharma N, O'Hare K, Antonelli RC, et al. Transition care: future directions in education, health policy and outcomes research. Acad Pediatr 2014;14:120–7.

[25] Mennito S. Resident preferences for a curriculum in healthcare transitions for young adults. South Med J 2012;105(9):462–6.

[26] Knowles MS. The adult learner. 5th edition. Houston (TX): Gulf Publishing; 1998.

[27] Rimer BK, Glanz K. Theory at a glance: a guide for health promotion practice. 2nd edition. Bethesda (MD): National Cancer Institute; U.S. Department of Health and Human Services; 2005 NIH Publication No. 05–3896.

[28] McLeroy KR, Bibeau D, Steckler A, et al. An ecological perspective on health promotion programs. Health Educ Behav 1988;15:351–77.

[29] Glasgow RE, Vogt TM, Boles SM. Evaluating the public health impact of health promotion intervention: the RE-AIM framework. Am J Public Health 1999;89(9):1322–7.

[30] Klesges JM, Estabrooks PA, Dzewaltowski DA, et al. Beginning with the application in mind: designing and planning health behavior change interventions to enhance dissemination. Ann Behav Med 2005;29(2):66–75.

[31] Sawicki GS, Lukens-Bull K, Yin X, et al. Measuring the transition readiness of youth with special healthcare needs: validation of the TRAQ—Transition Readiness Assessment Questionnaire. J Pediatr Psychol 2009;36:1–12.

[32] Ferris ME, Harward DH, Bickford K, et al. A clinical tool to measure the components of health-care transition from pediatric care to adult care: the UNC TR(x)ANSITION scale. Ren Fail 2012;34(6):744–53.

[33] Florida Health and Transition Services, Children's Medical Services, Florida Department of Health. Available at: www.floridahats.org. Accessed January 1, 2014.

[34] Ulin PR, Robinson ET, Tolley EE. Qualitative methods in public health: a field guide for applied research. San Francisco (CA): Jossey-Bass; 2005.

[35] Robson C. Real world research: a resource for social scientists and practitioner researchers. 2nd edition. Malden (MA): Blackwell Publishers; 1993.

[36] Koh HK, Brach C, Harris LM, et al. A proposed 'health literate care model' would constitute a systems approach to improving patients' engagement in care. Health Aff 2013;32(2): 257–67.

Advances in Pediatrics 62 (2015) 165–184

ADVANCES IN PEDIATRICS

ELSEVIER
MOSBY

Evidence-Based Psychological Treatments of Pediatric Mental Disorders

Monica S. Wu, MA[a,b,*], Rebecca J. Hamblin, PhD[a,e],
Eric A. Storch, PhD[a,b,c,d,e,f]

[a]Department of Pediatrics, University of South Florida, 880 6th Street South, 4th Floor North, Box 7523, St. Petersburg, FL 33701, USA; [b]Department of Psychology, University of South Florida, 4202 East Fowler Avenue, PCD 4118G, Tampa, FL 33620-7200, USA; [c]Department of Psychiatry and Behavioral Neurosciences, University of South Florida, 3515 East Fletcher Avenue, Tampa, FL 33613, USA; [d]Department of Health Management and Policy, University of South Florida, 13201 Bruce B. Downs Boulevard, MDC 56, Tampa, FL 33612, USA; [e]Rogers Behavioral Health – Tampa Bay, 2002 North Lois Avenue, Suite 400, Tampa, FL 33607, USA; [f]Mind-Body Branch, All Children's Hospital, Johns Hopkins Medicine, 880 6th Street South, 4th Floor North, Box 7523, St. Petersburg, FL 33701, USA

Keywords

- Pediatric mental disorders • Psychological treatment • Internalizing disorders
- Externalizing disorders

Key points

- With many youth presenting to primary care settings for mental health difficulties, knowledge of the respective evidence-based psychotherapies is imperative in ensuring that these youth receive the appropriate interventions in a timely manner.

- Most frequently, children present with internalizing and/or externalizing disorders, which cover a broad range of common pediatric mental disorders.

- Treatments of these disorders generally incorporate cognitive and/or behavioral components, which are derived from theoretical underpinnings and empirical support.

- Although the interventions share common components, they are distinctive in nature and are further tailored toward the idiosyncratic needs of children and their families.

- Careful consideration of the apposite intervention and individual needs of the youth are pertinent to the effective amelioration of symptomology.

*Corresponding author. Department of Pediatrics, Rothman Center for Neuropsychiatry, University of South Florida, 880 6th Street South, Suite 460, Box 7523, St. Petersburg, FL 33701. E-mail address: MonicaWu@mail.usf.edu

0065-3101/15/$ – see front matter
http://dx.doi.org/10.1016/j.yapd.2015.04.007

With millions of youth affected by psychiatric illnesses each year [1], it is imperative that appropriate psychotherapeutic treatments are received in a timely manner. Because families often present at primary care settings for mental health difficulties [2–5], primary care physicians frequently serve as a gateway to receiving proper interventions. Knowledge about the most up-to-date, empirically supported therapies is pertinent. Numerous psychological treatments have proved efficacious for pediatric mental disorders. Empirically validated treatments are considered the gold-standard treatments for use with specific populations [6] because they must meet several rigorous criteria to be classified as such (eg, requiring efficacy beyond psychological control/placebo treatments in methodologically sound studies).

Based on the range of pediatric mental disorders, this article presents empirically supported psychological treatments of internalizing and externalizing disorders [7]. The theoretical perspectives of specific therapies are discussed, followed by descriptions of the typical components within the treatment. Lastly, explanations regarding the implementation of the interventions are provided, tailored for each specific mental disorder.

INTERNALIZING DISORDERS

Internalizing disorders (ie, anxiety disorders, obsessive-compulsive disorder [OCD], and depression) are characterized by difficulties concerning emotions and mood [8]. Although distinct, these disorders share similarities in mechanisms of maintenance, psychological theories of etiology, neurobiological pathways, and comorbidities [8–12]. The general theoretical basis for the cognitive-behavioral treatment of internalizing disorders is discussed, followed by a discussion of the typical components (eg, cognitive and behavioral) within the intervention. Thereafter, the implementation of a typical course of cognitive-behavioral therapy (CBT) for internalizing disorders is reviewed, with nuanced descriptions tailored for each disorder.

General theoretical perspective of treatment

Internalizing disorders are theoretically conceptualized under a cognitive-behavioral umbrella, emphasizing the interplay between thoughts, feelings, and behaviors [13]. Specifically, it is proposed that thoughts have an impact on feelings and behaviors, feelings influence thoughts and behaviors, and behaviors affect thoughts and feelings. The cognitive component involves the maladaptive thoughts that are experienced by an individual, often characterized by unrealistic appraisals of various situations. For instance, example negative cognitions include the worry that others may be negatively evaluating them (eg, social anxiety) or the thought that only bad things happen to individuals and they are unable to control these events (eg, depression). The feelings component, on the other hand, include somatic sensations as well as emotions. Under this operationalization, feelings can include heart palpitations and shortness of breath as well as sadness and anxiety. The behavioral component is defined by the actual actions and behaviors that are carried out by an individual. For example, avoidance is a common behavior observed in anxiety disorders, along with various safety behaviors (eg, needing to be accompanied by an adult for fear of being alone). Collectively, these 3 components of thoughts, feelings, and behaviors are postulated to affect one another, resulting in an interdependent cycle.

Historically, the cycle between thoughts, feelings, and behaviors is theorized to be maintained through various processes, namely classical and operant conditioning [11]. Specifically, the negative reinforcement cycle between cognitions and behaviors is highlighted, given its role in the maintenance of symptomology. Broadly, youth with internalizing disorders experience negative cognitions, resulting in negative valence states and behaviors that are designed to remove the experience of these negative feelings and thoughts. Behaviors, such as avoidance, serve to negatively reinforce the cycle; these actions allow a child to avoid experiencing (or mitigate) distress, thereby making it more likely that the child will engage in the maladaptive behaviors in the future. To illustrate this cycle, consider the negative reinforcement cycle for a socially anxious child. This youth may experience worries about doing something embarrassing in front of peers, causing the child to avoid going to social events. Because the behavior allows the child to avoid experiencing anxiety, the behavior is negatively reinforced and thereby more likely to occur in the future. Consequently, the child is unable to face the feared situation, disallowing any chances for experiencing firsthand that the feared outcome was unlikely to happen and making it difficult to form more realistic appraisals. As such, the goals of CBT serve to target the individual components that maintain the symptomology of internalizing disorders.

Implementation of treatment

Because thoughts, feelings, and behaviors are interrelated, targeting individual components in CBT results in consequent changes to the other components as well [14]. When using CBT for internalizing disorders, the intervention predominantly focuses on targeting the cognitive and behavioral components, with emphases on either/both components varying across different types of CBT; that is, some interventions focus primarily on the cognitive component or the behavioral component, whereas others are balanced across both components. When using behavior therapy with internalizing disorders, therapists are focused on targeting the actions that occur due to the negative thoughts and feelings. In anxiety disorders, behavior therapy is pivotal in having a child gradually and systematically confront the feared situations; these experiences allow the child to see that the feared outcome is unlikely to happen, which provides the opportunity to reframe maladaptive cognitions and thereby attenuate the negative reinforcement cycle. In mood disorders, the behavioral component places more emphasis on behavioral activation, which is designed to enhance the youth's mood through engagement in pleasurable activities [15].

When using cognitive therapy, therapists target maladaptive appraisals and work with children to formulate more realistic cognitions. In internalizing disorders, youth often have distorted views of the world, possessing negative and catastrophic thoughts about various situations. The cognitive component of CBT aims to help children identify and challenge these negative cognitions. This is typically accomplished by first increasing a youth's awareness of the presence of these thoughts, which can be achieved through thought logs, role-playing, and modeling. Once distorted cognitions are identified, a therapist works with the child to challenge and restructure the thoughts, using techniques such as gathering evidence from the past, considering the likelihood of the anticipated outcome, and remedying thinking traps (eg, catastrophizing).

Although the CBT package can be delivered in multiple ways, there are typically a few core steps that are consistent across treatment protocols. Treatment is typically time-limited and occurs in hour-long weekly sessions. First, psycho-education about the disorder and treatment is provided during the first session. Within that session, parents and their youth learn about the general etiology and maintenance of the disorders as well as the theoretical basis and components behind CBT. Thereafter, individualized information from the youth is garnered, and awareness-building activities commence. Specifically, a therapist works with a family to help identify the cognitive distortions, negative feelings, and specific situations that are feared or contribute to poorer mood. Depending on the developmental ability of the child, this portion of therapy also contains emotion education, because youth often have difficulties recognizing the emotional and physical attributes of various feelings. Once negative thoughts, feelings, and situations are identified, cognitive restructuring is used. These techniques are typically introduced and practiced in nonthreatening situations first, because it can be difficult to acquire information when in emotionally heightened states [14]. Problem-solving techniques are also introduced and practiced, allowing a child to independently formulate various solutions and select the most adaptive response. After repeated practice of these skills, real-life practice of these skills is pertinent to promote generalization of these newly acquired abilities. Once these therapeutic procedures have been mastered, the intervention typically concludes with a final session designed to review progress and provide skills for relapse prevention.

Depending on the developmental stage of the youth, parental involvement is highly encouraged in CBT [16–22]. Younger children may have more difficulty acquiring these cognitive-behavioral skills, necessitating parental guidance and oversight. CBT protocols require in-between session homework, which typically includes out-of-session practices of what was learned in the therapy session (eg, documenting use of cognitive restructuring or facing a feared situation outside of session). Additionally, parents can help model adaptive ways of coping and thinking, so parental involvement in treatment is imperative to help generalize these skills.

Disorder-specific treatment

Anxiety disorders

CBT is a well-established treatment of pediatric anxiety disorders, with many randomized controlled trials (RCTs) demonstrating its efficacy over placebo and other control groups (combined effect sizes ranging from 0.86–0.94) [23–27]. Like other internalizing disorders, CBT with anxious youth also includes the typical cognitive and behavioral therapies. There are certain aspects of CBT with this population, however, that are unique to anxiety disorders and not to other internalizing disorders.

The behavioral component of CBT for pediatric anxiety disorders involves exposing children to their feared situations, which is typically conducted in graduated manner. A fear hierarchy, which is a list of feared situations ranked in order of least distressing to most distressing, is constructed at the beginning of therapy. This fear hierarchy essentially serves as the general treatment plan for the rest of therapy, helping to guide the implementation of exposures. To encourage mastery and enhance self-confidence, low-anxiety situations are practiced first, and latter exposures are tackled in a gradated fashion. Exposure tasks can be conducted in an imaginal session or *in vivo* (ie, in session). Practicing exposures *in vivo* is typically preferred, because it allows a therapist to conduct the exposure in a real-life situation in session. An example *in vivo* exposure is having an arachnophobic child touch a spider with a hand. There are times, however, when it is unrealistic to conduct an exposure in-session (eg, fear of death), so exposures can also be done imaginally [28]. Imaginal exposures are meant to be conducted in a detailed fashion, because they are designed to replicate the real-life situation as closely as possible. Scripts are typically written with nuanced details to create the full experience within the session, incorporating the specific sights, textures, sounds, and smells of the feared stimulus.

When using cognitive therapy for anxiety disorders, there are typically several methods to help youth combat negative thoughts. Because anxious youth have a tendency to catastrophize situations and anticipate the worst possible outcomes, they are encouraged to consider the true likelihood of the event occurring and gather evidence from their surroundings (eg, "Has this ever happened before?" "Do I know anyone that this has happened to?" "How likely is it to really happen?"). Therapists should not, however, promise a child that a feared event is never going to happen, because that is also an unrealistic expectation. Instead, anxious youth typically hold cognitions that convince them that the feared event is likely to happen, so cognitive restructuring helps them achieve a more balanced and realistic appraisal of the situation. Additionally, given that the anxious apprehension is usually worse than the actual outcome, youth are also encouraged to ask themselves, "What is the worst that could happen?" Lastly, therapists are also encouraged to refrain from trying to convince a child that nothing bad is likely to happen. Instead, Socratic questioning and eliciting responses from a child helps better facilitate learning (eg, "Can you think of a time that this has happened before?").

CBT can be implemented in varying durations and in various formats depending on the specific anxiety disorder. For instance, a typical course of CBT for anxiety disorders can range anywhere from 12 to 20 weeks on average, but youth possessing specific phobias may be successfully treated under a truncated CBT protocol within 1 day [29–32]. Additionally, CBT can be delivered in an individual or a group format, with either modality achieving treatment gains and attenuation in childhood anxiety symptoms [17,25,33–37]. With the advent of technology, computerized CBT for anxious youth has also been examined in RCTs; similar to in-person CBT, computerized administration of CBT protocols has demonstrated reduction in anxiety symptomology and durability in treatment gains [38–40].

Obsessive-compulsive disorder
Based on recently published practice parameters [41], the first-line treatment of pediatric OCD is a behavior-based variant of CBT called exposure and response prevention (ERP). In ERP, youth are exposed to the feared thoughts and situations and are prevented from engaging in their compulsions thereafter. For instance, if a child presents with contamination fears, the child is asked to touch objects that were perceived as "dirty" or contaminated and then asked to refrain from any compulsive cleaning behaviors (eg, hand washing). Exposures should be gradual, repetitive, and prolonged; each of those components is discussed later.

Similar to the treatment protocol of anxiety disorders, ERP for OCD incorporates the use of a fear hierarchy to rank the feared obsessions and situations. Each feared stimulus can be broken down to further gradations as needed, falling in line with the aforementioned plan to gradually expose a child to feared stimuli; initial exposures elicit mild discomfort, and treatment eventually progresses to the top of the fear hierarchy, which includes high-anxiety stimuli. For instance, a child with contamination fears may first be asked to touch a "contaminated" door handle with a pinky finger, followed by 2 fingers, and exposures continue on until the child is able to touch the door handle with the whole hand without engaging in washing/cleaning compulsions. Once the anxiety elicited from those exposures has decreased considerably and/or the child has demonstrated the ability to tolerate the anxiety [42,43], the therapist and youth are able to move onto the next item on the fear hierarchy.

Also similar to CBT for anxiety disorders, exposures within ERP can also be done imaginally or *in vivo*. *In vivo* exposures are still the preferred method of exposures, but there are various subtypes of OCD that can limit opportunities to do so. For instance, obsessions of the aggressive, sexual, and/or religious nature may constrain the types of *in vivo* exposures that can be ethically carried out, necessitating the need for creative imaginal exposures. In these cases, the distressing obsession and feared outcome are written down in meticulous detail, and the child is asked to repeatedly read the script to induce repeated exposure, and thus habituation (or tolerance of anxiety), to the feared stimulus.

Cognitive techniques can also be used as a secondary component to treatment, serving as a motivating factor for children to resist giving into the obsessions and compulsions. In other words, cognitive tools are not purposed to attenuate a child's anxiety and are instead used to help build awareness into the symptoms and resist the OCD. Similar to CBT for anxiety, common thinking traps such as catastrophizing ("I am going to contract a deadly illness if I touch that doorknob"), over-responsibility ("If I don't move this eraser a certain way, something bad will happen to my sister"), and thought-action fusion ("If I think that I will hurt my mother, that is just as bad as actually doing it"), are identified [44,45]. To counteract maladaptive thinking patterns, children are taught to detach themselves from their OCD symptoms, build their self-confidence and motivation to combat OCD, and use cognitive restructuring techniques. There is a fine line, however, between effectively using these cognitive tools and turning them into a compulsion (eg, excessive self-reassurance), so clinicians must remain vigilant when using these techniques [46,47].

Many RCTs have demonstrated its efficacy in pediatric OCD, with effect sizes between 1.20 and 1.45 demonstrating that ERP achieves significantly greater attenuation in OCD symptoms than other placebo, pharmacotherapy, and control groups [20,48–54]. It remains unclear if CBT combined with an antidepressant is more effective than CBT alone, because findings have been mixed [49]. This treatment can be delivered in group or individual formats, with both modalities showing durable improvement in OCD symptoms [48]. Additionally, ERP for pediatric OCD is able to be delivered in an intensive format, occurring multiple times during the week instead of the standard weekly administration [50,55,56]. Because technology has been increasingly incorporated into mental health care, preliminary studies investigating the utility of providing ERP through telehealth mechanisms have also shown promise in decrease OCD symptom severity [57–59].

Depression
CBT is a well-established treatment of depression in both children and adolescents [11,60]. Depending on the treatment protocol and idiosyncratic needs of the child, CBT for depression may be more concentrated on the cognitive components, behavioral components, or both. Alternatively, adolescents may also benefit from interpersonal psychotherapy (IPT), given the emerging impact of social relationships within this developmental stage [61,62].

In CBT for depression, the cognitive components are used to target the negative cognitions that cyclically influence their negative affect. The first step in treatment involves the utilization of mood logs designed to document a baseline assessment of the types of thoughts and situations that have an impact on mood. Both positive and negative situations are recorded, because it is important to evaluate the types of situations and thoughts that can both enhance and diminish mood. Commonly observed types of negative cognitions include self-defeating ("I am worthless"), hopeless ("Things are never going to get better"), and catastrophizing ("Nothing could possibly get worse") thoughts [63]. Once the distorted thoughts are recognized, the therapist works with the child to identify, examine, challenge, and reframe the thoughts. The ultimate goal of the cognitive tools is for a child to be able to reevaluate the veracity of the thoughts and replace them with a more adaptive, realistic cognition.

On the other hand, the behavioral component in CBT for depression is more focused on behavioral activation. In this element of therapy, children are encouraged to engage in rewarding activities designed to augment mood. Typical pleasurable activities that are prescribed include exercise, social engagements, and participating in hobbies. Many youth with depression may feel increased lethargy and amotivation to engage in activities, so the behavioral activation component of CBT is designed to compete with the behavioral tendencies that maintain the negative mood. By activating and engaging these youth, they consequently have the opportunity to receive positive feedback and reinforcement from these activities, thereby increasing their mood [64].

For depressed adolescents, IPT may be a more appropriate choice of treatment. Specifically, IPT is predicated on the theory that interpersonal relationships have considerable impact on the development, maintenance, and protective effects against depression. Thus, this type of treatment focuses on evaluating and enhancing youths' interpersonal relationships as they relate to their depressive symptoms. First, a problem area is identified, which typically falls into 1 of 4 categories [65]: grief (eg, death of a loved one), role dispute (eg, conflicts in social relationships), role transition (eg, graduation or diagnosis of illness), or interpersonal deficits (eg, lack of friends). Once a problem area is identified, skill-building for developing effective communication and problem-solving skills are implemented. Thereafter, the skills are practiced in session, with the ultimate goal of generalizing the skills to be used in the adolescent's social relationships.

RCTs of psychotherapeutic interventions for pediatric depression have demonstrated their efficacy, exhibiting effect sizes between 0.34 and 0.72 [11,66–68]. These psychotherapeutic interventions can also be implemented in group formats with similar efficacy, with preliminary evidence in favor of their use in school systems [69–71]. Advances in technology have also made it possible to implement these treatments via telehealth mechanisms [72].

EXTERNALIZING DISORDERS
This section includes information on empirically supported psychosocial treatments of externalizing behavior disorders, including attention-deficit/hyperactivity disorder (ADHD), oppositional defiant disorder (ODD), and conduct disorder (CD). Collectively, externalizing disorders are the most common child psychiatric issues encountered in primary care settings [73]. Although etiologically and clinically distinct, these disorders are discussed together because of the similarity and overlap of empirically supported treatment options and the high comorbidity among them. The theoretical underpinnings of the treatments are reviewed as well as research supporting their use, and a description and outline of the course of treatment are provided.

General theoretical perspective of treatment
The most commonly implemented treatments of externalizing disorders are based on the principles of operant conditioning, a theory based on the premise

that behavior is learned and modified by way of antecedents and consequences. Antecedents are the events and circumstances in the environment that occur directly before a particular behavior, and consequences are the events that occur immediately afterwards. Behavior modification techniques, also known as contingency management, are most commonly delivered by training parents and teachers in the use of antecedent modification and systematic delivery of consequences to reduce unwanted behavior and increase desired behavior. Antecedent modifications are changes made to the environment designed to change the probability of a behavior; examples include visual and verbal prompts and using effective commands. Caregivers are taught to identify and reward positive behavior through the use of praise, attention, preferred activities, tangible rewards, or point systems. Appropriate punishment is used sparingly to reduce problems, such as aggression; common punishments include time-out for young children and loss of privileges for older children and adolescents. A combination of behavioral strategies implemented across home and school settings may be used to maximize effectiveness and generalize gains.

Cognitive and interpersonal skills training may be delivered directly to a child in conjunction with parent and teacher training to remediate cognitive distortions and deficits related to interpersonal interactions [74,75]. Cognitive interventions are based on the theoretical and empirical basis that children with conduct problems, in particular aggression, often misperceive others as hostile and lack skills to inhibit negative responses and generate effective solutions to interpersonal problems [75,76]. They may also have delays in the development of perspective taking and social skills necessary to achieve positive peer relationships [77]. Child cognitive skills training programs use modeling, didactic instruction, role-play, and rewards for participation and correct use of skills to teach children to more effectively handle distressing interpersonal situations and reduce aggression and other negative behaviors [75,77,78].

Implementation of treatment
Behavioral parent training
The most common delivery method of contingency management is through behavioral parent training (BPT) in which a child's caregivers are trained by a clinician to use operant conditioning techniques in the home. There are several manualized programs that teach parents how to effectively respond to and reduce problematic behavior, increase compliance, teach prosocial skills and attitudes, and develop strong relationships with their children. BPT programs may be delivered to individual families or in a group format and range from approximately 8 to 30 once-weekly sessions, depending on the age of the child, number of skills targeted in the specific program, and severity of problems. Individual family sessions are typically held for 50 minutes, and group training sessions are generally 2 to 2.5 hours in length.

BPT typically begins with a component aimed at increasing special time between parent(s) and child to improve the quality of the relationship, thereby reducing family conflict and increasing the likelihood of compliance. The format of the special time component varies by program but involves either teaching parents to engage in child-directed play, to set aside daily special time with the child, or to give nondirective attention by focusing on and narrating children's activities without judgment, instructions, or questions [79,80]. Parents subsequently are taught to increase desired behaviors (eg, compliance, assertiveness, task persistence, and sharing) by using verbal praise and giving attention immediately after desired actions. Avoidance of negative behavior is accomplished through increasing structure and clarity of expectations. Specific discipline techniques focused on reduction of negative behavior through aversive consequences are generally introduced only after increasing positive behaviors and modifying antecedents. Strategies include withdrawal of attention to minor behavior problems and brief loss of reinforcement (time out) or privileges (older children). Box 1 provides an example flow of skills that might be covered in a typical program.

Teaching methods for individual families consist of explanation and demonstration of skills, reading assignments, in-session role-play with a therapist, identification of child-specific problem areas and preferred rewards, in-session practice with the child, and weekly homework assignments for implementing strategies at home. Group format programs may also incorporate large and small group discussion and skills practice, role-play and practice with other parents, and a buddy system for at-home problem solving and increasing homework compliance [77]. Some programs also use prerecorded vignettes

Box 1: Example sessions for behavioral parent training

1. Psychoeducation regarding specific diagnosis and contingency management principles
2. Increasing positive attention and child-directed time with parent
3. Using praise and attention to and increase appropriate behavior (eg, compliance)
4. Procedures for ignoring minor inappropriate behaviors (eg, arguing)
5. Establishing structure and routines
6. Giving effective commands and redirecting behavior
7. Establishing rules and contingencies
8. Effective implementation of time-out for serious behavior
9. Using token economy or other reward systems
10. Enforcing rules and consequences in public; planning ahead for misbehavior
11. Implementing a daily school behavior report card
12. Troubleshooting specific behavior problems
13. Maintenance

modeling common behavior problems and effective and ineffective use of parenting skills as a basis for focused discussions and problem solving [77].

There are several BPT manuals available for children of various age groups. BPT may be implemented alone or in conjunction with classroom management training and behavior plans for school and/or child cognitive and interpersonal skills training. BPT is often a stand-alone treatment of preschool-aged children and has a high rate of success for this age group [81], whereas older children also need support in school and social environments [82].

School-based contingency management
School-based contingency management parallels behavior modification techniques taught in BPT in that a child's classroom teacher is trained in the use of token systems, praise, active ignoring, and so forth [83,84]. Most commonly, a mental health professional is contacted to provide a consultation and individualized behavior plan for a particular child who is displaying disruptive behavior [82,84]. To identify the most problematic behaviors, antecedents (eg, time of day, change in routine, and transitions), and consequences (eg, attention and avoidance of schoolwork), the consultant observes the child in the classroom and in an unstructured activity (eg, recess) and interviews teachers and parents. The consultant establishes a specific plan based on the child's needs and preferences and trains the teachers in timing and implementation of techniques. Antecedent modifications in the classroom may include giving cues for appropriate behavior, providing additional structure around transitions, seating the child near prosocial peers, breaking down assignments, and establishing clear expectations and contingencies. Point systems or token economies are used in conjunction with increasing praise and attending to desired behavior, and home-school report cards assist teachers and parents with communication and consistency in goals, expectations, and progress and facilitate parent implementation of rewards for positive behavior at school [85].

Some school-based behavioral programs implement school-wide training of teachers and programs and thus are inclusive of many children in the school with disruptive behavior and/or ADHD [77]. Such programs use behavioral training procedures similar to those used with parents in BPT. In addition, teachers are also provided targeted strategies for school-specific difficulties, such as transitions and peer rejection and aggression, as well as strategies for improving parent-teacher communication. Whether teacher interventions are delivered for an individual child or as part of a school-wide initiative, school-based contingency management is most effective when used in combination with parent interventions [86].

Cognitive and social skills training
Cognitive skills training for children with conduct problems involves teaching children how to more appropriately interpret social situations and cues, how to generate possible solutions and responses, and how to select from possible approaches. Problem-solving skills training is an example of such a program used to treat children with ODD and CD [87]. Problem-solving skills training

is delivered with children individually while a parent participates in BPT, maximizing both efficiency of skill mastery and generalization to a child's day-to-day interactions. First, the child is taught a series of problem-solving steps and then is encouraged to make self-talk statements to orient to the steps to cue and guide behavior. The first 4 sessions involve introducing the steps and how to apply them. In the fifth session, the child teaches the parents the steps within a mutual therapy session and parents are encouraged to cue and reinforce use of the steps in the child's natural environment using the reinforcement strategies they are concurrently learning in BPT. The next 5 sessions include role-playing using the steps in real-life scenarios with gradually increasing complexity. The 12th and final session is a wrap-up assessment in which the child teaches the steps to the therapist to check for understanding. Other cognitive and skills interventions follow a similar format, with some variation in skills taught and specific problems of focus [76], but all cognitive interventions are most effective when delivered in combination with parent and/or school-based behavioral interventions.

Disorder-specific treatments

Attention-deficit/hyperactivity disorder
BPT is the most frequently implemented behavioral intervention for ADHD. BPT programs were originally created to target disruptive and noncompliant behavior; as such, BPT has a substantial empirical basis of support for addressing disruptive behavior, noncompliance, and impaired family functioning associated with ADHD [88]. Recent adaptations of BPT for ADHD also include components focused on increasing sustained attention, task persistence, and other impairments related to the inattentive cluster of symptoms. Several studies evaluating BPT enhanced to target sustained attention and effort for parents of preschool-aged children with ADHD have shown efficacy at reducing inattentive and hyperactive/impulsive symptoms in addition to improvements in related functional impairments [89]. A significant portion of children achieve normalized functioning and approximately half no longer meet clinical threshold for ADHD post-treatment; most importantly, these gains are maintained at long-term follow-up [81,89–91]. Thus, it is possible that behavioral interventions delivered early may thwart an ADHD illness trajectory for many children and reduce the symptom severity and functional impairments for others.

School-based interventions similarly have historically focused on and shown short-term success in reducing disruptive behavior associated with ADHD, and several programs addressing impairments in academic performance, inattention, organization, and time management have recently been developed and explored [85,92]. The Collaborative Life and Attention Skills Program [93] focuses on school-related impairments for children with predominantly inattentive symptoms of ADHD. The program consists of BPT, behavioral teacher consultation with contingencies targeting attention and organizational skills, a school-home report card system, and social and cognitive skills training directly with the child. Results of an RCT showed greater teacher-rated improvements in inattention, organization, social skills, and global functioning for participants receiving the full treatment relative to those who received only the BPT component and those assigned to treatment as usual. Treatment gains were maintained at follow-up for parent- but not teacher-rated measures, highlighting the need for continuous monitoring and as-needed implementation of treatment boosters with behavioral interventions for ADHD [93].

Despite the fact that BPT and school-based interventions do not directly address internalizing problems, these interventions are effective in reducing comorbid anxiety and mood symptoms in children with ADHD. Additionally, in a large multisite RCT comparing interventions for school-aged children, behavioral interventions were as effective as pharmacologic interventions in reducing inattentive and hyperactivity/impulsivity symptoms for children with a comorbid anxiety disorder [94], which is noteworthy considering that approximately one-third of children with ADHD also have an anxiety disorder [95]. Anxiety in children with ADHD is also associated with heightened sensitivity to stimulant medication [96]; thus, it is important to conduct a thorough assessment when considering the first-line intervention approach for children with various clinical presentations.

Contingency management programs implemented at home, school, or both are effective interventions for reducing core symptoms of ADHD and related functional impairments [88,97,98]. Behavioral interventions in combination with psychostimulant medication are superior to medication alone for improvements in related impairments, including oppositional and disruptive behavior, parent-child relationships, and internalizing disorders [99]. A limitation of behavioral strategies is that treatment gains are not sustained long term in the absence of continuous implementation of contingency management, and benefits may not be conferred to settings in which contingencies are not directly used [83,99]. On balance, psychostimulants are ineffective unless taken daily and do not result in improved academic achievement, and long-term studies show that psychostimulants do not result in long-term improvements in functioning [100]. Parents tend to prefer behavioral interventions over stimulant medication as a first line of treatment [101] and report greater satisfaction with treatment of behavioral interventions delivered alone or in conjunction with psychostimulants compared with medication alone [102]. Overall, behavior contingency management likely is beneficial for nearly all children who have ADHD, particularly for preschool-aged children and those with comorbid anxiety disorders and/or ODD/CD. To achieve long-term functional improvements and maintain symptom reduction, treatment boosters should be delivered and contingencies maintained across settings.

Oppositional defiant disorder and conduct disorder
BPT has the largest base of empirical support of any intervention for the treatment and prevention of ODD and CD and is the first-line treatment of children in all age ranges [103]. Gains made from BPT interventions for

children with ODD are likely be maintained long term. For example, children in families treated with Helping the Noncompliant Child curriculum were functioning equally as well as community peers 14 years after treatment [104], and other programs have demonstrated maintenance of treatment gains 1 year after treatment [77,89]. As with ADHD treatment, early intervention is key to attaining the greatest benefits for children with ODD or CD [76].

Children of different ages and symptom severity may require differing levels of intervention [76,105,106]. BPT is likely to be effective for very young children with ODD; however, older children and those with CD or severe ODD are likely to need school-based and/or cognitive skills interventions along with BPT. As children are exposed to negative peer influences at school and continued reinforcement of negative behavior, conduct problems may become more deeply entrenched. School-based contingency management for conduct problems is similar to ADHD in procedures and format and confers additional benefits when delivered in conjunction with BPT [86].

Children with severe conduct problems and/or aggression, in particular those with deficits in social and perspective taking skills, may require individual cognitive skills treatment in combination with contingency management. Problem-solving skills training is effective at reducing CD and aggression and increasing prosocial behavior when delivered as a stand-alone treatment [78] and confers additional benefits over and above BPT alone for 5 to 13 year olds with CD [107].

For adolescents with severe, intractable antisocial behavior, multisystemic therapy is a comprehensive approach that applies a combination of evidence-based interventions tailored to meet the specific needs of an individual family [108]. An assessment is conducted within all relevant social contexts to determine ecological factors maintaining the problematic behavior. Once specific antecedents and consequences have been determined, a multisystemic intervention plan targeting all relevant contingencies and influences is designed and implemented. The treatment is based in a child's home and, when indicated, includes intensive BPT, empirically supported therapy for parental psychopathology, school-based contingency management, and individual CBT for aggression, skill deficits, and internalizing problems. Barriers to treatment are addressed with support from a therapist and case manager, who assist the family in availing resources and communicating with schools and community members with whom the adolescent is involved. The therapist and case manager identify and draw on strengths of the family and available social support (neighbors, coaches, and extended family) to support the family and overcome challenges. The therapist meets with the family in the home at least once weekly and is available by phone 24 hours per day. Effects of interventions are monitored and the treatment plan is revised as necessary throughout. Multisystemic therapy has been shown to reduce recidivism rates for juvenile offenders, improve family relations, increase school attendance, and decrease externalizing and internalizing symptomology [108–111].

Overall, cognitive-behavioral interventions are effective at reducing common behavior problems in children, such as noncompliance, rule-breaking, and minor aggression. Early intervention is more likely effective than later intervention because behavior problems may worsen over time, and treatment is likely to result in long-term improvement. Unimodal treatment, such as BPT, may be sufficient for mild problems, those occurring only in 1 environment, and very young children. Older children and those displaying greater symptom severity are likely to need behavioral interventions implemented across settings. Children demonstrating aggressive behavior and those with deficits in social problem-solving skills are likely to benefit from individual cognitive and social skills training. Thus, the treatment package should be tailored to meet the needs of individual children and families.

SUMMARY

With many youth presenting to primary care settings for mental health difficulties, knowledge of the respective evidence-based psychotherapies is imperative in ensuring that these youth receive the appropriate interventions in a timely manner. Most frequently, children present with internalizing and/or externalizing disorders, which cover a broad range of common pediatric mental disorders. Treatments of these disorders generally incorporate cognitive and/or behavioral components, which are derived from theoretical underpinnings and empirical support. Although the interventions share common components, they are distinctive in nature and are further tailored toward the idiosyncratic needs of children and their families. Careful consideration of the apposite intervention and individual needs of youth are pertinent to the effective amelioration of symptomology.

References

[1] Centers for Disease Control and Prevention. Mental health surveillance among children - United States. 2005–2011. MMWR Morb Mortal Wkly Rep 2013;62(Suppl):1–35, May 16, 2013.

[2] Goldberg ID, Roghmann KJ, McInerny TK, et al. Mental health problems among children seen in pediatric practice: prevalence and management. Pediatrics 1984;73(3):278–93.

[3] Goldberg ID, Regier DA, McInerny TK, et al. The role of the pediatrician in the delivery of mental health services to children. Pediatrics 1979;63(6):898–909.

[4] Lavigne JV, Arend R, Rosenbaum D, et al. Mental health service use among young children receiving pediatric primary care. J Am Acad Child Adolesc Psychiatry 1998;37(11): 1175–83.

[5] Briggs-Gowan MJ, Horwitz SM, Schwab-Stone ME, et al. Mental health in pediatric settings: distribution of disorders and factors related to service use. J Am Acad Child Adolesc Psychiatry 2000;39(7):841–9.

[6] Chambless DL, Baker MJ, Baucom DH, et al. Update on empirically validated therapies, II. Clin Psychol 1998;51(1):3–16.

[7] Cicchetti D, Toth SL. A developmental perspective on internalizing and externalizing disorders. In: Cicchetti D, Toth SL, editors. Internalizing and externalizing expressions of dysfunction, vol. 2. New York: Psychology Press; 2014. p. 1–19.

[8] Kovacs M, Devlin B. Internalizing disorders in childhood. J Child Psychol Psychiatry 1998;39(1):47–63.

[9] Ressler KJ, Nemeroff CB. Role of serotonergic and noradrenergic systems in the pathophysiology of depression and anxiety disorders. Depress Anxiety 2000;12(S1):2–19.

[10] Eison MS. Serotonin: a common neurobiologic substrate in anxiety and depression. J Clin Psychopharmacol 1990;10(3):26S–30S.

[11] Compton SN, March JS, Brent D, et al. Cognitive-behavioral psychotherapy for anxiety and depressive disorders in children and adolescents: an evidence-based medicine review. J Am Acad Child Adolesc Psychiatry 2004;43(8):930–59.

[12] Cryan JF, Kaupmann K. Don't worry 'B'happy!: a role for GABAB receptors in anxiety and depression. Trends Pharmacol Sci 2005;26(1):36–43.

[13] Brewin CR. Theoretical foundations of cognitive-behavior therapy for anxiety and depression. Annu Rev Psychol 1996;47:33–57.

[14] Kendall PC, Panichelli-Mindel SM. Cognitive-behavioral treatments. J Abnorm Child Psychol 1995;23(1):107–24.

[15] Hopko DR, Lejuez CW, Ruggiero KJ, et al. Contemporary behavioral activation treatments for depression: procedures, principles, and progress. Clin Psychol Rev 2003;23(5): 699–717.

[16] Barrett PM, Duffy AL, Dadds MR, et al. Cognitive–behavioral treatment of anxiety disorders in children: long-term (6-year) follow-up. J Consult Clin Psychol 2001;69(1):135.

[17] Kendall PC, Hudson JL, Gosch E, et al. Cognitive-behavioral therapy for anxiety disordered youth: a randomized clinical trial evaluating child and family modalities. J Consult Clin Psychol 2008;76(2):282.

[18] Wood JJ, Piacentini JC, Southam-Gerow M, et al. Family cognitive behavioral therapy for child anxiety disorders. J Am Acad Child Adolesc Psychiatry 2006;45(3):314–21.

[19] Podell JL, Kendall PC. Mothers and fathers in family cognitive-behavioral therapy for anxious youth. J Child Fam Stud 2011;20(2):182–95.

[20] Piacentini J, Bergman RL, Chang S, et al. Controlled comparison of family cognitive behavioral therapy and psychoeducation/relaxation training for child obsessive-compulsive disorder. J Am Acad Child Adolesc Psychiatry 2011;50(11):1149–61.

[21] Lewin AB, Park JM, Jones AM, et al. Family-based exposure and response prevention therapy for preschool-aged children with obsessive-compulsive disorder: a pilot randomized controlled trial. Behav Res Ther 2014;56:30–8.

[22] Lewin AB, Piacentini J. Obsessive-compulsive disorder in children. In: Sadock BJ, Sadock VA, Ruiz P, editors. Kaplan & Sadock's comprehensive textbook of psychiatry, vol. 2, 9th edition. Philadelphia: Lippincott Williams & Wilkins; 2009. p. 3671–8.

[23] Silverman WK, Pina AA, Viswesvaran C. Evidence-based psychosocial treatments for phobic and anxiety disorders in children and adolescents. J Clin Child Adolesc Psychol 2008;37(1):105–30.

[24] Connolly SD, Bernstein GA, Work Group on Quality Issues. Practice parameter for the assessment and treatment of children and adolescents with anxiety disorders. J Am Acad Child Adolesc Psychiatry 2007;46(2):267–83.

[25] Walkup JT, Albano AM, Piacentini J, et al. Cognitive behavioral therapy, sertraline, or a combination in childhood anxiety. N Engl J Med 2008;359(26):2753–66.

[26] Ishikawa SI, Okajima I, Matsuoka H, et al. Cognitive behavioural therapy for anxiety disorders in children and adolescents: a meta-analysis. Child Adolesc Ment Health 2007;12(4):164–72.

[27] In-Albon T, Schneider S. Psychotherapy of childhood anxiety disorders: a meta-analysis. Psychother Psychosom 2007;76(1):15–24.

[28] Podell JL, Mychailyszyn M, Edmunds J, et al. The coping cat program for anxious youth: the FEAR plan comes to life. Cogn Behav Pract 2010;17(2):132–41.

[29] Davis TE III, Ollendick TH, Öst LG. Intensive treatment of specific phobias in children and adolescents. Cogn Behav Pract 2009;16(3):294–303.

[30] Öst LG, Svensson L, Hellström K, et al. One-session treatment of specific phobias in youths: a randomized clinical trial. J Consult Clin Psychol 2001;69(5):814.

[31] Ollendick TH, Öst LG, Reuterskiöld L, et al. One-session treatment of specific phobias in youth: a randomized clinical trial in the United States and Sweden. J Consult Clin Psychol 2009;77(3):504.

[32] Zlomke K, Davis TE III. One-session treatment of specific phobias: a detailed description and review of treatment efficacy. Behav Ther 2008;39(3):207–23.

[33] Flannery-Schroeder EC, Kendall PC. Group and individual cognitive-behavioral treatments for youth with anxiety disorders: a randomized clinical trial. Cognit Ther Res 2000;24(3):251–78.

[34] Liber JM, Van Widenfelt BM, Utens EM, et al. No differences between group versus individual treatment of childhood anxiety disorders in a randomised clinical trial. J Child Psychol Psychiatry 2008;49(8):886–93.

[35] Muris P, Meesters C, van Melick M. Treatment of childhood anxiety disorders: a preliminary comparison between cognitive-behavioral group therapy and a psychological placebo intervention. J Behav Ther Exp Psychiatry 2002;33(3–4):143–58.

[36] Wergeland GJ, Fjermestad KW, Marin CE, et al. An effectiveness study of individual vs group cognitive behavioral therapy for anxiety disorders in youth. Behav Res Ther 2014;57:1–12.

[37] Manassis K, Mendlowitz SL, Scapillato D, et al. Group and individual cognitive-behavioral therapy for childhood anxiety disorders: a randomized trial. J Am Acad Child Adolesc Psychiatry 2002;41(12):1423–30.

[38] Adelman CB, Panza KE, Bartley CA, et al. A meta-analysis of computerized cognitive-behavioral therapy for the treatment of DSM-5 anxiety disorders. J Clin Psychiatry 2014;75(7):e695–704.

[39] Khanna MS, Kendall PC. Computer-assisted CBT for child anxiety: the coping cat CD-ROM. Cogn Behav Pract 2008;15(2):159–65.

[40] Khanna MS, Kendall PC. Computer-assisted cognitive behavioral therapy for child anxiety: results of a randomized clinical trial. J Consult Clin Psychol 2010;78(5):737.

[41] American Academy of Child and Adolescent Psychiatry. Practice parameters for the assessment and treatment of children and adolescents with obsessive-compulsive disorder. J Am Acad Child Adolesc Psychiatry 2012;51(1):98–113.

[42] Abramowitz JS. The practice of exposure therapy: relevance of cognitive-behavioral theory and extinction theory. Behav Ther 2013;44(4):548–58.

[43] Arch JJ, Craske MG. Addressing relapse in cognitive behavioral therapy for panic disorder: methods for optimizing long-term treatment outcomes. Cogn Behav Pract 2011;18(3):306–15.

[44] Amir N, Freshman M, Ramsey B, et al. Thought-action fusion in individuals with OCD symptoms. Behav Res Ther 2001;39(7):765–76.

[45] Shafran R, Rachman S. Thought-action fusion: a review. J Behav Ther Exp Psychiatry 2004;35(2):87–107.

[46] Williams MT, Farris SG, Turkheimer E, et al. Myth of the pure obsessional type in obsessive–compulsive disorder. Depress Anxiety 2011;28(6):495–500.

[47] Newth S, Rachman S. The concealment of obsessions. Behav Res Ther 2001;39(4):457–64.

[48] Barrett PM, Healy-Farrell L, March JS. Cognitive-behavioral family treatment of childhood obsessive-compulsive disorder: a controlled trial. J Am Acad Child Adolesc Psychiatry 2004;43(1):46–62.

[49] The Pediatric OCD Treatment Study (POTS) Team. Cognitive-behavior therapy, sertraline, and their combination with children and adolescents with obsessive-compulsive disorder: the Pediatric OCD Treatment Study (POTS) randomized controlled trial. JAMA 2004;292(16):1969–76.

[50] Storch EA, Geffken GR, Merlo LJ, et al. Family-based cognitive-behavioral therapy for pediatric obsessive-compulsive disorder: comparison of intensive and weekly approaches. J Am Acad Child Adolesc Psychiatry 2007;46(4):469–78.

[51] Lewin AB, Wu MS, McGuire JF, et al. Cognitive behavior therapy for obsessive-compulsive and related disorders. Psychiatr Clin North Am 2014;37(3):415–45.

[52] Watson HJ, Rees CS. Meta-analysis of randomized, controlled treatment trials for pediatric obsessive-compulsive disorder. J Child Psychol Psychiatry 2008;49(5):489–98.

[53] Olatunji BO, Davis ML, Powers MB, et al. Cognitive-behavioral therapy for obsessive-compulsive disorder: a meta-analysis of treatment outcome and moderators. J Psychiatr Res 2013;47(1):33–41.

[54] Sanchez-Meca J, Rosa-Alcazar AI, Iniesta-Sepulveda M, et al. Differential efficacy of cognitive-behavioral therapy and pharmacological treatments for pediatric obsessive-compulsive disorder: a meta-analysis. J Anxiety Disord 2014;28(1):31–44.

[55] Franklin ME, Kozak MJ, Cashman LA, et al. Cognitive-behavioral treatment of pediatric obsessive-compulsive disorder: an open clinical trial. J Am Acad Child Adolesc Psychiatry 1998;37(4):412–9.

[56] Lewin AB, Storch EA, Merlo LJ, et al. Intensive cognitive behavioral therapy for pediatric obsessive compulsive disorder: a treatment protocol for mental health providers. Psychol Serv 2005;2(2):91.

[57] Storch EA, Caporino NE, Morgan JR, et al. Preliminary investigation of web-camera delivered cognitive-behavioral therapy for youth with obsessive-compulsive disorder. Psychiatry Res 2011;189(3):407–12.

[58] Comer JS, Furr JM, Cooper-Vince CE, et al. Internet-delivered, family-based treatment for early-onset OCD: a preliminary case series. J Clin Child Adolesc Psychol 2014;43(1): 74–87.

[59] Goetter EM, Herbert JD, Forman EM, et al. Delivering exposure and ritual prevention for obsessive–compulsive disorder via videoconference: clinical considerations and recommendations. J Obsessive Compuls Relat Disord 2013;2(2):137–45.

[60] David-Ferdon C, Kaslow NJ. Evidence-based psychosocial treatments for child and adolescent depression. J Clin Child Adolesc Psychol 2008;37(1):62–104.

[61] Mufson L, Weissman MM, Moreau D, et al. Efficacy of interpersonal psychotherapy for depressed adolescents. Arch Gen Psychiatry 1999;56(6):573–9.

[62] Mufson L, Dorta KP, Wickramaratne P, et al. A randomized effectiveness trial of interpersonal psychotherapy for depressed adolescents. Arch Gen Psychiatry 2004;61(6): 577–84.

[63] Kazdin AE. Evaluation of the automatic thoughts questionnaire: negative cognitive processes and depression among children. Psychol Assess 1990;2(1):73.

[64] Jacobson NS, Dobson KS, Truax PA, et al. A component analysis of cognitive-behavioral treatment for depression. J Consult Clin Psychol 1996;64(2):295–304.

[65] Markowitz JC, Weissman MM. Interpersonal psychotherapy: principles and applications. World Psychiatry 2004;3(3):136–9.

[66] Weisz JR, McCarty CA, Valeri SM. Effects of psychotherapy for depression in children and adolescents: a meta-analysis. Psychol Bull 2006;132(1):132–49.

[67] TADS Team. The treatment for adolescents with depression study (TADS): long-term effectiveness and safety outcomes. Arch Gen Psychiatry 2007;64(10):1132–43.

[68] Michael KD, Crowley SL. How effective are treatments for child and adolescent depression? A meta-analytic review. Clin Psychol Rev 2002;22(2):247–69.

[69] Chu BC, Colognori D, Weissman AS, et al. An initial description and pilot of group behavioral activation therapy for anxious and depressed youth. Cogn Behav Pract 2009;16(4): 408–19.

[70] Clarke GN, Rohde P, Lewinsohn PM, et al. Cognitive-behavioral treatment of adolescent depression: efficacy of acute group treatment and booster sessions. J Am Acad Child Adolesc Psychiatry 1999;38(3):272–9.

[71] Clarke GN, Hawkins W, Murphy M, et al. Targeted prevention of unipolar depressive disorder in an at-risk sample of high school adolescents: a randomized trial of a group cognitive intervention. J Am Acad Child Adolesc Psychiatry 1995;34(3):312–21.

[72] Nelson EL, Barnard M, Cain S. Treating childhood depression over videoconferencing. Telemed J E Health 2003;9(1):49–55.

[73] Arndorfer RE, Allen KD, Aljazireh L. Behavioral health needs in pediatric medicine and the acceptability of behavioral solutions: implications for behavioral psychologists. Behav Ther 1999;30:137–48.

[74] de Castro BO, Veerman JW, Koops W, et al. Hostile attribution of intent and aggressive behavior: a meta-analysis. Child Dev 2002;73:916–34.

[75] Lochman JE, Dodge KA. Social-cognitive processes of severely violent, moderately aggressive and nonaggressive boys. J Consult Clin Psychol 1994;62:366.

[76] Kazdin AE. Problem-solving skills training and parent management training for oppositiona defiant disorder and conduct disorder. In: Weisz JR, Kazdin AE, editors. Evidence-based psychotherapies for children and adolescents. 2nd edition. New York: Guilford Press; 2010. p. 211–26.

[77] Webster-Stratton C, Reid MJ. The incredible years parents, teachers, and children training series: a multifaceted treatment approach for young children with conduct disorders. In: Weisz JR, Kazdin AE, editors. Evidence-based psychotherapies for children and adolescents. 2nd edition. New York: Guilford Press; 2010. p. 194–210.

[78] Kazdin AE, Esveldt-Dawson K, French NH. Problem-solving skills training and relationship therapy in the treatment of antisocial child behavior. J Consult Clin Psychol 1987;55:76–85.

[79] Barkley RA. Defiant children: a clinician's manual for assessment and parent training. New York: Guilford Publications; 2013.

[80] McMahon RJ, Forehand RL. Helping the noncompliant child: family-based treatment for oppositional behavior. 2nd edition. New York: Guilford Press; 2003.

[81] Thompson MJ, Laver-Bradbury C, Ayres M, et al. A small-scale randomized controlled trial of the revised new forest parenting programme for preschoolers with attention deficit hyperactivity disorder. Eur Child Adolesc Psychiatry 2009;18(10):605–16.

[82] Abramowitz AJ, O'Leary SG. Behavioral interventions for the classroom: implications for students with ADHD. School Psych Rev 1991;20(2):220.

[83] Antshel KM, Barkley R. Psychosocial interventions in attention deficit hyperactivity disorder. Child Adolesc Psychiatr Clin N Am 2008;17(2):421–37.

[84] DuPaul GJ. School-based interventions for students with ADHD: current status and future directions. School Psych Rev 2007;36(2):183–94.

[85] DuPaul GJ, Weyandt LL, Janusis GM. ADHD in the classroom: effective intervention strategies. Theory Pract 2011;50(1):35–42.

[86] Webster-Stratton C, Reid MJ, Hammond M. Treating children with early-onset conduct problems: intervention outcomes for parent, child, and teacher training. J Clin Child Adolesc Psychol 2004;33(1):105–24.

[87] Kazdin AE, Esveldt-Dawson K, French NH, et al. Effects of parent management training and problem-solving skills training combined in the treatment of antisocial child behavior. J Am Acad Child Adolesc Psychiatry 1987;26(3):416–24.

[88] Fabiano GA, Pelham WE Jr, Coles EK, et al. A meta-analysis of behavioral treatments for attention-deficit/hyperactivity disorder. Clin Psychol Rev 2009;29(2):129–40.

[89] Bor W, Sanders MR, Markie-Dadds C. The effects of the Triple P-Positive Parenting Program on preschool children with co-occurring disruptive behavior and attentional/hyperactive difficulties. J Abnorm Child Psychol 2002;30:571.

[90] Webster-Stratton C, Reid MJ, Beauchaine TP. One-year follow-up of combined parent and child intervention for young children with ADHD. J Clin Child Adolesc Psychol 2013;41(2):251–61.

[91] Webster-Stratton CH, Reid MJ, Beauchaine T. Combining parent and child training for young children with ADHD. J Clin Child Adolesc Psychol 2011;40(2):191–203.

[92] DuPaul GJ, Weyandt LL. School-based intervention for children with attention deficit hyperactivity disorder: effects on academic, social, and behavioural functioning. Intl J Disabil Dev Educ 2006;53(2):161–76.

[93] Pfiffner LJ, Hinshaw SP. A two-site randomized clinical trial of integrated psychosocial treatment for ADHD-inattentive type. J Consult Clin Psychol 2014;82:1115.

[94] Jensen PS, Hinshaw SP, Kraemer HC, et al. ADHD comorbidity findings from the MTA study: comparing comorbid subgroups. J Am Acad Child Adolesc Psychiatry 2001;40(2):147–58.

[95] Biederman J. Attention-deficit/hyperactivity disorder: a selective overview. Biol Psychiatry 2005;57(11):1215–20.

[96] Urman R, Ickowicz A, Fulford P, et al. An exaggerated cardiovascular response to methylphenidate in ADHD children with anxiety. J Child Adolesc Psychopharmacol 1995;5(1): 29–37.

[97] Corcoran J, Dattalo P. Parent involvement in treatment for ADHD: a meta-analysis of the published studies. Res Soc Work Pract 2006;16(6):561–70.

[98] DuPaul GJ, Eckert TL, Vilardo B. The effects of school-based interventions for attention deficit hyperactivity disorder: a meta-analysis 1996–2010. School Psych Rev 2012;41(4):387–412.

[99] MTA Cooperative Group. A 14-month randomized clinical trial of treatment strategies for attention-deficit/hyperactivity disorder. Arch Gen Psychiatry 1999;56(12):1073–86.

[100] Molina BS, Hinshaw SP, Swanson JM, et al. The MTA at 8 years: prospective follow-up of children treated for combined-type ADHD in a multisite study. J Am Acad Child Adolesc Psychiatry 2009;48(5):484–500.

[101] Pelham WE Jr, Fabiano GA. Evidence-based psychosocial treatments for attention-deficit/hyperactivity disorder. J Clin Child Adolesc Psychol 2008;37(1):184–214.

[102] Swanson JM, Kraemer HC, Hinshaw SP, et al. Clinical relevance of the primary findings of the MTA: success rates based on severity of ADHD and ODD symptoms at the end of treatment. J Am Acad Child Adolesc Psychiatry 2001;40(2):168–79.

[103] Pliszka S, AACAP Work Group on Quality Issues. Practice parameter for the assessment and treatment of children and adolescents with attention-deficit/hyperactivity disorder. J Am Acad Child Adolesc Psychiatry 2007;46(7):894–921.

[104] Forehand R, Long N. Outpatient treatment of the acting out child: procedures, long term follow-up data, and clinical problems. Adv Behav Res Ther 1988;10(3):129–77.

[105] Patterson GR, Forgatch MS. Parents and adolescents living together - part 1: the basics. Eugene (OR): Castalia Publishing Co; 1987.

[106] Patterson GR, Forgatch MS. Predicting future clinical adjustment from treatment outcome and process variables. Psychol Assess 1995;7:275–85.

[107] Kazdin AE, Siegel TC, Bass D. Cognitive problem-solving skills training and parent management training in the treatment of antisocial behavior in children. J Consult Clin Psychol 1992;60:733–47.

[108] Huey SJ Jr, Henggeler SW, Brondino MJ, et al. Mechanisms of change in multisystemic therapy: reducing delinquent behavior through therapist adherence and improved family and peer functioning. J Consult Clin Psychol 2000;68(3):451–67.

[109] Henggeler SW, Melton GB, Smith L. Family preservation using multisystemic therapy: an effective alternative to incarcerating serious juvenile offenders. J Consult Clin Psychol 1992;60:953–61.

[110] Henggeler SW, Rowland MD, Randall J, et al. Home-based multisystemic therapy as an alternative to the hospitalization of youths in psychiatric crisis: clinical outcomes. J Am Acad Child Adolesc Psychiatry 1999;38(11):1331–9.

[111] Letourneau EJ, Henggeler SW, Borduin CM, et al. Multisystemic therapy for juvenile sexual offenders: 1-year results from a randomized effectiveness trial. J Fam Psychol 2009;23(1): 89–102.

Advances in Pediatrics 62 (2015) 185–210

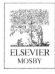

ADVANCES IN PEDIATRICS

Gene Therapy for Blinding Pediatric Eye Disorders

Alina V. Dumitrescu, MD[a,b], Arlene V. Drack, MD[c,*]

[a]KU Eye Department, Kansas University Medical School, 7400 State Line Road, Suite 100, Prairie Village, Kansas City, KS 66208, USA; [b]Department of Ophthalmology and Visual Sciences, University of Iowa, 11190-G PFP, Iowa City, IA 52242, USA; [c]Department of Ophthalmology and Visual Sciences, Stephen A. Wynn Institute for Vision Research, University of Iowa, 11190-G PFP, Iowa City, IA 52242, USA

Keywords
- Inherited eye disorders • Gene replacement therapy • Ocular disorders

Key points
- Inherited eye disorders are among the most common causes of pediatric blindness in the United States and usually manifest early in life.
- Until recently, genetic causes of blindness have been untreatable. Gene replacement therapy delivered to the retina by subretinal injections shows promise for treatment for some of these disorders.
- The first human subretinal gene therapy clinical trials using adeno-associated virus vectors to deliver genes for treatment of *RPE65* associated Leber congenital amaurosis reported their positive results in 2008.
- In all safety trials improvement in retinal and visual function was observed in some patients and it was maintained years after the treatment.

 Videos of subretinal injection for gene replacement therapy accompany this article at http://www.advancesinpediatrics.com/

INTRODUCTION

Inherited eye disorders are conditions that are genetically determined and present from birth although they may or may not be obvious to patients or observers at that time. They can be broadly categorized as exclusively ocular or systemic, based on extent of the disease (limited to the eye or involving additional organs or systems). Ocular disorders can be further categorized based on the part of the eye that is involved. This article discusses the

*Corresponding author. E-mail address: arlene-drack@uiowa.edu

0065-3101/15/$ – see front matter
http://dx.doi.org/10.1016/j.yapd.2015.04.012

current knowledge and future potential of using gene therapy for treatment of inherited eye disorders. Although, generally speaking, inherited eye disorders are not common, taken as a group they are among the most common causes of pediatric blindness in the United States, after retinopathy of prematurity.

A simple algorithm, which can be applied to all inherited eye disorders, starts with a clinical diagnosis, followed by a molecular diagnosis; genetic counseling for the affected individuals, families, and relatives at risk; and from there exploring the possibilities for treatment. The clinical diagnosis is based on symptoms (eg, decreased vision, light sensitivity, difficulty seeing in the dark), ocular examination (evaluating function and biomicroscopic appearance of various parts of the eye), and ancillary testing, such as optical coherence tomography (OCT), electroretinogram (ERG), and visual field. The molecular diagnosis confirms the specific genetic defect causing the disease. Taking a detailed family history may help to determine an inheritance pattern and identify other affected individuals, and individuals at risk of having affected offspring. DNA analysis should always begin with testing an affected person in the pedigree, preferably with samples from parents as well. Because many different genes can cause the same clinical appearance, and because not all genes causing inherited eye diseases have been discovered yet, a negative test result does not completely rule out a disorder and is not as helpful in patient management as a positive one. Even in cases in which a genetic mutation is found, careful vetting of the pathogenicity of each mutation must be done due to the variability of the human genome. In cases in which a novel mutation is found, analyzing parental or other family samples for the genetic variation in question can be illuminating and is often necessary to definitively prove causality. Genetic testing is now widely available but it is still not as simple as ordering a routine blood test like a white blood cell count and comparing the results with a nomogram. Genetic testing detects changes from the norm in the genetic code. It is known that only some of these changes (or mutations) cause diseases. The mutations with no clinical consequences are called benign polymorphisms and they represent natural variations in the genome. In interpreting genetic testing for patients with inherited disorders, it is vitally important that a multistep approach be taken to ensure correct interpretation of variations found in the genome of patients. Patients with benign polymorphisms (non–disease causing) detected in a gene known to be associated with their disease, but with true disease-causing mutations in some other, unidentified gene, may get inaccurate counseling, or be erroneously enrolled in gene replacement trials and may miss the opportunity for the appropriate treatment if each genetic change found is not carefully evaluated [1]. Accurate molecular genetic testing also can be helpful in predicting future health issues and for family planning. If a child is known to be at risk for certain ocular or systemic diseases, the intervals for various screening tests can be adjusted accordingly [2] and tests that are not routinely performed can be ordered.

For most of human existence, genetic causes of blindness have been completely untreatable and incurable; fortunately, this is starting to change. Attempts at treatment fall into 5 broad categories:

- Gene therapy (replacing or editing the defective gene to allow production of the necessary gene product that is lacking; or silencing a gene that is making a toxic product),
- Enzyme-replacement therapy (replace the gene product directly),
- Stem cell–derived ocular cells (replace the damaged, dead, or nonfunctional ocular cells),
- Use of neuroprotective molecules (help preserve the patient's own existing, functional cells and slow disease progression), and
- Use of prosthetic devices (various implants that bypass the damaged ocular structures and transmit visual stimuli to the brain).

This article is focused primarily on treating inherited retinal eye disorders using gene replacement therapy.

The American Society of Gene and Cell Therapy defines gene therapy as "a set of strategies that modify the expression of an individual's genes or that correct abnormal genes. Each strategy involves the administration of a specific DNA (or RNA)" [3]. Genes are delivered to cells with the purpose of replacing an abnormal gene or altering the way a gene is turned on or off, or other techniques are used to repair an abnormal gene [4]. Delivering genes to the cells is usually done using a vector virus. The virus's own genes are removed and replaced with a specific, normally functioning, human gene.

The best-studied and most commonly used viral vectors for ocular gene replacement therapy are adeno-associated viruses (AAVs). AAVs are non–disease-causing and cannot replicate. AAVs are members of the *Dependovirus* genus of the parvoviruses. They are helper-dependent viruses, which means they need coinfection with other viruses, such as adenovirus or herpes virus, to replicate. Approximately 80% of the population is seropositive for anti-AAV antibodies against serotypes 1, 2, 3, and 5. Sixty percent of the population has neutralizing antibodies by age 10 years [5]. Although the lack of pathogenicity is a plus for use as a therapeutic vector, the presence of antibody to the virus could be a negative. This has not proven to be an impediment in the eye, as will be discussed shortly. AAV2 is the most studied of the AAV serotypes, with a genome consisting of 4.7 kilobases (kb) of single-stranded DNA. Inverted terminal repeats are present at each end of the genome. Two genes, *REP* and *CAP*, encode 4 nonstructural proteins required for replication and capsid proteins. There are 3 viral promoters and a single intron. In brief, rAAV vectors can be produced by deleting the rep and cap genes and replacing the viral genes with gene of interest, leaving the flanking viral inverted terminal repeats in place [5].

Because virus particles are readily taken up into human cells, the desired genes are smuggled into cells very efficiently. Once inside the cells, the virus begins producing the protein product of the gene inside it, thus replacing the missing component (Fig. 1). Recombinant AAV is the most widely used vector for ocular gene delivery because of its ability to transduce efficiently in vivo various retinal cell types. Six different serotypes of AAV are currently used with different serotypes preferentially transfecting different layers of the retina; modifications of viral capsids can also direct transfection to specific retinal cell types [6].

AAV vectors have a limited cargo capacity, preventing their use for treatment requiring transfer of genes with a coding sequence larger than 5 kb. Vectors with larger capacity, like nanoparticles, lentivirus, and adenoviral vectors are being investigated for transfer of larger genes to the retina. However, adenovirus and lentivirus do not have the same safety profile as AAV, and nanoparticles are still unproven in clinical trials. Some viral vectors, such as lentivirus, insert the delivered gene into the genetic make-up of the cell rather than just directing production of its product in the nucleus [6]. Insertion into the host genome is not without risk; the location of insertion cannot be completely controlled, making the chance of altering nearby genes, including genes capable of causing cancer or other disorders, a concern. The penetration of vectors into the retinal cells also varies with the site of the injection with intravitreal delivery mainly targeting the inner retina and subretinal delivery preferentially targeting the photoreceptors and retinal pigment epithelium (RPE) (Fig. 2).

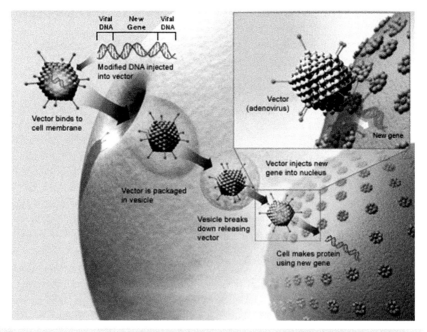

Fig. 1. Schematic of gene therapy delivery by AAV. (*From* US National Library of Medicine. Gene therapy using an adenovirus vector. Genetics Home Reference 2015. Available at: http://ghr.nlm.nih.gov/handbook/illustrations/therapyvector. Accessed January 8, 2015.)

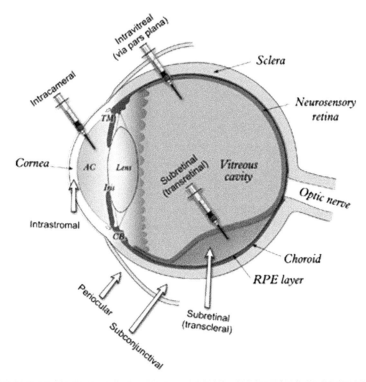

Fig. 2. Schematic of intravitreal and subretinal injections. TM, trabecular meshwork; AC, anterior chamber; CB, ciliary body. (*From* Balaggan KS, Ali RR. Ocular gene delivery using lentiviral vectors. Gene Ther 2012;19(2):145–53, with permission; and Original video of subretinal injection for gene replacement therapy - Steve Russell, MD. Available at: http://start.s-weetpacks.com/?barid={327C53A4-FC6B-11E2-AB6C-0030679F4C46}&src=97&crg=3.5000006.10042&st=23. Accessed January 14, 2015.)

Intravitreal injection was described for the first time in 1911 when an air bubble was used to tamponade a retinal detachment. Intravitreal injection is frequently used in clinical practice today to deliver highly targeted drug therapy to the retina, maximizing therapeutic drug delivery to that tissue while minimizing systemic toxicity. These injections can usually be performed with topical anesthesia in the clinic. Subretinal injections are used less commonly and require specialized equipment. They are performed in the operating room (Video 1) [7].

None of these procedures is risk free, although the frequency of complications is low particularly after intravitreal injections. The most commonly reported complications are infection, retinal detachment, and increased intraocular pressure.

Gene replacement therapy for inherited eye disorders is generally applicable for monogenic, autosomal recessive defects in which little or no normal protein is the cause of the disorder. Gene therapy has been studied and applied particularly for inherited retinopathies. In autosomal dominant disorders in which there is a gain of function or toxic effect of the mutant protein, other strategies, such as small-interfering RNA to silence the abnormal copy of the gene, must be used [8,9].They have been studied in neurodegenerative disorders [10]. A new technology, Clustered, Regularly Interspaced, Short Palindromic Repeats (CRISPR), which uses a Cas9 enzyme, may offer an alternative to gene replacement therapy [11,12]. CRISPR was first identified as an immune response in bacteria to invading viruses [13]; it has now been described as a way to directly correct or change genes. An RNA guide is made that is complementary to a strand of DNA of interest (eg, a deleterious mutation or a small deletion). This guides the Cas9 enzyme to the target site, where it causes a double-stranded break [13]. After cleavage by Cas9 enzyme, the target locus typically uses either nonhomologous end joining or homology-directed repair for DNA damage repair. Alternatively, a repair template can be provided to correct the portion of sequence that has been removed, or, double-stranded breaks can be re-ligated through the nonhomologous end-joining process. CRISPR/Cas9 can also be used to generate gene knockouts for research (Fig. 3) [12,13].

The eye is more amenable to gene therapy than other organs because of its accessibility with minor or relatively noninvasive procedures, immune privilege, small size, compartmentalization, the existence of a contralateral control, and because it is easy to examine directly to evaluate for side effects and complications [14]. In addition, the blood retinal barrier avoids the delivery of genes and virus vectors to the rest of the body.

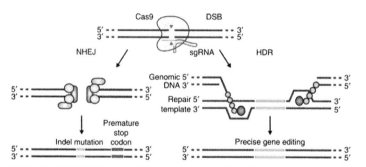

Fig. 3. DSB repair promotes gene editing. DSBs induced by Cas9 (*yellow*) can be repaired in 1 of 2 ways. In the error-prone NHEJ pathway, the ends of a DSB are processed by endogenous DNA repair machinery and rejoined, which can result in random indel mutations at the site of junction. Indel mutations occurring within the coding region of a gene can result in frameshifts and the creation of a premature stop codon, resulting in gene knockout. Alternatively, a repair template in the form of a plasmid or ssODN can be supplied to leverage the HDR pathway, which allows high fidelity and precise editing. Single-stranded nicks to the DNA can also induce HDR. DSB, double-stranded breaks; NHEJ, nonhomologous end joining; ssODN, single-stranded DNA oligonucleotides; HDR, homology-directed repair. (*From* Ran FA, Hsu PD, Wright J, et al. Genome engineering using the CRISPR-Cas9 system. Nat Protoc 2013;8(11):2281–308, with permission; and Jinek M, Chylinski K, Fonfara I, et al. A programmable dual-RNA-guided DNA endonuclease in adaptive bacterial immunity. Science 2012;337(6096):816–21.)

HISTORY OF SUBRETINAL GENE THERAPY

Gene therapy for ocular disorders has a long history. The first successful treatment was delivered in 1999 as an intravitreal injection for retinoblastoma in a murine model [15]. It proved that human retinoblastoma cells can be killed when transduced with an adenoviral vector containing the herpes simplex thymidine kinase gene (AdV-TK) followed by treatment with the prodrug ganciclovir. Later, in 2001, intravitreal adenoviral vector expressing human pigment epithelium–derived factor was shown to produce antiangiogenic activity that lasts for several months after a single injection for treatment of neovascular age-related macular degeneration (AMD) [16,17]. Successful subretinal gene therapy was first reported in 2001 for treatment of autosomal recessive Leber congenital amaurosis (LCA) caused by RPE-specific 65-kDa protein gene (*RPE65*) deficiency. The successful therapy was demonstrated first in a canine model that naturally develops the disease, the Swedish Briard dog, which carries a natural 4 base pair deletion of the *Rpe65* gene [18]. Gene therapy using AAV-mediated *RPE65* transfer was delivered as subretinal injection in 4-month-old animals. The treatment restored function in both rod and cone systems (as measured by ERGs, visually evoked potential, pupillary response, and vision-dependent behaviors) and was proven to be stable over time in the canine model [19].

The first human subretinal gene therapy clinical trials investigated the safety of subretinal delivery of a recombinant AAV carrying *RPE65* complementary DNA (cDNA) for treatment of *RPE65*-associated LCA, also called LCA2. Three simultaneous independent studies provided evidence that the subretinal administration of AAV vectors encoding *RPE65* in patients affected with LCA2 is safe [20–22]. All 3 of these studies used an AAV2 vector carrying a normal human *RPE65* cDNA delivered subretinally to the worse-seeing eye. A fourth study confirmed safety of the treatment shortly thereafter [23]. The results showed acceptable local and systemic safety.

After more than 15 years from the first reported success, subretinal gene therapy is still not largely available but multiple clinical trials are currently in progress.

CURRENT GENE THERAPY TRIALS

RPE65 gene therapy trials

LCA is a group of retinal dystrophies with onset in early childhood characterized by severely decreased vision at birth, loss of retinal function as evidenced by abnormal ERG and nystagmus, often with slow progressive degeneration of the retina, which destroys the limited vision present at birth [24]. Patients usually present in the first few months of life with decreased vision and nystagmus (shaking eyes). ERG responses, which record the electrical activity of photoreceptors in the retina to light stimuli, are usually nonrecordable for both cones and rods. Other clinical findings include high hypermetropia, photophobia, keratoconus, cataracts, oculodigital sign, and a variable appearance of the retina on fundus examination from normal to severe dystrophy [25]. LCA is estimated to affect 1 in 81,000 to 1 in 30,000 live births, although being primarily an autosomal recessive disease it may be more common in communities that are relatively genetically isolated or in countries with common consanguineous pairings. LCA accounts for more than 5% of all inherited retinopathies and 20% of children attending schools for the visually impaired [25]. To date, 19 different genes are known to cause LCA [26]. At least one of these, cone-rod homeobox gene (*CRX*), transmits the disease in an autosomal dominant fashion with most being autosomal recessive. *RPE65*-associated LCA (LCA2) is caused by mutations in the *RPE65* gene (RPE65; 180069) on chromosome 1p31. Mutations in this gene account for approximately 8% of patients with LCA. *RPE65* is almost exclusively expressed in the RPE cells and is responsible for converting *all-trans* retinoid to *11-cis* retinal during pigment regeneration in the photo-transduction pathway. Improper functioning, or absence, of this retinoid isomerase results in lack of *11-cis* retinal production and inability to form the visual pigments in photoreceptors. At the same time, accumulation of all-*trans*-retinyl esters in the RPE cells may lead to RPE cell death and photoreceptor degeneration.

 RPE65-associated LCA was an ideal first ocular disorder in which to try human gene therapy for several reasons. First, a spontaneously occurring large animal model (dog) exists. Second, the gene defect is in the RPE, the layer of cells below the photoreceptors, not in the photoreceptors themselves. Because of this, the anatomic structure of the retina itself is normal and is only lacking an enzyme needed for function. Finally, children have nystagmus and poor vision from infancy and usually lose what little vision they have over time, making the risk-benefit ratio appropriate.

 After the successful canine and mouse gene therapy of *RPE65*-associated LCA, 3 independent human studies provided solid evidence that the subretinal administration of AAV vectors encoding *RPE65* in patients affected with LCA2 is safe [20–22]. The area of retina targeted for treatment was selected based on clinical evaluations and retinal imaging studies to identify areas of retina with viable cells (Fig. 4).

 In all these safety trials, significant improvement in retinal and visual function was observed as early as 1 month after treatment and was maintained through 1.5 years after treatment [27]. In these initial studies, most patients were adults and the youngest patient at the time of the treatment was 8 years old. There were some differences in the promoters used, vector manufacturing, dose and volumes delivered, anesthesia during vector delivery, and postoperative steroid use; however, all studies concluded that AAV-mediated subretinal gene therapy is safe and well tolerated. No vector-related major adverse events or toxic immune responses, ocular or systemic, were noted. A recent review of the gene replacement therapy recapitulates these findings [28].

 In 2009, in the phase I dose-escalation trial that enrolled 12 patients (aged 8–44 years) with LCA2, patients were given 1 subretinal injection of AAV2-hRPE65v2 in the worst-seeing eye. After 2 years of follow-up, data showed that treatment was well tolerated. All patients showed sustained improvement

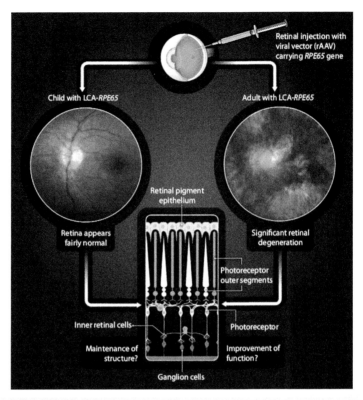

Fig. 4. Shown are retinas of a child and adult with RPE65-based LCA; a diagram of the gene delivery procedure and the RPE and multiple cell layers that form the neural retina. Photoreceptor nuclei are located in the outer nuclear layer (ONL). Photoreceptors initiate the process of vision and relay information to ganglion cells, which synapse in the brain through inner retinal cells. (*From* Wojno AP, Pierce EA, Bennett J. Seeing the light. Sci Transl Med 2013;5(175):175fs8, with permission.)

in subjective and objective measurements of visual function: dark adaptometry (rod-mediated response), pupil reactivity, nystagmus, and ambulatory behavior. Improvement in visual acuity did not correlate with dose. The greatest improvement was noted in the youngest patients (Videos 2–4) [29]. A second, open-label, dose-escalation phase I study of 15 patients (11–30 years) given 1 subretinal injection of rAAV2-hRPE65 to the worse-functioning eye demonstrated, after 3 years of follow-up, no systemic toxicity and improvement in visual function in all patients, to different degrees, localized to treated areas of the retina. The study concluded *RPE65*-LCA gene therapy is sufficiently safe and substantially efficacious to the extrafoveal retina and there is no benefit and some risk in treating the fovea. All ocular adverse events were related to surgery [30]. The long-term follow-up data (3 years) on a subgroup of 5 patients in an Italian cohort involved in the LCA2 gene therapy clinical trial showed stability of improvement in visual and retinal function that had been achieved a few months after treatment. Longitudinal data analysis showed that the maximum improvement was achieved within 6 months after treatment, and the visual improvement was stable up to the last observed time point [31].

The most significant adverse effect of surgery was formation of iatrogenic foveal hole during the injection of vector under the macula. The fovea is the anatomic center of the retina in which the retinal layers are thinnest and cone packing is most dense; it is the area of best visual acuity and the only part of the retina capable of 20/20 vision. In the 3-year study [30], approximately half the patients received a vector bleb that detached the fovea during surgery. Loss of foveal thickness, attributed to foveal cone loss, as assessed with follow-up OCT analysis, was observed. This suggests that foveal cones may be particularly sensitive to the potential damaging effects of foveal detachment during the procedure, and that this location for vector delivery should be approached with caution. In addition, Maguire and colleagues [22] after reporting that a foveal hole formed during injection in some patients, suggested a modified surgical approach to decrease the incidence of this complication. The technique is either to avoid the directly subfoveal region for injection or to tamponade the area with a bubble of Perfluoro-n-octane, a heavy liquid that is used as an aid for retinal surgical procedures. Although macular hole or decreased foveal thickness is an untoward event, patients who experienced it did not have a decrease in vision because the vision before surgery was so poor. Ostensibly, subfoveal transfection of cells would give the most benefit to patients if it can be done safely, as the fovea is the only area of the retina capable of detailed acuity and 20/20 vision. Additional findings concerning for safety were self-limited intraocular inflammation after surgery, nonspecific activation of T cells (which could have been attributed to corticosteroid withdrawal) in the postoperative period, antibodies to the AAV2 capsid that resolved after 90 days, and mildly increased lymphocyte stimulation index to the capsid protein. There was no immune response to the vector insert (*RPE65* gene) noted.

An important question for subretinal gene therapy was whether the second eye could be treated and/or whether a treated eye could be retreated either to augment treatment effect if it was noted to diminish over time, or to enlarge visual field (because only the retina directly over the injection bleb is transduced by virus and improves in function leaving the peripheral retina without improvement). Studies in animals and humans showed mild antibody response to the viral capsid but not to the gene cargo [32]. Early safety studies demonstrated very little viral shedding or escape to systemic circulation. By clinical examination, no significant inflammatory response has been attributed to the AAV or transgene product. Biodistribution studies have been part of each of the 3 initial trials and used polymerase chain reaction of AAV sequences in various compartments, including tears, serum, saliva, and semen. Results have generally been negative with the exception of transient positivity in serum and tears, which resolved within a few postoperative days [22,33]. The patients' antibody response did not decrease treatment effect, however.

Readministration of vector to the contralateral (initially untreated) eye was carried out in 3 adults with LCA2 1.7 to 3.3 years after they had received their initial subretinal injection of AAV2-hRPE65v2. Results, out to 6 months, indicated that retreatment to the initially untreated, contralateral eye did not trigger an immune response in either eye. The treatment was safe and efficacious with improvement in the visual parameters in the second eye (as expected) and unchanged vision in initially treated eye [34]. A phase III clinical trial is under way at this writing to evaluate safety and efficacy of bilateral treatment in patients with a lower age limit of 3 years (www.clinicaltrials.gov).

One of the challenges of a subretinal gene therapy trial for blind children was determining treatment endpoints that were acceptable to the Food and Drug Administration (FDA). The gold standard treatment endpoint in ophthalmology trials has always been visual acuity. For children blind from birth, it was understood early on by several investigators that visual acuity may not change sufficiently to show efficacy, or that it may not be measurable for many years in young children [35]. For this reason an obstacle course was specially designed for the early trials and was modified to include changeable obstacles and different light levels for subsequent trials. This endpoint has the additional benefit of being more relevant to activities of daily living. The subjects are videotaped navigating the course before and after treatment, and videos are scored and timed by masked observers. It is clear that after treatment, navigation through the course is faster and easier [28]. Another unexpected but welcome outcome of the study is the resolution of nystagmus in children who are treated. Nystagmus is a poorly understood phenomenon; lack of visual input in the first few months of life results in this involuntary shaking movement of the eyes, presumably due to lack of fixation in the fovea. Although other measures of visual function, such as sensitivity to light and pupillary reaction, showed more significant improvements with treatment than acuity, however, nystagmus was abolished in children after treatment. Another concern in treating a congenital form of blindness was whether amblyopia would limit treatment effect. Amblyopia is the failure of connection between the occipital cortex of the brain and the eye that occurs if there is visual deprivation in the first 9 years of life. It is well demonstrated that infants with dense congenital cataracts, for example, who have never had visual input, will not regain normal vision if cataract surgery is delayed beyond the first few months of life. However, despite the early visual impairment of these patients, functional MRI has demonstrated that the occipital cortex, which showed no signs of stimulation to vision before gene therapy, lights up afterward, proving there is enough plasticity in the system for vision to be restored years after birth [35]. The greater improvement in vision in the youngest patients, however, likely is due to a combination of denser amblyopia and greater loss of retinal cells in older patients.

RETINAL DISORDERS WITH GENE THERAPY TRIALS UNDER WAY

Choroideremia

Choroideremia (CHM) is a progressive chorioretinal degeneration caused by mutations in the *CHM* gene on chromosome Xq21. The *CHM* gene encodes Rab Escort Protein 1 (REP-1), which is necessary in the process of geranylgeranylation (or prenylation) of *ras*-related GTPases also called Rab protein. The Rab proteins are involved in exchanging of vesicles in endocytosis and exocytosis pathways. The prenylation process requires the presence and activity of REP-1 and a transferase called RabGGTase. The REP 1 protein presents the unprenylated Rab substrate to the transferase and then moves the final product to the cellular membrane. Patients with CHM express little or no REP-1, which affects opsin transport and the phagocytosis of photoreceptor outer segments by the RPE [36–39]. CHM is characterized by progressive chorioretinal degeneration in affected male individuals and milder signs in carrier female individuals. CHM has a prevalence of about 1:50,000, with northern Finland having the highest reported prevalence [40]. Patients have the characteristic fundus appearance of scalloped peripheral retinal pigment loss and night blindness in the first or second decade of life followed by progressive peripheral visual field loss. Central vision is preserved until late in life. Although carrier female individuals are generally asymptomatic, signs of chorioretinal degeneration can be observed with careful fundus examination after the second decade [41]. Some women "carriers" do develop true retinal degeneration and it can be mistaken for autosomal recessive or dominant retinitis pigmentosa (RP), which will lead to an inaccurate diagnosis.

In a multicenter phase 1/2 clinical trial, 6 male patients (aged 35–63 years) with CHM were treated with subfoveal injection of rAAV2.REP1. In the case of CHM, the only retina remaining in advanced cases is the retina in the foveal/macular area; therefore, this critical area had to be treated despite the concerns about foveal perforation (Fig. 5).

A special technique (2-step procedure) was developed to avoid having the injected fluid cause a foveal hole through the thin central retina, and it was largely successful in this study. The initial results of this trial found that 2 of 6 patients, in whom visual acuity was reduced at baseline, gained 21 letters and 11 letters, respectively, whereas 4 of 6 patients with near-normal visual acuity at baseline had a marginal loss of 1 to 3 letters by 6 months. All 6 patients showed improvement in maximal retinal sensitivity and 5 of 6 patients showed improvements in mean retinal sensitivity despite the detached fovea/macula necessary during surgery [42]. The treatment was overall safe and well tolerated with no ocular or systemic side effects. Further follow-up is necessary to determine whether the disease progression is changed after the treatment.

Currently, an open-label dose-escalation phase I clinical trial of retinal gene therapy for CHM using rAAV2.REP1 is recruiting patients (NCT01461213).

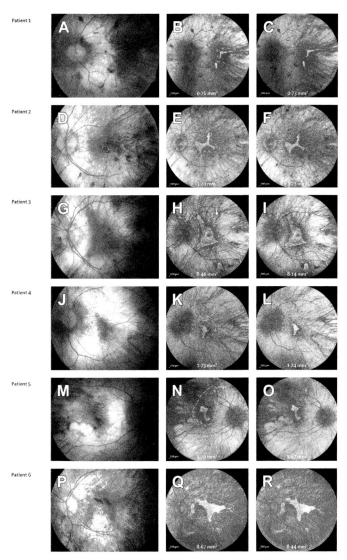

Fig. 5. Images show the retina in patients 1 to 6 (*A, D, G, J, M,* and *P,* respectively) and the corresponding baseline autofluorescent retina (*B, E, H, K, N,* and *Q,* respectively). The area of autofluorescent RPE exposed to vector is annotated on each panel in mm². The limits of the retinal detachment are indicated by the green dotted line and the injection site is indicated with a green dot. The corresponding autofluorescence images and measurements in the RPE at 6 months are shown in panels *C, F, I, L, O,* and *R.* The area of the RPE did not change substantially 6 months after surgery, although focal loss of autofluorescence superior to the injection site was noted in patient 3 (*I*). In patients 4 and 6, more than one injection was required to detach the fovea (additional *green lines*). (*From* MacLaren RE, Groppe M, Barnard AR, et al. Retinal gene therapy in patients with choroideremia: initial findings from a phase 1/2 clinical trial. Lancet 2014;383(9923):1129–37, with permission; and MacDonald IM, Russell L, Chan CC. Choroideremia: new findings from ocular pathology and review of recent literature. Surv Ophthalmol 2010;54(3):401–7.)

Stargardt disease

Stargardt macular degeneration (SMD) is an autosomal recessive disorder that causes progressive central (macular) vision loss usually beginning in mid to late childhood. Early in the course of the disease, the retina often appears normal, and children with decreased vision are often suspected of malingering. Careful examination shows decreased color vision when tested with Ishihara color plates, as well as central scotoma on visual field testing. Tiny yellow pisciform flecks may be barely visible in the macula or periphery early on and become more prominent over time. Changes can be detected sometimes on OCT and fundus autofluorescence imagines. Vision progressively worsens, and in a minority of patients with especially deleterious mutations, most vision is lost. Most patients retain peripheral vision, with central vision diminishing to the 20/200 (legally blind) range over time. SMD is caused by mutations in the adenosine triphosphate (ATP)-binding cassette transporter (*ABCA4*) gene. A clinically similar but less common disorder is inherited in an autosomal dominant fashion, which is caused by mutations in the *ELOVL4* gene [43,44].

The human photoreceptor rim (ABCR) protein expressed by the *ABCA4* gene is found in photoreceptors and is hypothesized to be involved in the clearance of a by-product of the retinoid cycle of vision. *ABCA4* functions as a transmembrane protein that changes its conformation to transport *N*- retinylidene-phosphatidyl ethanolamine (all-trans retinaldehyde bounded to phosphatidylethanolamine) from the lumen of photoreceptor outer segment disks to the cytoplasmic surface. Mutations in *ABCA4* result in decreased transport of *N*- retinylidene-phosphatidyl ethanolamine, which leads to accumulation in the RPE of lipidic debris, named lipofuscin. This is primarily composed of *N*-retinylidene-*N*-retinylethanolamine, also called A2E [45,46]. *ABCA4* mutations can lead to a wide spectrum of disease severity. Although the common feature of *ABCA4* disease is progressive degeneration of photoreceptors and RPE in the macula, there are notable extremes of *ABCA4* disease. At one end of the spectrum are individuals with mild retinopathy confined to the macula, and at the other end are those with severe retina-wide disease, including cone–rod dystrophy and even autosomal recessive RP [47]. Numerous disease-causing alleles are known and it has been hypothesized that each allele makes an independent and additive contribution to severity of the retinal disease [48]. In addition, the *ABCA4* gene is very polymorphic, with many benign and ethnicity-specific benign changes that do not cause disease. This makes proving that a given genetic deviation is disease-causing especially challenging; novel mutations must be compared with ethnically matched controls (Fig 6).

Because of the highly polymorphic nature of the gene and because many healthy people carry a benign polymorphism that may be novel, finding both disease-causing alleles is an important part of the diagnosis and an essential prognostic factor. Even when 2 likely disease-causing mutations are found, great care must be taken to be certain there is a mutation on both copies of the patient's gene. This is most easily done by analyzing parental samples but can also be achieved with markers. It is possible to have more than one change in the same allele (copy of the gene), while the remaining copy is normal. Because there are many years of normal vision preceding retinal degeneration in patients with Stargardt disease, there is real potential for genetic testing to identify patients before vision is lost, and provide preventive treatment [49].

StarGen is an equine infectious anemia virus (EIAV)-based lentiviral vector that expresses the photoreceptor-specific ABCA4 protein. EIAV vectors were proven to be able to efficiently transduce rod and cone photoreceptors in addition to RPE cells in the adult macaque and rabbit retina following subretinal delivery; self-limited inflammation was noted [50]. There are currently 2 active human clinical trials to evaluate the long-term safety, tolerability and biological activity of StarGen. A phase I/II dose-escalation safety study of subretinally injected StarGen administered to patients with SMD and an open-label study to determine the long-term safety, tolerability, and biological activity of StarGen in patients with SMD are ongoing (NCT01367444 and NCT01736592).

Age-related macular degeneration

Although not a childhood disease, macular degeneration is another ocular disorder being treated with gene therapy, but in a unique way that may have applicability for some pediatric disorders.

In the wet, exudative, or neovascular form of AMD, pathologic choroidal neovascular membranes (CNVM) develop under the retina. The CNVM can leak fluid and blood under the retina, which leads to decreased visual acuity. If left untreated, CNVM ultimately can cause a blinding disciform scar in the fovea. Approximately 10% to 20% of patients with nonexudative AMD will eventually progress to the exudative form. The exudative form of AMD is responsible for most advanced cases of AMD in the United States, which is currently estimated at 1.75 million cases [51,52]. Several growth factors have been implicated in disease pathology, including vascular endothelial growth factor (VEGF). Anti-VEGF therapy delivered as intravitreal injections has markedly changed the outcome of treatment for this blinding disorder, for the first time improving, rather than just stabilizing, vision. Therapies for exudative AMD are delivered as repeated, sometimes as frequently as monthly, intravitreal injections, which often must be continued throughout a patient's lifetime to maintain visual benefits. Despite their good visual results, these injections have risk of complications that occasionally can lead to permanent loss of vison. Gene therapy approaches have been described for AMD treatment using an AAV-expressing pigment epithelium–derived factor, a factor that inhibits angiogenesis. Preclinical studies in nonhuman primate with Ad5-pigment epithelium–derived factor have been promising for use of gene therapy vectors in neovascular macular degeneration [16].

Soluble fms-like tyrosine kinase-1 (sFlt-1) is a tyrosine kinase protein that inhibits the proteins that stimulate blood vessel growth. sFlt-1 is a splice variant of VEGF receptor 1 that is produced by a variety of tissues. These proteins act as a receptor of VEGF, which is a very potent angiogenic growth factor. In a large animal (cynomolgus monkey) study, AAV2 vector that expresses a portion of

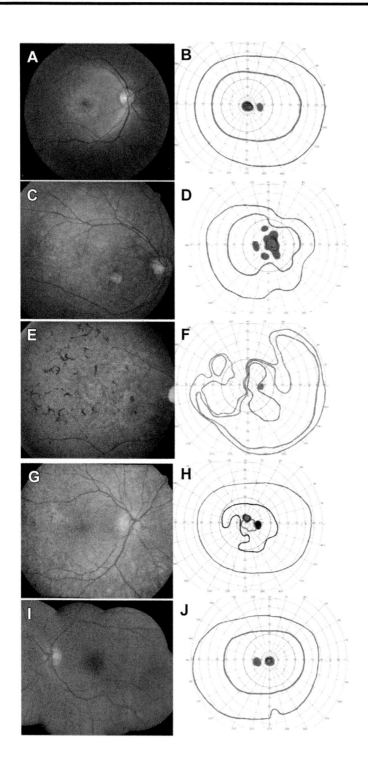

the sFlt1 VEGF receptor named AAV2-sFLT01 was administered intravitreally. A late-onset (1–3 months after the injection), mild, persistent inflammatory response that resolved by 5 months after treatment was noted, but otherwise the treatment proved to be safe. Efficiency was evaluated by expression of sFlt-1 protein in the eye. Protein expression proved to be variable and dose dependent and was detected in the aqueous humor and the vitreous humor up to 1 year in the treated animals [53].

Currently a phase I/II clinical research study is in progress to examine the baseline safety and efficacy of intravitreal rAAV.sFlt-1 for treatment of exudative AMD in humans (www.clinicaltrials.gov).

GENE THERAPY IN ANIMAL MODELS OF HUMAN DISEASE
Usher syndrome

Usher syndrome (USH) is a group of clinically variable and genetically heterogeneous autosomal recessive disorders. USH is characterized by early-onset sensorineural hearing loss and pigmentary retinopathy, which usually manifests in late childhood or adolescence and may lead to total blindness. Night blindness or difficulty seeing in dim light is the most frequent presenting visual symptom. The 2 most common types of USH are type I and II. Patients with Usher syndrome type I (USH1) have severe to profound congenital hearing impairment and vestibular dysfunction. Walking is often delayed until 18 months of age, and cochlear implant is often required to improve hearing. The retinal degeneration occurs later then the hearing problems, but it still starts during childhood. Patients with type II (USH2) have moderate to severe hearing impairment, normal vestibular function, and later onset of retinal degeneration [54]. USHIII is an intermediate form. The first USH1 gene identified was *myosinVIIa71* (*MYO7A*), which encodes an actin-based molecular motor that performs critical functions in both the inner ear and retina. Mutations

Fig. 6. Fundus photographs and Goldman visual fields of 5 patients with *ABCA4*-associated retinal disease. The patients depicted in the upper 10 panels have acuities and visual fields that are completely predicted by the additive effects of their *ABCA4* alleles. The patient depicted in (G) and (H) has better visual acuity and poorer visual fields than expected for her genotype, whereas the patient depicted in (I) and (J) has poorer visual acuity and better fields than expected. (A) and (B) depict the left eye of a 27-year-old woman with a mild *ABCA4* genotype, 20/30 acuity, and a visual field score of 37.5; (C) and (D) depict the right eye of an 24-year-old man with a moderate *ABCA4* genotype, 20/160 acuity, and a visual field score of 18.6; (E) and (F) depict the right eye of a 26-year-old man with a severe *ABCA4* genotype, 10/160 acuity, and a visual field score of 1.1; (G) and (H) depict the right eye of a 47-year-old woman with a moderate *ABCA4* genotype, 20/20 acuity, and a visual field score of 8.2; (I) and (J) depict the left eye of a 15-year-old woman with a moderate *ABCA4* genotype, 20/160 acuity, and a visual field score of 43.2. (From Schindler EI, Nylen EL, Ko AC, et al. Deducing the pathogenic contribution of recessive ABCA4 alleles in an outbred population. Hum Mol Genet 2010;19(19):3693–701, with permission; and Mullins RF, Kuehn MH, Radu RA, et al. Autosomal recessive retinitis pigmentosa due to ABCA4 mutations: clinical, pathologic, and molecular characterization. Invest Ophthalmol Vis Sci 2012;53(4):1883–94.)

in MYO7A cause Usher syndrome type 1b (Ush1b) and account for approximately 60% of all USH1 [55]. In the retina, MYO7A is expressed in RPE, photoreceptor synapses, and the cilia. It plays an important role in multiple cellular processes, including intracellular transport, endocytosis, and cell-cell adhesion [56,57].

Early cochlear implantation improves hearing significantly in patients with USH. Gene therapy with AAV vectors is limited by AAV cargo capacity because the USH1B gene is larger than the carrying capacity of 5 kb. Use of oversized, dual AAV overlapping, trans-splicing and hybrid vectors have shown some early success for large gene expression in the animal retina [58].

The mouse model of USH has a prominent vestibular phenotype leading to its name "twirler" or "shaker." However the retinal phenotype is much milder than in humans, making successful subretinal gene therapy difficult to quantify [59]. The protein products of Usher genes form a protein complex, however, which is abnormal in the Usher mouse, and can be assayed biochemically. The shaker-1 mouse carries a mutant *MYO7A* gene and is used as an animal model of USH1. Subretinal gene therapy using a lentiviral vector in *MYO7A*-null mice was shown to reconstitute the Usher protein complex in the retina, providing hope that subretinal gene therapy may be possible [60]. UshStat, a recombinant EIAV-based lentiviral vector expressing human *MYO7A* was safe and well tolerated after subretinal delivery and rescued photoreceptor phenotypes in the shaker1 mouse. In addition, subretinally delivered UshStat is safe and well tolerated in macaque safety studies [61]. Based on these results, 2 human studies are currently enrolling patients to examine the long-term safety of UshStat for treatment of RP associated with USH1b (NCT01505062 and NCT02065011).

Achromatopsia

Achromatopsia (ACHM) is a nonprogressive or very slowly progressive, hereditary visual disorder that is characterized by decreased vision, light sensitivity, and the absence of color vision. In the United States, it affects approximately 1 in every 33,000 people. Individuals with ACHM have impaired color discrimination along all 3 axes of color vision in various degrees. Most individuals have complete ACHM, with total lack of function of all 3 types of cones but some can have incomplete ACHM, in which 1 or more cone types may be partially functioning. The symptoms are similar in all patients but generally less severe in patients with incomplete ACHM [62]. Mutations in genes encoding subunits of the cone-specification channel, cyclic nucleotide gated channel α and β3 (*CNGA3* and *CNGB3*) are responsible for approximately 50% of cases of autosomal recessive ACHM, which is usually of the complete type. Each of these genes provides instructions for production of a protein that is involved in the normal function of retinal cones. Mutations in 2 genes associated with phototransduction in cones, cone-specific α subunit of transducin, *GNAT2*, and α subunit of cone-specific phosphodiesterase, *PDE6C*, are less common. Mutations in any of these genes affect the response to light stimulation in all 3 types of cones. As a result, most people with mutations in one of these genes must depend on rods alone for vision, thus they see better in dim light, or with tinted lenses, particularly with an orange-brown tint that blocks short wavelength blue and green light. In childhood, the foveal involvement in the disease is limited and milder than has been observed in older individuals with ACHM. This observation suggests that early therapeutic intervention may be more successful in preserving vision. Neither age alone nor genotype alone are predictive of the degree of photoreceptor loss or preservation, and because of that, the window for treatment is not yet well understood [63,64].

Animal studies have shown that gene replacement therapy with AAV is a viable treatment option for this disease [65]. To target cone photoreceptors it is necessary to optimize capsid proteins for increased specificity or to restrict expression via the use of cell type–specific promoters [66]. The ACHM mouse model is a Gnat2cpfl3 mouse that carries a recessive mutation in *Gnat2* resulting in little or no recordable light-adapted ERG response and poor visual acuity [67]. The first report of gene therapy for ACHM showed restored cone-mediated ERG amplitudes and cone-mediated behavioral responses to levels indistinguishable from age-matched wild-type mice after subretinal injection of AAV5 *Gnat2* under the control of the human red cone opsin promoter [68]. Gene replacement therapy has also been tested in 2 large animal models of ACHM. Two canine models of *CNGB3*-ACHM with either the $CNGB3^{-/-}$ or $CNGB3^{m/m}$ mutation are blind in bright light after approximately 8 weeks of age. At this age, cone-mediated function is absent, but rod responses are normal. AAV5 containing human *CNGB3* was delivered subretinally as a single injection. Vector-treated dogs exhibited restored cone function as measured by cone flicker ERGs. In dogs maintained for long-term follow-up, the rescued cone function was sustained for more than 1 year with the longest period of observation being approximately 2.5 years. Importantly, *GNAT2* and *CNGA3*, which are absent or mislocalized in untreated cones, showed normalization of protein expression and localization to cone outer segments in treated eyes [69].

There is another form of achromatopsia that is X-linked, caused by a different gene in which blue cone function is spared. Discussion of this form is beyond the scope of this article.

Bardet-Biedl syndrome

Bardet-Biedl syndrome (BBS) is an autosomal recessive disease from a class named "ciliopathy." BBS is characterized by progressive retinal dystrophy, early obesity, polydactyly (a completely developed extra finger or just a rudiment), renal dysfunction, learning difficulties, and hypogonadism [70]. BBS is a disorder with significant interfamilial and intrafamilial variation due to genetic pleiotropism. The reported prevalence of BBS varies markedly between populations, from 1:160,000 in northern European populations to 1:13,500 and 1:17,500, respectively, in isolated communities in Kuwait and Newfoundland [71].

The proteins encoded by BBS gene family members are structurally diverse and the similar phenotypes exhibited by mutations in BBS genes is likely due to their shared roles in cilia formation and function. These proteins participate in specific steps or aspects of pathways that control protein movement to and from cilia. BBS proteins also seem to be involved in intracellular trafficking via microtubule-related transport. The proteins encoded by 7 of these genes form a multiprotein BBSome complex [72]. The protein products of many different genes associated with BBS interact and malfunction or absence of any of them affect the structure and/or function of cilia [73]. At this writing, 19 causative genes have been identified [26]. Inheritance is autosomal recessive; there is some evidence that mutations in a second BBS gene may modify the expression of the disease [74]. An example of such interaction is that components of the BBSome, a protein complex composed of 7 BBS proteins, physically and genetically interact with *CEP290* (LCA-causing gene) and modulate the expression of disease phenotypes caused by *CEP290* mutations in mouse models [75].

In a knockin mouse model of the most common type of BBS1, Bbs1$^{M390R/M390R}$, subretinal delivery of AAV-*Bbs1* rescues BBSome formation and rhodopsin localization, and shows a trend toward improved ERG. However, the same dose of vector is toxic to wild-type (normal) retinas [75]. This overexpression toxicity also has been seen with another gene capable of causing BBS, *CEP290* [76]. Because of the stoichiometry of the BBSome protein complex and overexpression toxicity, BBS and other disorders from the ciliopathy group may be challenging to treat with gene therapy [76].

An AAV-BBS4 vector has been reported to rescue rhodopsin mislocalization, and to maintain more normal rod outer segments in the Bbs4-null mouse model; however, only a small portion of the retina (4%) was treated in this study [77]. Because breeding with transgenic Bbs4 mice also rescued the ocular phenotype [78], BBS4 may be more easily treatable by gene replacement than BBS1.

OTHER TREATMENTS: NONSURGICAL

Although the most definitive treatment would be replacing the deficient gene, enzyme, or cell in the retina, progress also has been made in developing noninvasive (nonsurgical) treatments to replace gene products.

RPE65 oral supplement trial

Replacing the product of the RPE65 gene by oral ingestion is possible and has demonstrated some improvement in visual field in treated patients. Patients were treated for 7 days with oral QLT091001 (10–40 mg/m^2 per day). Fourteen patients aged 6 to 38 years were enrolled in the trial and followed for 2 years. The trial reported 10 of 14 patients had an improvement in visual field testing and 6 patients had an improvement in visual acuity. After 2 years, 11 patients had returned to their baseline visual field and 10 had returned to baseline visual acuity letter values. No serious adverse events occurred, although the investigators noted transient headaches (11 patients), photophobia (11 patients), reduction in serum high-density lipoprotein concentrations (4 patients), increases in serum triglycerides (8 patients), and aspartate aminotransferase concentrations (2 patients) [79].

Other treatments

There is evidence supporting the use of oral supplements, neuroprotective molecules, and antioxidants for slowing the progression of retinal degeneration in certain animal models of retinal degeneration [80,81].

Stem cells

For patients in whom all or most of the photoreceptors have been lost, pluripotent stem cells may provide a mechanism to replace these cells, which are necessary for vision. The photoreceptors pass the visual signal on to the neural cells in the inner retina, and then on to the brain, so successful stem cell replacement will rely on an intact inner retina, and the ability to establish a neural connection between the implanted photoreceptor cells and this layer. Induced pluripotent stem cells (iPSCs) are cells that are harvested from a patient's skin keratinocytes, and then are de-differentiated using Yamanaka factors into pluripotent cells [82]. For use in the eye to replace lost retinal tissue, iPSCs need to be differentiated into retinal precursor cells. A stepwise differentiation protocol has been developed. This protocol combines different aspects of embryonic stem cells and iPSC differentiation to maximize the percentage of photoreceptor cells produced for transplantation. This protocol takes into account the role of bone morphogenic protein and Wnt signaling pathway inhibition in neuroectodermal development, as well as the role of insulinlike growth factor 1 in anterior neural/eye field development and Notch pathway inhibition in photoreceptor development. These cells express the retinal progenitor cell genes Chx10 and Lhx2 and the photoreceptor cell genes CRX, recoverin, rhodopsin, blue-opsin, red/green-opsin, and ROM-1 after 33 days of differentiation and even form a rudimentary eyecup in culture [83]. These cells can be used to study patients' diseases, and eventually to replace the cells lost to disease [84].

Retinal "chip"

For patients in whom no photoreceptive cells remain but the optic nerve is still functional, an electrical array implanted on the retina may stimulate some vision. The Argus II retinal prosthesis system ("Argus II") is the first FDA-approved device intended to restore some functional vision for people suffering from blindness. The principle of the device is bypassing the damaged photoreceptors in the retina and using the still functional bipolar and retinal ganglion cells. A miniature video camera attached to a pair of spectacles captures the images. The video is sent to a small, patient-worn, computer called the video processing unit, where it is processed and transformed into signals that are sent back to the glasses via a cable. These processed signals are transmitted wirelessly to an antenna in the implant. The signals are then sent to the electrode

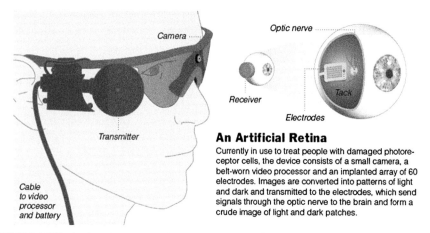

An Artificial Retina

Currently in use to treat people with damaged photore-ceptor cells, the device consists of a small camera, a belt-worn video processor and an implanted array of 60 electrodes. Images are converted into patterns of light and dark and transmitted to the electrodes, which send signals through the optic nerve to the brain and form a crude image of light and dark patches.

Fig. 7. Approval for an artificial retina. The FDA approved a system that allows people with a severe type of retinal deterioration to see patches of light and dark. Camera images are processed and transferred to electrodes implanted in the back of the eye. (*Courtesy of* Second Sight Medical Products, Sylmar, CA, *The New York Times*, with permission; *From* The Argus II retinal prosthesis system. Available at: http://www.2-sight.eu/ee/patients-and-families. Accessed January 9, 2015, with permission; and Tucker BA, Mullins RF, Streb LM, et al. Patient-specific iPSC-derived photoreceptor precursor cells as a means to investigate retinitis pigmentosa. Elife 2013;2:e00824.)

array, which emits small pulses of electricity. In the retina, the impulses are taken by the bipolar and ganglion cells and transmitted through the optic nerve to the brain. The patients see patterns of light and they learn to interpret these visual patterns (Fig. 7).

The process is lengthy and very involved for patients but it holds promise. The first group of implanted adult patients, who had vision loss from RP, showed improvement in visual tasks after the surgery, and the device was well tolerated and functional over a 1-year follow-up period [85].

THE FUTURE

Genetically caused blindness has been untreatable to this point in history. Thanks to subretinal gene therapy that is no longer true for a few of these conditions and potentially for many more in the future. Patients and parents have reason to hope, and practitioners have reason to offer genetic testing to their patients. Gene therapy is gene specific, so accurate molecular diagnosis is the key to unlocking the potential of this treatment.

SUPPLEMENTARY DATA

Supplementary data related to this article can be found online at http://dx.doi.org/10.1016/j.yapd.2015.04.012.

References

[1] Drack AV, Johnston R, Stone EM. Which Leber congenital amaurosis patients are eligible for gene therapy trials? J AAPOS 2009;13(5):463–5.

[2] Drack AV, Lambert SR, Stone EM. From the laboratory to the clinic: molecular genetic testing in pediatric ophthalmology. Am J Ophthalmol 2010;149(1):10–7.

[3] Gene therapy and cell therapy defined. ASGCT- American Society of Gene & Cell Therapy. Available at: http://www.asgct.org/general-public/educational-resources/gene-therapy–and-cell-therapy-defined. Accessed October 19, 2014.

[4] Torpy JM, Lynm C, Glass RM. Genetics: the basics. JAMA 2008;299(11):1388.

[5] Matthew D, Weitzman RM. Adeno-associated virus biology. In: Snyder RO, Moullier P, editors. Totowa (NJ): Humana Press; 2011; http://dx.doi.org/10.1007/978-1-61779-370-7.

[6] Carvalho LS, Vandenberghe LH. Promising and delivering gene therapies for vision loss. Vision Res 2014; http://dx.doi.org/10.1016/j.visres.2014.07.013.

[7] Original video Dr Steve Russell MD. Available at: http://start.sweetpacks.com/?barid={327C53A4-FC6B-11E2-AB6C-0030679F4C46}&src=97&crg=3.5000006.10042&st=23. Accessed January 14, 2015.

[8] Ramachandran PS, Bhattarai S, Singh P, et al. RNA interference-based therapy for spinocerebellar ataxia type 7 retinal degeneration. PLoS One 2014;9(4):e95362.

[9] Amarzguioui M, Lundberg P, Cantin E, et al. Rational design and in vitro and in vivo delivery of Dicer substrate siRNA. Nat Protoc 2006;1(2):508–17.

[10] Miller VM, Xia H, Marrs GL, et al. Allele-specific silencing of dominant disease genes. Proc Natl Acad Sci U S A 2003;100(12):7195–200.

[11] Ran FA, Hsu PD, Wright J, et al. Genome engineering using the CRISPR-Cas9 system. Nat Protoc 2013;8(11):2281–308.

[12] Jinek M, Chylinski K, Fonfara I, et al. A programmable dual-RNA-guided DNA endonuclease in adaptive bacterial immunity. Science 2012;337(6096):816–21.

[13] Gasiunas G, Barrangou R, Horvath P, et al. Cas9-crRNA ribonucleoprotein complex mediates specific DNA cleavage for adaptive immunity in bacteria. Proc Natl Acad Sci U S A 2012;109(39):E2579–86.

[14] Petrs-Silva H, Linden R. Advances in gene therapy technologies to treat retinitis pigmentosa. Clin Ophthalmol 2014;8:127–36.

[15] Hurwitz MY, Marcus KT, Chévez-Barrios P, et al. Suicide gene therapy for treatment of retinoblastoma in a murine model. Hum Gene Ther 1999;10(3):441–8.

[16] Campochiaro PA, Nguyen QD, Shah SM, et al. Adenoviral vector-delivered pigment epithelium-derived factor for neovascular age-related macular degeneration: results of a phase I clinical trial. Hum Gene Ther 2006;17(2):167–76.

[17] Campochiaro PA. Gene transfer for neovascular age-related macular degeneration. Hum Gene Ther 2011;22(5):523–9.

[18] Acland GM, Aguirre GD, Ray J, et al. Gene therapy restores vision in a canine model of childhood blindness. Nat Genet 2001;28(1):92–5.

[19] Acland GM, Aguirre GD, Bennett J, et al. Long-term restoration of rod and cone vision by single dose rAAV-mediated gene transfer to the retina in a canine model of childhood blindness. Mol Ther 2005;12(6):1072–82.

[20] Bainbridge JW, Smith AJ, Barker SS, et al. Effect of gene therapy on visual function in Leber's congenital amaurosis. N Engl J Med 2008;358(21):2231–9. Available at: http://www.nejm.org/doi/full/10.1056/NEJMoa0802268. Accessed October 20, 2014.

[21] Hauswirth WW, Aleman TS, Kaushal S, et al. Treatment of Leber congenital amaurosis due to RPE65 mutations by ocular subretinal injection of adeno-associated virus gene vector: short-term results of a phase I trial. Hum Gene Ther 2008;19(10):979–90.

[22] Maguire AM, Simonelli F, Pierce EA, et al. Safety and efficacy of gene transfer for Leber's congenital amaurosis. N Engl J Med 2008;358(21):2240–8.

[23] Cideciyan AV, Aleman TS, Boye SL, et al. Human gene therapy for RPE65 isomerase deficiency activates the retinoid cycle of vision but with slow rod kinetics. Proc Natl Acad Sci U S A 2008;105(39):15112–7.

[24] Fulton AB, Hansen RM, Mayer DL. Vision in Leber congenital amaurosis. Arch Ophthalmol 1996;114(6):698–703. Available at: http://www.ncbi.nlm.nih.gov/pubmed/8639081. Accessed October 20, 2014.

[25] Chung DC, Traboulsi EI. Leber congenital amaurosis: clinical correlations with genotypes, gene therapy trials update, and future directions. J AAPOS 2009;13(6):587–92.

[26] RetNet. Retinal information Network, a service of the Laboratory for the Molecular Diagnosis of Inherited Eye Diseases. Available at: https://sph.uth.edu/retnet/. Accessed April 29, 2015.

[27] Simonelli F, Maguire AM, Testa F, et al. Gene therapy for Leber's congenital amaurosis is safe and effective through 1.5 years after vector administration. Mol Ther 2010;18(3): 643–50.

[28] Boye SE, Boye SL, Lewin AS, et al. A comprehensive review of retinal gene therapy. Mol Ther 2013;21(3):509–19.

[29] Maguire AM, High KA, Auricchio A, et al. Age-dependent effects of RPE65 gene therapy for Leber's congenital amaurosis: a phase 1 dose-escalation trial. Lancet 2009;374(9701): 1597–605.

[30] Jacobson SG, Cideciyan AV, Ratnakaram R, et al. Gene therapy for Leber congenital amaurosis caused by RPE65 mutations: safety and efficacy in 15 children and adults followed up to 3 years. Arch Ophthalmol 2012;130(1):9–24.

[31] Testa F, Maguire AM, Rossi S, et al. Three-year follow-up after unilateral subretinal delivery of adeno-associated virus in patients with Leber congenital amaurosis type 2. Ophthalmology 2013;120(6):1283–91.

[32] Amado D, Mingozzi F, Hui D, et al. Safety and efficacy of subretinal readministration of a viral vector in large animals to treat congenital blindness. Sci Transl Med 2010;2(21): 21ra16.

[33] Willett K, Bennett J. Immunology of AAV-mediated gene transfer in the eye. Front Immunol 2013;4:261.

[34] Bennett J, Ashtari M, Wellman J, et al. AAV2 gene therapy readministration in three adults with congenital blindness. Sci Transl Med 2012;4(120):120ra15.

[35] Wojno AP, Pierce EA, Bennett J. Seeing the light. Sci Transl Med 2013;5(175):175fs8.

[36] Alory C, Balch WE. Organization of the Rab-GDI/CHM superfamily: the functional basis for choroideremia disease. Traffic 2001;2(8):532–43. Available at: http://www.ncbi.nlm.nih.gov/pubmed/11489211. Accessed October 25, 2014.

[37] Sergeev YV, Smaoui N, Sui R, et al. The functional effect of pathogenic mutations in Rab escort protein 1. Mutat Res 2009;665(1–2):44–50.

[38] Pylypenko O, Rak A, Reents R, et al. Structure of Rab escort protein-1 in complex with Rab geranylgeranyltransferase. Mol Cell 2003;11(2):483–94. Available at: http://www.ncbi.nlm.nih.gov/pubmed/12620235. Accessed October 25, 2014.

[39] Zerial M, McBride H. Rab proteins as membrane organizers. Nat Rev Mol Cell Biol 2001;2(2):107–17.

[40] Sankila EM, Tolvanen R, van den Hurk JA, et al. Aberrant splicing of the CHM gene is a significant cause of choroideremia. Nat Genet 1992;1(2):109–13.

[41] MacDonald IM, Russell L, Chan CC. Choroideremia: new findings from ocular pathology and review of recent literature. Surv Ophthalmol 2010;54(3):401–7.

[42] MacLaren RE, Groppe M, Barnard AR, et al. Retinal gene therapy in patients with choroideremia: initial findings from a phase 1/2 clinical trial. Lancet 2014;383(9923):1129–37.

[43] Walia S, Fishman GA. Natural history of phenotypic changes in Stargardt macular dystrophy. Ophthalmic Genet 2009;30(2):63–8.

[44] Molday RS, Zhang K. Defective lipid transport and biosynthesis in recessive and dominant Stargardt macular degeneration. Prog Lipid Res 2010;49(4):476–92.

[45] Molday L, Rabin A, Molday R. ABCR expression in foveal cone photoreceptors and its role in Stargardt macular dystrophy. Am J Ophthalmol 2000;130(5):689. Available at: http://www.ncbi.nlm.nih.gov/pubmed/11078864. Accessed October 20, 2014.

[46] Molday RS, Zhong M, Quazi F. The role of the photoreceptor ABC transporter ABCA4 in lipid transport and Stargardt macular degeneration. Biochim Biophys Acta 2009;1791(7):573–83.

[47] Mullins RF, Kuehn MH, Radu RA, et al. Autosomal recessive retinitis pigmentosa due to ABCA4 mutations: clinical, pathologic, and molecular characterization. Invest Ophthalmol Vis Sci 2012;53(4):1883–94.

[48] Schindler EI, Nylen EL, Ko AC, et al. Deducing the pathogenic contribution of recessive ABCA4 alleles in an outbred population. Hum Mol Genet 2010;19(19):3693–701.

[49] Cideciyan AV, Swider M, Aleman TS, et al. ABCA4 disease progression and a proposed strategy for gene therapy. Hum Mol Genet 2009;18(5):931–41.

[50] Binley K, Widdowson P, Loader J, et al. Transduction of photoreceptors with equine infectious anemia virus lentiviral vectors: safety and biodistribution of StarGen for Stargardt disease. Invest Ophthalmol Vis Sci 2013;54(6):4061–71.

[51] Tielsch JM, Javitt JC, Coleman A, et al. The prevalence of blindness and visual impairment among nursing home residents in Baltimore. N Engl J Med 1995;332(18):1205–9.

[52] Friedman DS, O'Colmain BJ, Muñoz B, et al. Prevalence of age-related macular degeneration in the United States. Arch Ophthalmol 2004;122(4):564–72.

[53] Maclachlan TK, Lukason M, Collins M, et al. Preclinical safety evaluation of AAV2-sFLT01: a gene therapy for age-related macular degeneration. Mol Ther 2011;19(2):326–34; http://dx.doi.org/10.1038/mt.2010.258.

[54] Keats B, Corey D. The Usher syndromes. Am J Med 1999;89:158–66. Available at: http://corey.med.harvard.edu/PDFs/new/r1999 Keats Corey usher.pdf. Accessed October 20, 2014.

[55] Petit C. Usher syndrome: from genetics to pathogenesis. Annu Rev Genomics Hum Genet 2001;2:271–97.

[56] Hasson T, Heintzelman MB, Santos-Sacchi J, et al. Expression in cochlea and retina of myosin VIIa, the gene product defective in Usher syndrome type 1B. Proc Natl Acad Sci U S A 1995;92(21):9815–9. Available at: http://www.pubmedcentral.nih.gov/articlerender.fcgi?artid=40893&tool=pmcentrez&rendertype=abstract. Accessed October 25, 2014.

[57] Liu X, Vansant G, Udovichenko IP, et al. Myosin VIIa, the product of the Usher 1B syndrome gene, is concentrated in the connecting cilia of photoreceptor cells. Cell Motil Cytoskeleton 1997;37(3):240–52.

[58] Trapani I, Colella P, Sommella A, et al. Effective delivery of large genes to the retina by dual AAV vectors. EMBO Mol Med 2014;6(2):194–211.

[59] Lyon MF. Twirler: a mutant affecting the inner ear of the house mouse. J Embryol Exp Morphol 1958;6(1):105–16. Available at: http://www.ncbi.nlm.nih.gov/pubmed/13539273. Accessed October 25, 2014.

[60] Hashimoto T, Gibbs D, Lillo C, et al. Lentiviral gene replacement therapy of retinas in a mouse model for Usher syndrome type 1B. Gene Ther 2007;14(7):584–94.

[61] Zallocchi M, Binley K, Lad Y, et al. EIAV-based retinal gene therapy in the shaker1 mouse model for Usher syndrome type 1B: development of UshStat. PLoS One 2014;9(4): e94272.

[62] Kohl S, Jägle H, Wissinger B. Achromatopsia. In: Pagon RA, Adam MP, Ardinger HH, et al, editors. GeneReviews. Seattle (WA): Seattle University Washington; 1993–2014 [Internet]. Available at: http://www.ncbi.nlm.nih.gov/books/NBK1418/. Accessed October 20, 2014.

[63] Yang P, Michaels KV, Courtney RJ, et al. Retinal morphology of patients with achromatopsia during early childhood: implications for gene therapy. JAMA Ophthalmol 2014;132(7): 823–31.

[64] Sundaram V, Wilde C, Aboshiha J, et al. Retinal structure and function in achromatopsia: implications for gene therapy. Ophthalmology 2014;121(1):234–45.

[65] Mühlfriedel R, Tanimoto N, Seeliger MW. Gene replacement therapy in achromatopsia type 2. Klin Monbl Augenheilkd 2014;231(3):232–40 [in German].

[66] Dyka FM, Boye SL, Ryals RC, et al. Cone specific promoter for use in gene therapy of retinal degenerative diseases. Adv Exp Med Biol 2014;801:695–701.

[67] Chang B, Dacey MS, Hawes NL, et al. Cone photoreceptor function loss-3, a novel mouse model of achromatopsia due to a mutation in Gnat2. Invest Ophthalmol Vis Sci 2006;47(11):5017–21.

[68] Alexander JJ, Umino Y, Everhart D, et al. Restoration of cone vision in a mouse model of achromatopsia. Nat Med 2007;13(6):685–7.

[69] Komáromy AM, Alexander JJ, Rowlan JS, et al. Gene therapy rescues cone function in congenital achromatopsia. Hum Mol Genet 2010;19(13):2581–93.

[70] Forsythe E, Beales PL. Bardet-Biedl syndrome. Eur J Hum Genet 2013;21(1):8–13.

[71] Katsanis N, Ansley SJ, Badano JL, et al. Triallelic inheritance in Bardet-Biedl syndrome, a Mendelian recessive disorder. Science 2001;293(5538):2256–9.

[72] Zhang Q, Yu D, Seo S, et al. Intrinsic protein-protein interaction-mediated and chaperonin-assisted sequential assembly of stable Bardet-Biedl syndrome protein complex, the BBSome. J Biol Chem 2012;287(24):20625–35.

[73] Estrada-Cuzcano A, Roepman R, Cremers FP, et al. Non-syndromic retinal ciliopathies: translating gene discovery into therapy. Hum Mol Genet 2012;21(R1):R111–24.

[74] Zaghloul NA, Katsanis N. Mechanistic insights into Bardet-Biedl syndrome, a model ciliopathy. J Clin Invest 2009;119(3):428–37.

[75] Zhang Y, Seo S, Bhattarai S, et al. BBS mutations modify phenotypic expression of CEP290-related ciliopathies. Hum Mol Genet 2014;23(1):40–51.

[76] Seo S, Mullins RF, Dumitrescu AV, et al. Subretinal gene therapy of mice with Bardet-Biedl syndrome type 1. Invest Ophthalmol Vis Sci 2013;54(9):6118–32.

[77] Simons DL, Boye SL, Hauswirth WW, et al. Gene therapy prevents photoreceptor death and preserves retinal function in a Bardet-Biedl syndrome mouse model. Proc Natl Acad Sci U S A 2011;108(15):6276–81.

[78] Chamling X, Seo S, Bugge K, et al. Ectopic expression of human BBS4 can rescue Bardet-Biedl syndrome phenotypes in Bbs4 null mice. PLoS One 2013;8(3):e59101.

[79] Koenekoop RK, Sui R, Sallum J, et al. Oral 9-cis retinoid for childhood blindness due to Leber congenital amaurosis caused by RPE65 or LRAT mutations: an open-label phase 1b trial. Lancet 2014;384(9953):1513–20.

[80] Drack AV, Dumitrescu AV, Bhattarai S, et al. TUDCA slows retinal degeneration in two different mouse models of retinitis pigmentosa and prevents obesity in Bardet-Biedl syndrome type 1 mice. Invest Ophthalmol Vis Sci 2012;53(1):100–6.

[81] Fernández-Sánchez L, Lax P, Pinilla I, et al. Tauroursodeoxycholic acid prevents retinal degeneration in transgenic P23H rats. Invest Ophthalmol Vis Sci 2011;52(8):4998–5008.

[82] Tanabe K, Takahashi K, Yamanaka S. Induction of pluripotency by defined factors. Proc Jpn Acad Ser B Phys Biol Sci 2014;90(3):83–96. Available at: http://www.pubmedcentral.nih.gov/articlerender.fcgi?artid=3997808&tool=pmcentrez&rendertype=abstract. Accessed October 26, 2014.

[83] Tucker BA, Park I-H, Qi SD, et al. Transplantation of adult mouse iPS cell-derived photoreceptor precursors restores retinal structure and function in degenerative mice. PLoS One 2011;6(4):e18992.

[84] Tucker BA, Mullins RF, Streb LM, et al. Patient-specific iPSC-derived photoreceptor precursor cells as a means to investigate retinitis pigmentosa. Elife 2013;2:e00824.

[85] Rizzo S, Belting C, Cinelli L, et al. The Argus II Retinal Prosthesis: 12-month outcomes from a single-study center. Am J Ophthalmol 2014;157(6):1282–90.

Advances in Pediatrics 62 (2015) 211–226

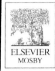

ADVANCES IN PEDIATRICS

ELSEVIER
MOSBY

Screening for Critical Congenital Heart Disease in Newborns

Christie J. Bruno, DO, Thomas Havranek, MD*

Department of Pediatrics, The Children's Hospital at Montefiore, Albert Einstein College of Medicine, 1601 Tenbroeck Avenue, 2nd Floor, Bronx, NY 10461, USA

Keywords

- Critical congenital heart disease • Newborns • Screening

Key points

- Routine newborn screening for critical congenital heart disease (CCHD) is becoming standard of care.
- Pulse oximetry screening for CCHD is reliable and cost-effective.
- Effective follow-up for screens with positive results must be implemented in order for screening programs to be successful.
- Determination of previously implemented screening programs effectiveness is preliminary and ongoing.

INTRODUCTION

Congenital heart disease affects approximately 40,000 neonates in the United States each year or about 1% of all US national births. It is the most common form of birth defect. The most common type of congenital heart disease lesion is the ventricular septal defect (VSD). A VSD is a noncyanotic heart lesion and is not considered a form of CCHD [1,2]. CCHD, on the other hand, is a heart lesion for which neonates require early surgical intervention to survive. Without intervention, the mortality and rates of survival with significant disability are extremely high. CCHD accounts for 20% of deaths in the neonatal period and is therefore a significant cause of mortality for infants in the first month of life [3].

*Corresponding author. E-mail address: thavrane@montefiore.org

0065-3101/15/$ – see front matter
http://dx.doi.org/10.1016/j.yapd.2015.04.002

EPIDEMIOLOGY

There are several types of congenital heart disease that are included in CCHD. These defects are listed in Box 1. Of the defects listed in Box 1, the detection of 7 is believed to potentially contribute to an improvement in overall survival with decreased morbidity for CCHD. These defects include hypoplastic left heart syndrome (HLHS), pulmonary atresia, tetralogy of Fallot (TOF), total anomalous pulmonary venous return (TAPVR), transposition of the great arteries (TGA), tricuspid atresia, and truncus arteriosus. It is estimated that CCHD affects 2 to 3 per 1000 live births in the United States. The prevalence of CCHD varies based on geographic area as well as the type of CCHD defect. For example, the literature demonstrates that TOF was the most prevalent type of CCHD in all ethnic groups in one study out of New York State [4]. Another study, within New York State as well, reported a variety of CCHD lesions with no true predominance of one lesion. In the former study, HLHS, TAPVR, and coarctation of the aorta were reported, among others [5].

Neonates born with CCHD are often well appearing for the first 12 to 24 hours of life and may be asymptomatic for a day or two beyond that period. Infants with CCHD typically present with physiologic compromise beyond 24 hours of life related to the type of CCHD lesion. Patients with right- and left-sided obstructive heart lesions are listed in Box 1. Patients typically present with symptoms at the time of closure of the ductus arterious. Those with right-sided obstructive lesions lose pulmonary blood flow when the ductus closes,

---

Box 1: Critical congenital heart disease defects

Left-sided obstructive lesions
1. Hypoplastic left heart syndrome
2. Interrupted aortic arch
3. Critical coarctation of the aorta
4. Critical aortic stenosis

Right-sided obstructive lesions
5. Pulmonary atresia with intact septum
6. Tricuspid atresia
7. Critical pulmonary stenosis
8. Tetralogy of Fallot

Mixing lesions
9. Total anomalous pulmonary venous return
10. Transposition of the great arteries
11. Truncus arteriosus communis

leading to profound cyanosis in the newborn. Those with left-sided obstructive lesions lose systemic blood flow as the ductus closes, leading to a presentation of neonatal shock. Before closure, the ductus arteriosus had been supplying pulmonary and systemic blood flow in these patients, respectively [6,7].

Given the window of time for potential intervention before an infant develops signs of compromise, many have examined the benefits of screening asymptomatic neonates for CCHD. If CCHD is confirmed in a patient, then various interventions may be undertaken to prevent physiologic compromise and possible neurologic injury. Potential interventions for these patients include administration of prostaglandin infusion to maintain the patency of the ductus arteriosus to increase systemic or pulmonary blood flow. In addition, patients may be transferred to tertiary facilities for valvuloplasty and atrial septostomy procedures, among others [8,9]. These interventions may improve neonatal survival.

The case for screening asymptomatic newborns for CCHD can be made as several studies indicate that earlier diagnosis can lead to improved outcomes. One-year survival rates for neonates born with CCHD have improved in the last 10 years from 67% pre-1993 to approximately 83% post-1994. However, mortality remains high for this group [10]. A recent study indicated that up to 35% of neonates with CCHD are not referred to a cardiac specialty center by day of life 4, accounting for higher mortality rates in these patients [11]. A recent population study in Texas demonstrated that neonates with HLHS have improved survival if they are born closer to a cardiac surgical center, supporting the case for early screening and evaluation of these children to transport them quickly to a hospital with adequate specialty support [12]. Optimizing the care of these infants early on is especially important because, at baseline, they have been reported to have abnormal presurgical brain development when compared with patients without CCHD [13]. In addition, patients with CCHD, particularly those with single ventricle physiology, such as HLHS, have poorer neurodevelopmental outcomes [14]. Prompt intervention may improve neurodevelopmental outcomes.

Ideally, if a mother has adequate prenatal care, a diagnosis of CCHD can be made using prenatal ultrasonography. Patients who are diagnosed with CCHD prenatally have demonstrated improved cardiac function, lower mechanical ventilation time, and a shorter length of stay in the intensive care unit postoperatively [15,16]. If a prenatal diagnosis of CCHD is not achieved, then early detection of CCHD postnatally may be helpful to improve overall outcomes.

FETAL ULTRASONOGRAPHY, PHYSICAL EXAMINATION, PULSE OXIMETRY, AND THEIR ROLE IN DETECTING CRITICAL CONGENITAL HEART DISEASE

Newborn physical examination has been traditionally used to detect CCHD before the onset of physiologic compromise. Although first invented in the 1950s, over the last few decades, obstetric ultrasonography has become standard of care at 18 to 20 weeks' gestation to evaluate for congenital defects, including heart disease. More recently, pulse oximetry screening has become a standard in many states in the United States to screen for CCHD. In the absence of a prenatal diagnosis, attempting to detect CCHD by newborn physical examination has its limitations. Although newborns may present with cyanosis and shock after the ductus arterious closes, most newborns are asymptomatic before ductus arterious closure. In the absence of abnormal heart sounds or perfusion, it can be challenging to accurately diagnose CCHD before ductal closure, especially if arterial and venous blood mixing is present [17,18]. In fact, many neonates with congenital heart disease do not have a murmur on physical examination [19]. An exception to those CCHD lesions that present with a delay in presentation is TAPVR, in which neonates are extremely ill shortly after birth as they present with profound cyanosis and respiratory distress. In this situation, newborn physical examination would be helpful.

Many infants with CCHD can be diagnosed prenatally after abnormalities on obstetric ultrasonography prompt a fetal echocardiogram to confirm the diagnosis. In order for a prenatal diagnosis to occur, there must be adequate and timely prenatal care. A barrier to prenatal diagnosis is that the Centers for Disease Control reports that up to 11% of women of various backgrounds do not receive prenatal care [20]. Even with adequate prenatal care, there are limitations to obtaining a prenatal diagnosis. The limitations are related to the quality of ultrasound imaging, which is operator dependent, and the types of cardiac views analyzed. These limitations have lead to somewhat low prenatal diagnosis rates in some areas. In a recent study, community centers had prenatal CCHD detection rates as low as 23%, whereas tertiary care centers had rates of 80% [21]. There is growing evidence demonstrating that a 4-chamber prenatal ultrasonographic view of the heart alone may miss several forms of CCHD, because, in many forms of CCHD, the 4-chamber heart view is within normal limits. One study demonstrated that the addition of outflow tract views can increase the detection of CCHD by as much as 25% [22], resulting in the detection of most ductal-dependent CCHD lesions.

Evidence shows that there are certain CCHD lesions that are much more likely to be diagnosed prenatally with ultrasonography and/or echocardiography than others. Fetuses with abnormal 4-chamber heart views, such as those with single ventricle physiology like HLHS and atrioventricular canal defects, in which the 4 chambers are not distinctly separate, are diagnosed from 50% to 80% of the time. On the other hand, heart lesions with seemingly normal 4-chamber heart views are less likely to be detected. These conditions include TOF and TGA. In these cases, 2 vessels enter and exit the heart, and the anatomic differences can be more easily missed. Prenatal diagnosis of these lesions has been reported to be as low as 19% to 31%. The same could be said for heart lesions with potentially more subtle prenatal signs, such as TAPVR and coarctation of the aorta [21].

Pulse oximetry screening has been introduced as an adjunct to newborn physical examination to help detect CCHD that has not been diagnosed prenatally. Most US states have now mandated that pulse oximetry screening for

CCHD be completed before a newborn is discharged from the hospital after birth. In January 2011, New Jersey was the first state to legally adopt this mandate [23]. As of October 2014, all states except for Mississippi and Idaho have either mandated CCHD pulse oximetry screening in the newborn or piloted programs for pulse oximetry screening for CCHD [24].

The general principle behind screening for CCHD with pulse oximetry is that healthy newborns beyond 24 hours of life should have pulse oximetry readings of greater than or equal to 95%. Saturations less than 95% are cause for concern. Screening is recommended to be delayed until after 24 hours of life to allow for a transition from fetal circulation and to avoid false-positive results. A pulse oximetry reading of less than 95% at that time is considered abnormal, and those patients are at risk for having CCHD or some other pathologic condition. The recent literature recommends objective pulse oximetry screening versus subjective visual appreciation of cyanosis; this is because one study demonstrated that, depending on the hemoglobin level of the patient, visual cyanosis may not be recognized until a patient has oxygen saturations of less than 78% [25]. In another study of delivery room personnel assessing neonates for cyanosis, there was a wide range of inconsistency between subjective assessment of cyanosis and actual pulse oximetry readings. The range of subjective resolution of cyanosis was reported at pulse oximetry reading levels of 10% to 100%, demonstrating that objective measures should be used for better accuracy [26].

Some of the pulse oximetry screening guidelines that were initially instituted on a state level went through some modifications early on to attain the most appropriate guidelines; this was true in Tennessee, as initially, a 94% oxygen saturation was considered a normal oxygen saturation level. It was then determined that changing the threshold of normal oxygen saturation to 95% improved the positive predictive value of the screen by decreasing the number of false-positive results. In the first evaluation of Tennessee's pulse oximetry screening for CCHD in 2011, it was determined that a 1% false-positive rate was quite burdensome and resulted in thousands of dollars in additional costs. In addition, the need for the development of a comprehensive follow-up plan for a screen with positive result was realized, as many were unsure of how to methodically evaluate those neonates with positive screen results. An infant was noted in Tennessee's initial evaluation of the screening program to have screened positive for CCHD but did not have appropriate follow-up. Therefore, the need for appropriate follow-up was addressed [27].

The state of Tennessee has taken an approach to the screening algorithm that is different from the algorithm recommended by the American Academy of Pediatrics (AAP). Instead of screening both upper and lower extremity oxygen saturations simultaneously, Tennessee guidelines start with screening the left or right foot first. An oxygen saturation in the lower extremity of greater than or equal to 97% results in a passed screen. An oxygen saturation between 90% and 96% warrants the addition of the right upper extremity to be screened simultaneously with the lower extremity. From this point onward, the

Tennessee screening mirrors many of the other state-mandated screens and that recommended by the AAP [28,29]. The reason that Tennessee physicians give for a mild deviation from other protocols is quite sound and rational. It would be impossible for a neonate to have a greater than 3% higher oxygen saturation in the upper extremities with a lower extremity saturation of 97% or higher. In the rare case of reverse differential cyanosis such as with TGA with interrupted aortic arch, there would have to be thousands of unnecessary upper extremity pulse oximetry readings performed to potentially detect 1 of these cases. According to Tennessee officials, this would not make clinical or economic sense.

PULSE OXIMETRY AND BASIC CRITERIA FOR SCREENING TEST

An ideal screening tool is one that fulfills certain criteria in the setting of disease detection and intervention. An ideal screening tool detects a condition before a patient becomes symptomatic from that condition. It is a test that can detect a disease at a stage when treatment can be effective to improve outcomes. An ideal screening test is safe to administer, reasonably low in cost, and widely available for use in a desired population [30]. Pulse oximetry screening in newborns fulfills these criteria for detecting CCHD by possessing several desired traits. Pulse oximetry screening has a high specificity for detecting CCHD (99%), low cost ($6.28 per newborn), and high availability in the United States, and screening after 24 hours of life can lead to detection of CCHD during a critical period when potentially life-saving intervention may occur [31].

The superior role of pulse oximetry in improving the detection of CCHD when compared with physical examination alone has been demonstrated in several studies. Pulse oximetry sensitivity in detecting CCHD has been demonstrated to be high with a specificity up to 99% with a very low false-positive rate, making it a strong test [32,33]. Pulse oximetry works as a probe is placed on a newborns finger, hand, foot, or ear lobe. The probe contains 3 important components that aid in calculating the percentage of hemoglobin that is saturated with oxygen in the newborn's blood. These components include a light source, light detector, and microcompressor. Understanding that oxygen-saturated blood is red and oxygen-desaturated blood is dark, there is a differential absorption of the light source (infrared and red) in the pulse oximetry probe. Based on the light detector absorption, the microcompressor determines the differences in the absorption of oxygen saturated versus desaturated blood and the percentage of oxygenated hemoglobin is calculated [34].

Several studies have demonstrated that pulse oximetry screening beyond 24 to 48 hours of life decreases false-positive results and that using 2 limbs (right hand and either foot) are best for improving the accuracy of CCHD screening. When a working group, consisting of members of the Secretary's Advisory Committee on Heritable Disorders in Newborns and Children, the AAP, the American College of Cardiology Foundation, and the American Heart Association, recommended universal screening for CCHD in newborns, there were certain criteria for screening that were required. The basic criteria include that pulse oximetry screening should be based on an algorithm and should be performed by trained health care professionals. In addition, any newborn with an abnormal pulse oximetry screen result should be evaluated by a licensed clinician. If an abnormal screen finding cannot be explained by other reasons, then the newborn must be evaluated for CCHD with an echocardiogram read by a pediatric cardiologist before being discharged home. In addition, follow-up should be arranged for these patients [35].

A sample basic pulse oximetry screening protocol is listed in Fig. 1. This sample protocol encompasses most of the screening guidelines based on recommended protocols at both the state and national level in the United States. The general principle is that a newborn infant should have a pulse oximetry reading of greater or equal to 95% after 24 hours of life. A newborn with a pulse oximetry reading of less than 90% warrants an immediate evaluation. A newborn with a pulse oximetry reading of 90% to 94% may be screened for up to 2 hours to determine if these differences are real or transient. In addition, any difference in upper and lower extremity oxygen saturations greater than 3% also warrants further evaluation, but rescreening these differences for up to 2 hours is acceptable as well [35]. An example of a decision tree for a pulse oximetry screen positive for CCHD used by the authors' institution is demonstrated in Fig. 2.

PULSE OXIMETRY SCREENING: PRACTICAL CONSIDERATIONS

A positive screening test result warrants an echocardiogram to evaluate for CCHD after the newborn has been evaluated for other causes of hypoxemia.

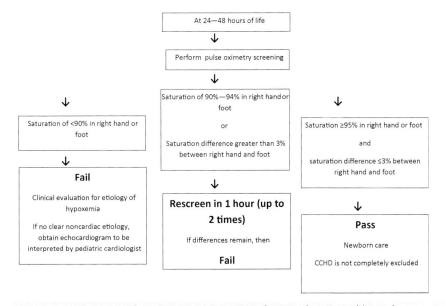

Fig. 1. Sample protocol for pulse oximetry screening for critical congenital heart disease.

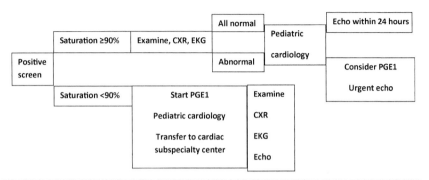

Fig. 2. Decision tree for positive CCHD screen. CXR, chest radiography; Echo, echocardiography; EKG, electrocardiography; PGE1, prostaglandin E1. (*Courtesy of* Sarah Chambers, MD, The Children's Hospital at Montefiore.)

However, there are several important considerations that must be addressed before the pulse oximetry screening process for CCHD at a given institution is considered legitimate or reliable. In addition to technical factors that must be refined to eliminate false-positive and false-negative screen results as much as possible, the skill of the staff in performing pulse oximetry screening must also be addressed. Finally, the availability of an echocardiogram with pediatric cardiology consultation is another real consideration and potential challenge.

Reich and colleagues [36] in 2008 demonstrated that there are several technical factors that can lead to errors in pulse oximetry readings. This group concluded that routine pulse oximetry screening was not reliable in their cohort for several reasons. However, they did demonstrate that reliability and accuracy could be improved. There are several factors that need to be noted and addressed that could lead to false-positive or false-negative results. For example, if a newborn has acrocyanosis in the absence of central cyanosis, this may lead to false-positive results related to poor distal perfusion. In this case, the ear lobe as a pulse oximeter screening site may be useful. In addition, in a newborn who is moving continuously or is crying and agitated, the pulse oximetry reading may not be accurate. One must then try to console the newborn to attempt to obtain an accurate reading. The pulse oximeter probe must be attached firmly to gain the most accurate reading. A partially attached or detached probe may result in an inaccurate oximetry reading. Given that a light source and light detector are used in the process of the generation of a pulse oximeter reading, external light sources such as those from overhead warmers may need to be turned down as they may interfere with the generated pulse oximeter readings. Finally, several pulse oximeter manufacturers exist, and the products themselves may have different accuracy and reliability. Regarding human factors that may interfere with reliable CCHD pulse oximetry screening, Reich and colleagues noted some important human factors that could be addressed to improve reliability. Between phase 1 and phase 2 of their study, they were able to improve the reliability of screening by 22%. They also noted that reliability could be improved to greater than 95% with 2 important factors. Administration of the pulse oximetry screening by a nurse with a licensed practical nursing degree or higher and administration of the screening for greater than 6 minutes also improved the reliability of the screening.

Understanding that quality-improvement projects may help to improve the process of CCHD screening, Oster and colleagues [37] hoped to improve the system of pulse oximetry screening. It has been established by several health care organizations that initiation of an algorithm may best help with the consistency of the administration of screening [20]. Oster and colleagues demonstrated that paper-based algorithms were still significantly susceptible to human error. The implementation of computer-based algorithms was demonstrated to improve the accuracy of the screening and significantly improve the ease of use. This study makes the case that refining the process can only further improve the pulse oximetry screening process.

There are several abnormalities for which a newborn may screen positive for CCHD but have another pathologic condition. For example, disorders of both the upper and lower airway may result in hypoxemia. These disorders include choanal atresia, severe micrognathia, laryngomalacia, vocal cord abnormalities, and tracheal compression by a mass or anatomic variant. In addition, lung pathology such as pneumothorax and pneumonia can cause hypoxemia in addition to anatomic variants such as congenital cystic adenomatoid malformation and congenital diaphragmatic hernia. Finally, infection and pulmonary hypertension must also be considered when a screen result is positive, among other pathologies.

In less densely populated states with larger geographic areas, challenges exist when a newborn has a positive screen result for CCHD. In these rural areas, access to those who can perform an accurate echocardiogram, as well as pediatric cardiology evaluation, may be limited. In contrast to a state like New Jersey, which has a large population in a smaller geographic area, a state like Wisconsin may encounter the situation of limited access to further evaluation for CCHD more readily. Approximately one-quarter of hospitals in the state of Wisconsin would have to transport newborn infants an average of more than 50 miles to obtain further cardiology evaluation after a positive pulse oximetry screen result [38]. This situation would result in potentially additional stress for the family in addition to separating a mother and child shortly after birth.

To prevent the transport of a newborn with solely a positive pulse oximetry screen result who ends up being healthy, some have advocated for the use of telemedicine. Telemedicine would allow for interpretation of echocardiography results by a pediatric cardiologist from afar as the images are transmitted to the interpreting cardiologist. One study demonstrated that the use of telemedicine resulted in faster diagnosis time, lesser number of neonatal transports, and shorter stays in the hospital [39]. One of the limitations of this approach is that many hospitals do not have echocardiographers who are trained in obtaining useful neonatal images for interpretation. The state of Wisconsin has implemented a system to educate adult echocardiographers in the technique of neonatal echocardiography as part of their Wisconsin SHINE (Screening Hearts in Newborns) Project. Wisconsin's education program introduces the technicians to 10 echocardiography findings that could indicate CCHD. The goal of the program is to screen for those newborns who warrant a more complete evaluation. This solution seems to be helpful to combat the challenges of screening in rural settings [40].

ECONOMIC CONSIDERATIONS AND COST

To estimate the cost-effectiveness of routine pulse oximetry screening for CCHD in the United States, several factors must be considered. The costs do vary based on the protocol being used. For example, the state of Tennessee performs pulse oximetry screening on one lower extremity first and proceeds based on those results. Tennessee's screening program may save several dollars per patient when compared with other states taking into account the cost of lesser time spent on screening as well as cost of second probe placement. Rural states with larger geographic areas, on the other hand, may need to deal with the additional costs of longer transports of infants over larger geographic areas, which must be accounted for on an individual state level.

The factors that contribute to the cost of pulse oximetry screening for CCHD include the time for staff to perform pulse oximetry screening along with time to educate and train the staff before implementation of screening. Other factors that contribute to overall cost are the costs of purchasing screening equipment (probes) and cost of keeping supply steady as needed. Additional costs associated with ensuring that all neonates are screened, following up results, and discussing results with families must also be considered. Finally, the costs associated with confirming a positive screen result as well as treatment and potential transport to a tertiary facility must also be addressed [35].

Costs for pulse oximetry screening for CCHD have been reported to range from as little as less than $5 per patient to as much as $10 per patient. Peterson and colleagues [31] reported that screening incurs an additional cost of $6.28 per newborn. The group reports that the incremental cost of screening may be as low as 50 cents per newborn if reusable pulse oximetry probes are used. In addition to the reported costs, it is estimated that almost 1200 neonates with CCHD will be detected yearly in the United States with screening and 20 neonatal deaths avoided with pulse oximetry screening for CCHD. In comparison to universal newborn hearing screening for neonates, which costs approximately 30 dollars per neonate, the costs for screening for CCHD are low [41,42]. Another large Swedish study examined pulse oximetry screening for CCHD detection in nearly 40,000 newborns. More than evaluating the overall cost of screening, they examined how much money is being saved by detecting CCHD cases earlier. The Swedish group reported that the cost of preventing 1 unrecognized case of CCHD would actually be more than the cost of screening more than 2000 neonates for CCHD [33]. Based on the existing literature, the cost-effectiveness of pulse oximetry screening for identifying CCHD has been demonstrated.

LIMITATIONS OF PULSE OXIMETRY SCREENING

There are several limitations to pulse oximetry screening for CCHD in neonates. One of the most important limitations is that pulse oximetry screening does not exclude all types of CCHD and other congenital heart disease lesions. Given that the sensitivity of pulse oximetry screening for CCHD is 75%, approximately 25% of neonates with CCHD are not detected by pulse oximetry screening alone. Therefore, clinicians and caretakers must be educated about these potential patients with false-negative results, so that other clinical characteristics of CCHD are not ignored.

Characteristics of severe congenital heart disease that are not detected or may be missed by pulse oximetry screening are distinct. These characteristics include that the defects do not always depend on a patent ductus arteriosus for systemic or pulmonary blood flow, they do not necessarily have mixing of arterial and venous blood, and they may have normal oxygen saturations in room air. Box 2 lists the types of congenital heart disease lesions that could be potentially missed by pulse oximetry screening for CCHD with the most frequently missed lesion listed first (coarctation of the aorta) [32,43].

Coarctation of the aorta and interrupted aortic arch are the most commonly missed CCHD lesions by pulse oximetry screening after 24 hours of life. Unfortunately, these same lesions are often missed during anatomy ultrasonographic scans at 18 to 20 weeks gestation as well as during neonatal physical examinations. A recent study out of the United Kingdom described their

---

Box 2: Congenital heart disease lesions that may be missed by pulse oximetry screening in order of frequency

1. Coarctation of the aorta
2. Pulmonic stenosis
3. Tetralogy of Fallot
4. Ventricular septal defect
5. Atrial septal defect
6. Patent ductus arteriosus
7. Atrioventricular canal
8. Interrupted aortic arch
9. Double outlet right ventricle
10. Single ventricle
11. Truncus arteriosus
12. Total anomalous pulmonary venous return
13. Aortic stenosis

experience with CCHD diagnoses missed by neonatal pulse oximetry screening. This group reported that 75% of the neonates who had missed CCHD diagnoses had some form of aortic obstruction [44].

Before implementation of pulse oximetry screening for CCHD in newborns, a population-based study out of California demonstrated that coarctation of the aorta was frequently not diagnosed before newborn discharge. In addition, this group reported that TOF and HLHS were also frequently missed. The median age of death for these neonates was before 2 weeks of age. It is unclear, before CCHD screening, if these neonates could have been diagnosed by routine pediatric physical examination as part of a well-child check. If these neonates were demonstrating signs of congestive heart failure (Box 3) at the time of their follow-up appointment, a diagnosis may have been possible [45,46]. Since the implementation of CCHD screening, one would expect to see that TOF and HLHS would be diagnosed with increased frequency, but the challenge still remains with diagnosing aortic obstruction in a timely manner [17].

CURRENT STATUS OF EXISTING SCREENING PROGRAMS
New Jersey was the first state to mandate pulse oximetry screening for CCHD in newborns in 2011. Clinicians from New Jersey published their experience of screening during the first 9 months after implementation of the program. New Jersey was successful in screening more than 99% of the more than 75,000 neonates who were born during this period. Three neonates were diagnosed with CCHD solely based on pulse oximetry screening. The 3 diagnoses captured included TGA, tricuspid atresia, and coarctation of the aorta with aortic arch hypoplasia. In total, 49 neonates failed the pulse oximetry screening with an overall failure rate of 0.067%. A total of 30 infants required a diagnostic evaluation for CCHD based on screening alone. A total of 17 infants had significant findings other than CCHD. These diagnosis included VSD (non-CCHD), pulmonary hypertension, pneumonia, and sepsis. The 10 other neonates who screened positive did not have any other abnormalities. Overall, in

---

Box 3: Characteristics of neonatal congestive heart failure

Poor weight gain

Poor feeding

Respiratory distress

Hypoxemia

Cyanosis

Irritability

Sweating

Decreased activity/lethargy

Delay in milestones

the first 9 months of the screening program in New Jersey, the false-positive rate was very low at 0.04%. The demonstrated success in New Jersey's pulse oximetry screening program for CCHD has been an example for other programs throughout the United States.

New Jersey has published their initial data, whereas other states remain in the early stages of implementation. On perusal of the existing literature, several states have generally available Web sites to give the public information about their individual state programs. Information on state programs that include Utah, Michigan, Tennessee, and others are readily available on the Internet.

MODEL CHARACTERISTICS OF CRITICAL CONGENITAL HEART DISEASE SCREENING PROGRAMS

As many states are in the early stages of implementing CCHD screening programs, several important characteristics of a successful screening program should be noted. In order for a CCHD pulse oximetry screening program to be effective, there should be formal education programs at individual institutions. Nurses and physicians in the well-baby nursery and neonatal intensive care unit must understand what the screening entails. All clinicians must achieve a level of competency in performing the screening and should take part in continuing medical educational sessions to ensure that at least a minimum level of competency is maintained. In addition, appropriate information must be distributed to and reviewed with families around the time of the screening. The importance of communication between families and clinicians as well as among clinicians themselves cannot be overestimated; this is especially true about communication between the clinicians caring for the baby and the consulting cardiologists and family pediatricians. In addition, the process of CCHD screening should be standardized among individual institutions with the goal of standardizing care between health care institutions. Box 4 lists the characteristics of a CCHD screening program that are essential to centralizing and standardizing CCHD screening in newborns to allow for information sharing [35].

Box 4: Goals of a standardized CCHD screening program

Use standardized screening algorithm

Use consistent equipment and supplies

Screen all eligible newborns

Maintain consistent educational programs

Establish a CCHD database

Link screening to medical record

Link positive screen results to health department

Communication with outpatient caregiver

SUMMARY

CCHD affects more than 25% of neonates born with congenital heart disease. Patients with CCHD require timely intervention in the form of surgery or cardiac catheterization to survive. These interventions may improve survival and outcomes for these patients. There is strong evidence that performing newborn pulse oximetry screening after the first 24 hours of life may help to detect more than 1200 neonates in the United States each year with CCHD.

Pulse oximetry screening for CCHD has been demonstrated to be reasonable to implement and seems to be cost-effective. There is evidence that asymptomatic patients with CCHD can be diagnosed before clinical presentation or cardiovascular collapse with this screening. Pulse oximeter screening has been endorsed by several national organizations as a valuable newborn screening tool.

Implementation of pulse oximetry screening programs in a standardized manner with strong communication among all involved parties will likely improve outcomes as well. As we move forward, we as clinicians should work to have a centralized system of reporting positive CCHD results, prompt patient evaluation, and good follow-up for the families of those neonates with positive screening results. Achieving these objectives will likely help us to achieve the goal of improving outcomes of the most critical neonates with CCHD.

References

[1] Hoffman JL, Kaplan S. The incidence of congenital heart disease. J Am Coll Cardiol 2002;39(12):1890–900.

[2] Reller MD, Strickland MJ, Riehle-Colarusso T, et al. Prevalence of congenital heart defects in Atlanta, 1998–2005. J Pediatr 2008;153:807–13.

[3] Lee K, Khoshnood B, Chen L, et al. Infant mortality from congenital malformations in the United States, 1970–1997. Obstet Gynecol 2001;98:620–7.

[4] Mai CT, Riehle-Colarusso T, O'Halloran A, et al. Selected birth defects from population-based birth defects surveillance programs in United States, 2005–2009: featuring critical congenital heart defects targeted for pulse oximetry screening. Birth Defects Res A Clin Mol Teratol 2012;94:970–83.

[5] Koppel RI, Druschel CM, Carter T. Effectiveness of pulse oximetry screening for congenital heart disease in asymptomatic newborns. Pediatrics 2003;111:451–5.

[6] Schultz AH, Localio AR, Clark BJ, et al. Epidemiologic features of the presentation of critical congenital heart disease: implications for screening. Pediatrics 2008;121(4):751–7.

[7] Pickert CB, Moss MM, Fiser DH. Differentiation of systemic infection and congenital obstructive left heart disease in the very young infant. Pediatr Emerg Care 1998;14:263.

[8] Boneva RS, Botto LD, Moore CA, et al. Mortality associated with congenital heart defects in the United States: trends and racial disparities 1979–1997. Circulation 2001;103(19):2376–81.

[9] Mahle WT, Martin GR, Beekman RH III, et al. Endorsement of health and human services recommendation for pulse oximetry screening for critical congenital heart disease. Pediatrics 2012;129(1):190–2.

[10] Oster ME, Lee KA, Honein MA, et al. Temporal trends in survival among infants with critical congenital heart defects. Pediatrics 2013;131:e1502–8.

[11] Fixler DE, Xu P, Nembhard WM, et al. Age at referral and mortality from CCHD. Pediatrics 2014;134:e95–105.

[12] Morris SA, Ethen MK, Penny DJ, et al. Prenatal diagnosis, birth location, surgical center, and neonatal mortality in infants with hypoplastic left heart syndrome. Circulation 2014;129: 285–92.
[13] Forbess JM, Visconti KJ, Hancock-Friesen C, et al. Neurodevelopmental outcome after congenital heart surgery. Circulation 2002;106:I95–102.
[14] Miller SP, McQuillen PS, Hamrick S, et al. Abnormal brain development in newborns with congenital heart disease. N Engl J Med 2007;357(19):1928–38.
[15] Blyth M, Howe D, Gnanapragasam J, et al. The hidden mortality of transposition of the great arteries and survival advantage provided by prenatal diagnosis. BJOG 2008;115: 1096–100.
[16] Fuchs B, Muller H, Abdul-Khaliq H, et al. Immediate and long-term outcomes in children with prenatal diagnosis of selected isolated congenital heart defects. Ultrasound Obstet Gynecol 2007;29:38–43.
[17] Chang RK, Gurvitz M, Rodriguez S. Missed diagnosis of critical congenital heart disease. Arch Pediatr Adolesc Med 2008;162:969.
[18] Wren C, Richmond S, Donaldson L. Presentation of congenital heart disease in infancy: implications for routine examination. Arch Dis Child Fetal Neonatal Ed 1999;80:F49.
[19] Ainsworth S, Wyllie JP, Wren C. Prevalence and clinical significance of cardiac murmurs in neonates. Arch Dis Child Fetal Neonatal Ed 1999;80:F43.
[20] United States Department of Health and Human Services (US DHHS), Centers for Disease Control and Prevention (CDC), National Center for Health Statistics (NCHS), Division of Vital Statistics, Natality public-use data 2007–2012, on CDC WONDER Online Database. Available at: http://wonder.cdc.gov/natality-current.html. Accessed December 12, 2014.
[21] Friedburg MK, Silverman NH, Moon-Grady AJ, et al. Prenatal detection of congenital heart disease. J Pediatr 2009;155:26–31.
[22] Ogge G, Gaglioti P, Maccanti S, et al. Prenatal screening for congenital heart disease with four-chamber and outflow-tract views: a multicenter study. Ultrasound Obstet Gynecol 2006;28:779–84.
[23] Garg LF, Van Naarden Braun K, Knapp MM, et al. Results from the New Jersey statewide critical congenital heart defects screening program. Pediatrics 2013;132:e314–23.
[24] Newborn Foundation Coalition, distributed under a creative commons license CC BY-ND. Available at: www.cchdscreeningmap.org. Accessed December 12, 2014.
[25] Jopling J, Henry E, Wiedmeier SE, et al. Reference ranges for hematocrit and blood hemoglobin concentration during the neonatal period: data from a multihospital healthcare system. Pediatrics 2009;123:e333–7.
[26] O'Donnell CP, Kamlin CO, Davis PG, et al. Clinical assessment of infant colour at delivery. Arch Dis Child Fetal Neonatal Ed 2007;92:F465–7.
[27] Walsh W. Evaluation of pulse oximetry screening in Middle Tennessee: cases for consideration before universal screening. J Perinatol 2011;31:125–9.
[28] Available at: https://health.state.tn.us/MCH/NBS/PDFs/CCHD_Screening_Protocol_Algorithm.pdf. Accessed December 12, 2014.
[29] Available at: http://www.aap.org/en-us/advocacy-and-policy/aap-health-initiatives/PEHDIC/Pages/Newborn-Screening-for-CCHD.aspx. Accessed December 12, 2014.
[30] Herman CR, Gill HK, Eng J, et al. Screening for preclinical disease: test and disease characteristics. Am J Roentgenol 2002;179:825–31.
[31] Peterson C, Grosse SD, Oster ME, et al. Cost-effectiveness of routine screening for critical congenital heart disease in US newborns. Pediatrics 2013;132:e595–603.
[32] Thangaratinam S, Brown K, Zamora J, et al. Pulse oximetry screening for critical congenital heart defects in asymptomatic newborn babies: a systematic review and meta-analysis. Lancet 2012;379(9835):2459–65.
[33] De-Wahl Granelli A, Wennergren M, Sandberg K, et al. Impact of pulse oximetry screening on the detection of duct dependent congenital heart disease: a Swedish prospective screening study in 39,821 newborns. BMJ 2009;338:a3037.

[34] Fahy B, Lareau S, Sockrider M. Pulse oximetry. Am J Respir Crit Care Med 2011;184:P1–2.

[35] Kemper AR, Mahle WT, Martin GR, et al. Strategies for implementing screening for critical congenital heart disease. Pediatrics 2011;128:e1–11.

[36] Reich JD, Connolly B, Bradley G, et al. The reliability of a single pulse oximetry reading as a screening test for congenital heart disease in otherwise asymptomatic newborn infants. Pediatr Cardiol 2008;29:885–9.

[37] Oster ME, Kuo KW, Mahle WT. Quality improvement in screening for critical congenital heart disease. J Pediatr 2014;164:67–71.

[38] Beissel DJ, Goetz EM, Hokanson JS. Pulse oximetry screening in Wisconsin. Congenit Heart Dis 2012;7:460–5.

[39] Webb CL, Waugh CL, Grisby J, et al. Impact of telemedicine on hospital transport, length of stay, and medical outcomes in infants with suspected heart disease: a multicenter study. J Am Soc Echocardiogr 2013;26:1090–8.

[40] Peterson AL, Srinivasan S, Hokanson J. Evaluating newborns for critical congenital heart disease: expanding the availability of diagnostic echocardiography. Neonatology Today 2014;9:1–6.

[41] Ewer AK, Middleton LJ, Furmston AT, et al. Pulse Ox Study Group. Pulse oximetry for screening for congenital heart disease in newborn infants (Pulse Ox): a test accuracy study. Lancet 2011;378:785–94.

[42] Thilo EH, Park-Moore B, Berman ER, et al. Oxygen saturation by pulse oximetry in healthy infants at an altitude of 1610 m (5280 ft): what is normal? Am J Dis Child 1991;145:1137–40.

[43] Ewer AK. Pulse oximetry screening for critical congenital heart disease in newborn infants: should it be routine? Arch Dis Child Fetal Neonatal Ed 2014;99(1):F93–5.

[44] Prudhoe S, Abu-Harb M, Richmond S, et al. Neonatal screening for critical cardiovascular anomalies using pulse oximetry. Arch Dis Child Fetal Neonatal Ed 2013;98:F346–50.

[45] Aisenberg RB, Rosenthal A, Nadas AS, et al. Developmental delay in infants with congenital heart disease. Correlation with hypoxemia and congestive heart failure. Pediatr Cardiol 1982;3:133.

[46] Sharma M, Nair MN, Jatana SK, et al. Congestive heart failure in infants and children. Med J Armed Forces India 2003;59:228–33.

Advances in Pediatrics 62 (2015) 227–255

ADVANCES IN PEDIATRICS

ELSEVIER
MOSBY

Vascular Anomalies in Pediatrics

Lisa S. Foley, MD, Ann M. Kulungowski, MD*

Division of Pediatric Surgery, Department of Surgery, Children's Hospital Colorado, University of Colorado School of Medicine, 13123 East 16th Avenue, Aurora, CO 80045, USA

Keywords

- Hemangioma • Vascular anomaly • Vascular malformation • Venous malformation
- Lymphatic malformation • Arteriovenous malformation
- Kaposiform hemangioendothelioma

Key points

- A standardized classification system allows improvements in diagnostic accuracy.
- Vascular anomalies are divided into two groups: vascular tumors and vascular malformations.
- Multidisciplinary vascular anomaly centers combine medical, surgical, radiologic, and pathologic expertise.

INTRODUCTION

For centuries, vascular birthmarks were referred to by vernacular names derived from the belief that a mother's emotions can affect her child's appearance. The modern era of vascular anomalies started in 1982 when Mulliken and Glowacki divided the field into hemangiomas and malformations [1]. The classification was refined to tumors and malformations in 1996 and updated by the International Society for the Study of Vascular Anomalies in 2014 (Tables 1 and 2) [2]. Vascular anomalies are confusing due to imprecise terminology and similar appearance of distinct lesions [3]. Vascular anomalies affect the endothelium of capillaries, arteries, veins, or lymphatics. The estimated prevalence is 4.5% [3,4]. Vascular tumors are characterized by endothelial hyperplasia. This group consists of hemangiomas and less common pediatric tumors. Vascular malformations occur due to errors in morphogenesis and exhibit normal endothelial turnover. The current classification system provides a clinically useful method for diagnosis, prognosis, and treatment of

*Corresponding author. Division of Pediatric Surgery, 13123 East 16th Avenue, B323, Aurora, CO 80045. E-mail address: ann.kulungowski@childrenscolorado.org

0065-3101/15/$ – see front matter
http://dx.doi.org/10.1016/j.yapd.2015.04.009

Table 1		
Vascular tumors		
Benign	Locally aggressive or borderline	Malignant
IH	KHE	Angiosarcoma
CH	—	—
Rapidly involuting		
Noninvoluting		
Partially involuting		
Tufted angioma	—	—

vascular anomalies. An accurate diagnosis is made in 90% of infants and children with history and physical examination. Vascular anomalies are often apparent in infancy as the skin and soft tissues are affected. More and more, vascular anomalies are diagnosed antenatally due to advances in fetal medicine. Pediatricians may be called on to assist with the diagnosis of a vascular anomaly.

VASCULAR TUMORS
Vascular tumors are divided into 3 groups: benign, locally aggressive, and malignant [2]. Malignant vascular tumors is beyond the scope of this text.

Benign vascular tumors
The term, *hemangioma*, has been indiscriminately applied to many different types of vascular lesions. In general, there are 2 types of hemangioma: infantile and congenital.

Infantile hemangioma
Clinical features. Infantile hemangioma (IH) is the most common tumor of infancy and childhood, occurring in approximately 4% of children [5]. The incidence is lower in dark-skinned infants. Increased risk factors for IH include

Table 2		
Vascular malformations		
Simple	Combined	Associated with other anomalies
CM	CM + VM	Klippel-Trenaunay syndrome
	CM + LM	
	CM + AVM	
LM	LM + VM	CLOVES syndrome
	CM + LM + VM	
VM	—	Parkes Weber syndrome
AVM	CM + LM + VM + AVM	—
	CM + VM + AVM	
Arteriovenous fistula	—	—

white race, female gender, prematurity, low birth weight, and multiple gestations. The exact etiology and pathogenesis of IH is yet to be determined. Evidence suggests that IH may arise due to a defect in an endothelial or progenitor cell as either a somatic (postzygotic) or germline mutation [6]. Other hypotheses include a clonal origin of the endothelial cells involved in IHs [7].

IHs appear approximately 1 to 4 weeks after birth (Fig. 1). Deep IH presents later, between 2 and 3 months of age. Many IHs have a premonitory mark at birth, such as a faint macular stain, small pale spot, or ecchymotic area [8]. IHs may be classified by their depth of soft tissue involvement: superficial, deep, and mixed [9,10]. Additionally, IHs are divided by whether they are spatially confined (localized) or whether they cover a territory (regional or segmental) [10,11]. The appearance of IH changes with location. Superficial IHs may be bright erythematous macules, papules, or plaques; deep IHs appear as blue nodules or a combination thereof [12]. IHs are usually small and localized and do not involve aesthetically or functionally vital structures [8,13].

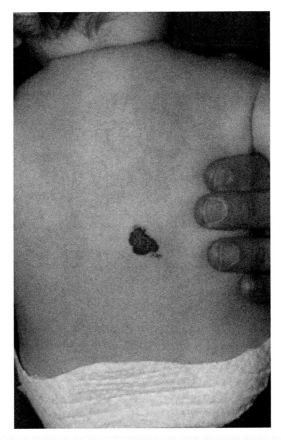

Fig. 1. Typical appearance of IH on the back of a 4-month-old infant.

IHs have a classic pattern of growth in infancy followed by spontaneous involution. Maximal tumor proliferation often is achieved by 3 months [10]. Superficial IHs have accelerated growth between 4 and 7 weeks [14]; deep IHs present 1 month later and proliferate longer than superficial lesions. Growth may be observed until 10 months of age. Based on these characteristics of tumor growth, therapies, if indicated, are ideally commenced prior to 3 months of age. Tumor involution occurs over several years and is nearly complete by 4 years of age [15,16]. IHs are found in the head and neck, trunk, extremities, and perineum; they may also be found in the viscera, most commonly the liver. Patients with multiple IHs, 5 or more, are screened for associated hepatic lesions by abdominal ultrasonography.

Because IHs are so diverse in size, location, and growth characteristics, decisions regarding when to treat them require an organized approach. IHs can be divided into 3 distinct groups based on risk of complications and location (Table 3) [17]. Regional (also referred to as segmental) IHs are frequently associated with complications, including ulceration, bleeding, infection, airway obstruction, visual impairment, and cardiac compromise. The most common complication of IH is ulceration, occurring in 10% to 15% of patients.

Approximately half of patients with IH have permanently damaged or redundant skin, scarring, telangiectasias, discoloration, or a fibrofatty residuum at the end of involution [8]. Permanent tissue destruction and distortion can result from an ulcerated IH involving the eyelid, nasal tip, lip, ear, or perineum. Patients with regional IHs of the lower face (beard distribution) may have associated upper airway and subglottic involvement. An infant may present with poor feeding, noisy breathing, hoarseness, and later with biphasic stridor at approximately 6 to 12 weeks of age [8]. A small periorbital IH can deform the cornea, causing astigmatism, or even block the visual axis and cause

Table 3
Risk stratification of infantile hemangomia

Risk group	Clinical features	Rationale for intervention
Low	Trunk, arms, legs (nonvisible) <5 cm	Low risk of disfigurement or functional compromise
Intermediate	Lateral face, scalp, hands, feet	Lower risk of disfigurement
	Body folds (neck, perineum, axilla)	Risk of ulceration
	Segmental >5 cm—trunk, arms, legs	Risk of ulceration, permanent residual skin changes
High	Segmental >5 cm—face, lumbosacral/perineal area	Possible PHACE, LUMBAR, scarring, ulceration, visual/airway compromise
	Early white discoloration	Marker of ulceration
	Central face, periorbital/nasal/oral	High risk of disfigurement; functional compromise
	Bulky lesion—face	Tissue distortion, scarring, risk of disfigurement

deprivation amblyopia. Other severe complications from IHs include cardiac failure, gastrointestinal (GI) bleeding, hypothyroidism, or abdominal compartment syndrome.

Associated syndromes. Most IHs occur solely as a cutaneous disease; however, segmental IHs confined to an anatomic territory deserve attention. There are 2 major groupings: PHACE and LUMBAR association. The acronym PHACE refers to posterior fossa abnormalities, hemangiomas, arterial cerebrovascular anomalies (eg, aneurysm, occlusion, stenosis, or persistent intra- and extracranial embryonic arteries), cardiac defects (eg, aortic coarctation or right-sided aortic arch), and eye abnormalities (eg, microphthalmia, cogenital cataract, or optic nerve hypoplasia). PHACES is the appropriate term when ventral defects, such as sternal clefting or supraumbilical raphe, are present [18–20]. More girls are affected with PHACE association, as high as 9:1, compared with 3:1 in IH [21]. Many patients with PHACE association do not have all the findings. The evaluation for a patient with PHACE(S) association includes an MRI and magnetic resonance angiography, echocardiogram, and ophthalmologic evaluation [17,22].

Large segmental IHs overlying the lumbosacral or perineal regions can be associated with structural anomalies. The acronym LUMBAR refers to lower-body IH, urogenital anomalies, ulceration, myelopathy, bony deformities, arterial and renal anomalies, and anorectal malformations [23–25]. The initial findings may be the anorectal malformations or genitourinary anomalies. Cutaneous involvement with IH may present days to weeks later. IHs involving the perineum are prone to ulceration. Furthermore, 50% of patients with a large lumbosacral IH have an associated intraspinal abnormality, such as tethered cord or intraspinal hemangioma [26]. Ultrasonography is used to screen infants less than 4 months of age for the presence of occult spinal dysraphism; MRI may be necessary in older children [27].

Radiologic features. A majority of IHs can be diagnosed by history and physical examination. Ultrasonography can assist with the diagnosis in deep and hepatic IHs. Ultrasonographic features of IH include a discrete soft tissue mass, decreased arterial resistance, and increased venous flow [28]. A proliferating IH on MRI demonstrates a well-circumscribed densely lobulated mass with uniform enhancement. Dilated feeding and draining vessels may be observed. IHs are isointense on T1 and hyperintense on T2 [29].

Pathology. Histologically, IHs are comprised of densely packed plump endothelial cells that form small capillaries. Endothelial proliferation is present during tumor expansion. Endothelial cells of IHs are immunopositive for glucose transporter-1 protein (GLUT-1). GLUT-1 is absent in other vascular anomalies [30].

Management. Observation and parental reassurance are the mainstay of management because most IHs are small and localized [8]. Active nonintervention can distress many parents. Numerous discussions with the family may be necessary to counsel the family about a tumor's natural history. Disfiguring hemangiomas may evoke parental emotions of loss and grief [31]. Frequent follow-up with serial photographs is useful to follow progress.

Ulceration is the most frequent complication of IHs. Local treatments include nonadherent occlusive dressings, topical or oral antibiotics, and pain medications. Superficial ulceration usually heals within days to weeks; a deep ulceration may take longer [8]. Pulsed dye laser may accelerate healing but carries the risk of ulceration. Topical timolol or intralesional corticosteroid (triamcinolone acetonide) may be used for small IHs of the nasal tip, cheek, lip, or eyelid during the proliferative phase [32]. Intralesional corticosteroid injections may be repeated every 4 weeks. Periorbital injection of corticosteroid is rarely associated with blindness due to embolic debris occluding the retinal or ophthalmic arteries [33,34].

Systemic pharmacologic intervention to treat IHs may be necessary for those lesions that are ulcerated, threaten vital function, or risk permanent disfigurement. The challenge is determining which infants are at risk. Oral propranolol has replaced oral corticosteroid as first-line therapy (Fig. 2). Since the initial report of propranolol for the use of IH, there have been numerous additional publications all with different protocols describing its administration [35,36]. Current recommendations include outpatient initiation of propranol for infants older than 8 weeks of age (corrected for gestation and no comorbidities), pretreatment electrocardiogram, and a target dose of 1 to 3 mg/kg/d divided 3 times daily [37]. Patients are monitored with heart rate and blood pressure measurements for the first 2 hours after receiving the initial dose and for

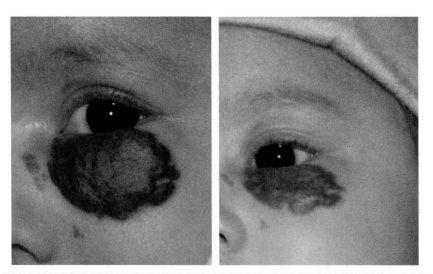

Fig. 2. IH. (*Left*) Two-month-old infant with an IH near the left eye. (*Right*) Appearance of the IH 1 month after initiation of propranolol.

dose increase (>0.5 mg/kg/d) [37]. Reported serious adverse effects of propranolol include hypoglycemia, bronchospasm, and hypotension [38–40]. Hypoglycemia is avoided by frequent feeding, avoiding prolonged periods or sleep, and medication cessation during fasting or illness [37]. Duration of treatment is 1 year, corresponding to the growth phase of the tumor. Relapse occurs in 25% of tumors especially for deep and segmental IHs [41].

Other systemic medications include corticosteroid, vincristine, and interferon. Side effects of corticosteroid include cushingoid facies, irritability, *Pneumocystis carinii*, GI reflux, delayed growth, cardiomyopathy, and hypertension [42–44]. Vincristine mandates a central venous catheter and may cause peripheral neuropathy, anemia, and leukopenia. Interferon is associated with spastic diplegia [45,46].

Surgical indications for excision of an IH vary by patient age and tumor stage. In infancy, a proliferative lesion that obstructs function, like an eyelid or airway hemangioma, may be excised. Excision during the involuting phase may be needed if scarring has occurred. Because many IHs involute completely, waiting until the involuted phase is a reasonable approach as long as there are no complications. Amazingly, the skin of an involuted IH can look normal. Excision of an involuted IH is indicated for damaged skin, for contour deformity, or to treat fibrofatty residua. Telangiectasia or superficial discoloration can be addressed in the involuted phase with pulsed dye laser therapy.

Congenital hemangioma

Congenital hemangiomas (CHs) present fully formed at birth and do not undergo postnatal expansion. They are usually solitary and present as a thickened plaque or exophytic mass of the head, neck, or extremities. There is no gender bias. There are at least 2 subtypes of lesions: rapidly involuting CH (RICH) and noninvoluting CH (NICH) (Fig. 3). Recently, an additional subtype, a partially involuting CH (PICH) has been described [47].

The incidence of CHs is unknown, but they are much less common than IHs. CHs are further distinguished from IHs by their lack of immunostaining

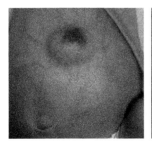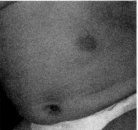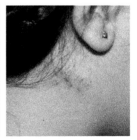

Fig. 3. CH. (*Left*) Three-week-old infant with abdominal wall mass consistent with CH. (*Middle*) Three months later, there is evidence of tumor regression confirming a RICH. (*Right*) Eight-year-old girl with an NICH of the neck.

for GLUT-1. Histopathologically, RICH and NICH appear as small to large lobules of capillary proliferations embedded in a dense fibrous stroma with surrounding large dysplastic vessels [48,49].

As the name implies, RICHs are characterized by earlier onset of involution, often beginning before birth and completing their involution on average between 6 and 14 months of age [50]. There are several morphologic variants described: a raised violaceous soft tissue mass with a prominent draining vein; a soft tissue mass with overlying telangiectasias with a surrounding peripheral pale halo; or a pink to violaceous soft tissue tumor with a deeper dermal or subcutaneous infiltration [12,49]. RICHs can range in size from a few centimeters to greater than 10 cm. Ulceration is problematic because it can result in hemorrhage. Thrombocytopenia and coagulopathy may be observed in the first 2 weeks of life with large RICHs. In contrast to Kasabach-Merritt phenomenon (KMP) associated with other vascular tumors, these laboratory abnormalities are self-limited and usually not complicated by bleeding [51]. After tumor involution, the residual area can appear deflated and lacks the usual fatty component of IHs [49].

NICHs and RICHs can present similarly, but NICHs are flatter and present as pink to purple plaques with overlying telangiectasia. They average 5 cm in size [52]. NICHs do not regress, rather persist and grow commensurate with somatic growth [52]. PICHs begin as RICHs but fail to completely involute and persist as an NICH-like lesion [47].

CHs are mostly diagnosed based on clinic findings. MRI and ultrasonography may help clarify the diagnosis. RICHs and NICHs show a predominant heterogeneous vascular structure with visible vessels. On MRI, RICHs exhibit large flow voids, heterogenous enhancement, and hyperintensity on T2-weighted sequences [53]. Prenatal detection of CHs is possible because these lesions form in utero [50,54,55].

CHs can be confused with infantile fibrosarcoma, vascular malformations, or other vascular tumors [56]. A biopsy is indicated when the diagnosis is unclear. The biopsy should be performed in a controlled setting due to the risk of bleeding. The specimen should include the periphery of the lesion because the lobular architecture is preserved in CHs [49].

Management of CHs is similar to IHs. Active observation and anticipatory guidance is a common therapy. Some CHs may require intervention based on location or bleeding. Disfigurement is managed with surgical excision of redundant skin or pulsed dye laser for telangiectasia. Surgical excision is the treatment of choice for larger, symptomatic lesions [12].

Hepatic hemangioma

Hepatic hemangiomas (HHs) must be differentiated from misnamed HHs observed in adulthood; these are venous malformation (VMs). HHs of infancy are true vascular tumors. The life cycle of HHs parallels their cutaneous counterparts. HHs are classified based on morphology: focal, multifocal, and diffuse [57]. Each category exhibits its own unique imaging, histopathologic, and physiologic characteristics [57]. Most HHs are not clinically significant and involute entirely without altering the hepatic parenchyma.

Focal HH is likely the hepatic equivalent of the cutaneous rapidly involuting congential hemangioma (RICH) (Fig. 4). Like a cutaneous RICH, focal HHs are fully formed at birth and involute faster than typical IHs. Focal HHs exhibit no gender predilection and are infrequently associated with cutaneous IHs [58]. Focal HHs, like a cutaneous RICH, can be detected on antenatal imaging [59]. Transient anemia and thrombocytopenia are related to intralesional central thrombosis and are self-limited. Focal HHs are GLUT-1 negative. Focal HHs usually present as an abdominal mass in an otherwise healthy infant. High-output cardiac failure due to the presence of shunts (arteriovenous or portovenous) is observed in some lesions. As the tumor involutes, the shunts usually close. Embolization may be necessary to occlude the larger shunts in the face of heart failure while protecting major hepatic vessels. Pharmacologic therapy is likely of no benefit. Focal HHs involute rapidly and are biologically distinct from IHs. Resection or hepatic transplantation is rarely necessary. Focal HHs are centrally hypodense due to thrombosis or necrosis on CT. They exhibit centripetal enhancement. The peripheral rim HH is more dense with contrast than the normal hepatic parenchyma. This is in distinction to hepatoblastoma. Hepatoblastoma also exhibits peripheral enhancement but is more similar to normal liver [60]. Dilation of the proximal abdominal aorta and hepatic arteries and veins is observed particularly if there are macrovascular shunts. A reduced caliber aorta is seen distally. Calcifications can also be evident and become more prominent with tumor involution [61]. Focal HH on MRI reveals a well-defined, solitary, spherical tumor that is hypointense relative to liver on T1-weighted sequences and hyperintense on T2-weighted sequences. The solid, noninvoluted portions, usually at the periphery of the

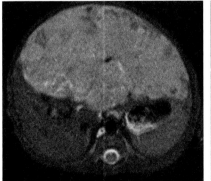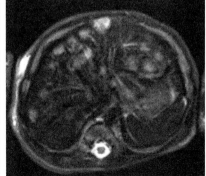

Fig. 4. Axial T2-weighted fat-saturation MRI of HHs. (*Left*) A focal HH is identified in the left lobe of the liver that is solitary and hyperintense relative to liver. (*Right*) Multifocal HH shows that tumors are hyperintense relative to liver.

lesion, demonstrate intense homogeneous enhancement, especially on gadolinium sequences. The center exhibits heterogeneous enhancement where areas of necrosis, thrombosis, or intralesional hemorrhage have occurred [57].

Multifocal HH and diffuse HH are true IHs both by histopathology and natural history. They occur in a spectrum. Multifocal HHs are randomly distributed throughout the liver; they are widely spaced with intervening normal hepatic parenchyma (see Fig. 4). Diffuse HHs exhibit near-total hepatic parenchymal replacement by innumerable, densely packed nodular lesions. There is a female preponderance in both groups. These lesions are GLUT-1 positive. Many infants with multifocal HH are asymptomatic. A diagnosis of multifocal HH is often made while screening for visceral hemangioma based on the finding of multiple cutaneous IHs. Shunting causing high-output cardiac failure is more frequent in multifocal HHs than in focal lesions. Infants with diffuse HH are more likely to have a serious clinical course. Massive hepatomegaly causes compression of the inferior vena cava and thoracic cavity leading to abdominal compartment syndrome and respiratory failure. All his express type-3 iodothyronine deiodinase, which inactivates biologically active thyroid hormone [62]. The rapid breakdown of thyroid hormone in multifocal and more commonly diffuse HH results in profound hypothyroidism, which can exacerbate cardiac failure and lead to developmental delay [62]. Exogenous thyroid replacement and endocrinologic consultation are imperative. Thyroid-stimulating hormone level should be evaluated in multifocal and diffuse HH. Propranolol has become the pharmacologic agent of choice for symptomatic multifocal and diffuse HH patients with cardiac failure, abdominal distention, or hypothyroidism [63]. Propanolol hastens tumor involution thus ameliorating cardiac failure and hypothyroidism. In more severe cases, embolization can be used to improve heart failure but carries considerable risk. Infants with HH should be followed closely with serial abdominal ultrasonography until involution of their hemangioma. Multifocal and diffuse HH on CT appear as well-defined, spherical lesions. The lesions are hypodense compared with liver without contrast; they enhance centripetally with contrast. Multifocal HHs have normal liver parenchyma between lesions. Diffuse HHs exhibit total parenchymal replacement with tumor. The hepatic arteries and veins and supraceliac aorta are large, indicative of shunting [61]. The aorta is narrowed distally. Flow-voids may be seen in and adjacent to the lesions. On MRI, tumors enhance homogenously and are hypointense relative to liver on T1-weighted sequencing and hyperintense on T2 (see Fig. 10) [61].

A liver hemangioma management treatment algorithm improves outcomes for infants with HH [57]. Close follow-up and frequent monitoring is mandatory for patients with HH because these infants can rapidly decompensate. If the diagnosis is unclear, percutaneous needle biopsy may be necessary to evaluate for malignancy. The differential diagnosis of HH includes arteriovenous malformation (AVM), arterioportal fistula, mesenchymal hamartoma, hepatoblastoma, angiosarcoma, and metastatic neuroblastoma.

Locally aggressive vascular tumor
Kaposiform hemangioendothelioma and Kasabach-Merritt phenomenon

Kaposiform hemangioendothelioma (KHE) is an uncommon vascular tumor often associated with KMP (Fig. 5). The cardinal features of KMP include an enlarging vascular lesion, thrombocytopenia, microangiopathic hemolytic anemia, and a mild consumptive coagulopathy [64]. The term, *KMP*, is regularly misused to describe thrombocytopenia associated with HH as well as a localized intravascular coagulopathy seen with some extensive VMs and lymphatic malformations (LMs).

KHE classically presents as a solitary lesion at birth or early infancy with an equal gender ratio. They are often a large (>5 cm), tense, edematous, violaceous, ill-defined plaque. KHEs typically occur on the trunk, extremities, axilla, groin, and retroperitoneum. KHEs exhibit episodic engorgement. Palpation reveals a warm lesion. Not all KHEs present with KMP. Smaller lesions may be spared [65]. It is generally accepted that tufted angioma (TA) and KHE are synonymous tumors. TAs present similarly; KMP may be evident [66,67]. The thrombocytopenia seen in KMP can be profound (<50 × 10⁹/mL). These infants are at risk for intracranial, pleural, pulmonary, peritoneal, and GI hemorrhage. Platelets become sequestered within the tumor. KHE may regress with time but complete involution is infrequent. The residual KHE often appears as a firm and fibrotic capillary malformation (CM).

Histopathology shows aggressive infiltration of normal tissues by sheets or lobules of spindled endothelial cells and dilated lymphatic channels. The vascular spaces are filled with hemosiderin and erythrocytes suggestive of stasis [68]. Unlike common IH, the endothelial cells of KHE do not express GLUT-1 [67]. MRI with and without gadolinium is the imaging modality of choice [37]. The tumor demonstrates enhanced signal on T2-weighted images. Additional characteristics include an infiltrative ill-defined tumor involving multiple contiguous layers with small feeding and draining vessels relative to tumor size. The

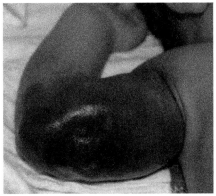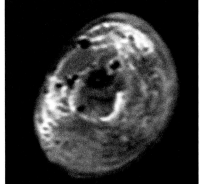

Fig. 5. KHE of the right arm. (*Left*) Two-day-old infant with KHE. (*Right*) Axial STIR images of the same infant's KHE revealing a diffusely infiltrative tumor that does not respect tissue planes.

skin thickening and edema appear as stranding in the subcutaneous fat due to lymphatic obstruction or invasion. Osteolysis may be apparent when KHE abuts the bone [68].

The treatment of KHE with KMP is primarily medical because the tumor is usually too extensive for surgical resection. First-line therapy for KHE with KMP includes with intravenous vincristine (0.05 mg/kg once weekly) and oral prednisolone (2 mg/kg/d) or intravenous methylprednisolone (1.6 mg/kg/d) [37]. For KHE not associated with KMP in need of intervention because of tumor growth or expansion, oral prednisolone (2 mg/kg/d) is recommended. Treatment with aspirin (at an antiplatelet dose of 2–5 mg/kg/d) may be administered as an adjunct [37]. Sirolimus is showing early promise for the treatment of KHE. In general, platelet transfusion is avoided. Platelets are indicated for active bleeding and around surgical procedures. Heparin is not indicated because of bleeding risk and minimal platelet effects. Cryoprecipitate or fresh frozen plasma is given for hypofibrinogenemia (<100 mg/dL). Careful monitoring is essential for patients with KHE.

VASCULAR MALFORMATIONS

Vascular malformations occur in up to 1.5% of the population and consist of lesions derived from aberrant embryonic development of vascular channels [69]. Distinct from vascular tumors, which exhibit postnatal growth due to endothelial proliferation, vascular malformations tend to exhibit growth commensurate with that of the child. These anomalies can be discrete or diffuse. Vascular malformations are divided into simple and combined based on type of vessels involved [2]. Simple malformations are further subdivided into subtypes. Combined vascular malformations are named according to involved vessels. Vascular malformations associated with anomalies are categorized separately [2].

Capillary malformation

CMs are commonly known as port-wine stains. CMs can be confused with the common vascular birthmarks of infancy, called nevus flammeus neonatorum, more popularly called angel kiss (on the forehead) and stork bite (on the nuchal area). CMs usually present as a sporadic, singular, red, flat, localized macule with a propensity for the head and neck (Fig. 6). There is an equal gender distribution. Histopathologic features include vessels within the superficial dermis with a relative paucity of surrounding nerves [70]. The lack of sympathetic innervation leads to ectatic vessels and accounts for the darker color and nodular expansion observed with aging [71]. CMs are also associated with soft tissue and bony overgrowth [72]. Radiographic features of cutaneous CM are nonspecific; soft tissue and skeletal hypertrophy is apparent on CT or MRI.

CMs may herald underlying abnormalities. CMs overlying the cervical or lumbar cord may signal an occult spinal dysraphism. CMs of the occiput can cover an encephalocele. A CM of the ophthalmic and maxillary distribution

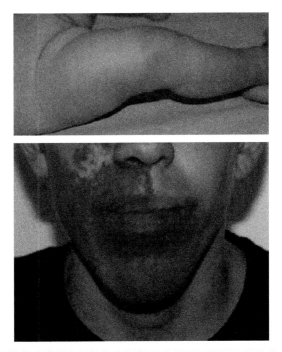

Fig. 6. Variable appearance of CM. (*Top*) CM of the right lower extremity. (*Bottom*) CM of the face associated with overgrowth of the lower lip.

warrants an evaluation for Sturge-Weber syndrome. This syndrome is composed of a facial CM with ipsilateral ocular and leptomeningeal vascular anomalies. Extensive leptomingeal involvement can manifest as seizures, contralateral hemiplegia, and developmental delays. Sturge-Weber syndrome is suggested by MRI, which reveals pial vascular enhancement. In later stages, gyriform cortical calcifications and cerebral atrophy are apparent.

Treatment of CMs is focused on lightening the stain. Pulsed dye laser treatment is the treatment of choice. Thin CMs of early infancy respond well to pulsed dye lasers, in particular lesions of the face, neck, and trunk. Complete eradication of CMs is unrealistic. Multiple pulsed dye laser sessions are necessary to achieve lightening. Treatment can be initiated at any age, including infancy [73]. Most CMs continue to darken with age.

Lymphatic malformation

LMs arise from embryologic disturbances of the developing lymphatic system. The embryonic lymphatics or lymphatic jugular sacs fail to connect or drain into the venous system. LMs are seen in a variety of forms, including cystic lymphatic lesions, angiokeratoma, chylous leak conditions, osseous lesions of Gorham-Stout disease, generalized lymphatic anomaly, and lymphedema.

LMs are usually identified at birth but may be discovered at any age (Fig. 7). There is no gender bias. LMs, unlike IHs, persist and do not involve. Some

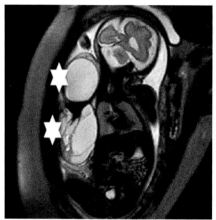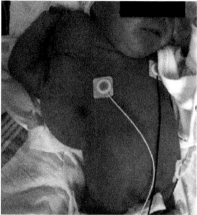

Fig. 7. LM. (*Left*) MRI T2-weighted sequences of a fetus with a large macrocystic LM of the right neck and shoulder (*stars*). (*Right*) Postnatal appearance of the same infant with an LM of the neck, shoulder, axilla, and chest wall.

lesions are localized whereas others exhibit diffuse infiltration of a single or multiple anatomic locations. LMs are more commonly seen in lymphatic-rich areas, such as the neck, axilla, groin, mediastinum, and retroperitoneum. There are 3 morphologic types of LMs: marocystic, microcystic, and combined (macrocystic and microcystic). In general, size is distinguished by whether or not the cystic cavity can be successfully aspirated to accomplish visible decompression. The usual presentation of a macrocystic lesion is a large mass that ranges from soft to firm. The overlying skin is normal with a deep blue hue. Microcystic lesions of the subcutis or submucosa appear as tiny variegated fluid filled vesicles. Intravesicular bleeding changes vesicles that are clear or white to red. In general, macrocystic LMs are located below the mylohyoid, whereas microcystic LMs are found above the mylohyoid muscle [74].

Histologically, LMs are composed of thin-walled vascular channels lined by a single layer of flattened endothelium. Lymphatic endothelial cells comprising the wall of the LM are immunopositive for podoplanin (D2-40) and lymphatic vessel endothelial hyaluronan receptor (LYVE)-1 [75]. The lumens may be empty or filled with eosinophilic and protein-rich fluid containing macrophages and lymphocytes [76]. Blood can also fill the channels, indicating spontaneous intralesional bleeding or trauma.

Increasingly, macrocystic LMs are detected on antenatal ultrasound [54]. The term, *cystic hygroma*, should not be applied to cystic lymphatic masses. The suffix, *-oma*, implies a tumor, which it is not. Furthermore, perinatologists use the term, *cystic hygroma*, to denote a posterior cervical cystic lesion associated with often lethal chromosomal abnormalities. Some families may receive misinformation regarding their true diagnosis and incorrectly believe that their fetus cannot survive. Amniocentesis and chromosomal analysis can be offered.

Antenatal consultation with pediatric specialists familiar with vascular anomalies can be beneficial and educational for families when a diagnosis of an LM is made in utero. This also allows planning for delivery and postnatal care especially when a large cervicofacial LM is diagnosed [54]. LM is not associated with chromosomal derangement or developmental disorders.

Some LMs present in certain anatomic patterns cause diagnostic and treatment challenges [77]. Consequences are anticipated depending on anatomic location and extent. One anatomic pattern is an LM, which involves the tongue, floor of mouth, neck, and mediastinum. These cervicofacial LMs can cause chronic airway problems, recurrent infection, and functional issues related to speech, oral hygiene, and malocclusion [78]. Large cervicofacial LMs diagnosed in utero should raise concern about potential airway obstruction leading to asphyxia in postnatal life. Fetal ultrasound and MRI allow evaluation of the airway. If the airway is deemed precarious, consideration should be given to deliver the fetus via an ex utero intrapartum treatment procedure [79]. Nevertheless, experience has shown that cervicofacial LMs are soft, which usually allows the infant to breathe spontaneously. Periorbital and orbital LMs can lead to proptosis. Hemorrhage or infection can cause swelling in the orbit leading to visual compromise. Thoracic lymphatic anomalies or rare abnormalities of the thoracic duct or cisterna chyli can manifest as chylous pericardial and pleural effusions and chylous ascites. GI LMs may present as a protein-losing enteropathy. Intrapelvic LMs can cause recurrent infections, constipation, and bladder outlet obstruction. LMs of the extremity can result in overgrowth and limb length discrepancy.

Lymphedema is also a type of LM. Lymphedema is the chronic, progressive swelling of tissue due to inadequate lymphatic function. The accumulation of protein-rich fluid in the interstitial space is followed by the deposition of fat and fibrous tissue [80]. Primary lymphedema occurs primarily from anomalous lymphatic development or secondarily from injury to lymphatic vessels or nodes. Lymphedema mostly affects the extremities followed by the genitalia [81]. Primary lymphedema is usually idiopathic, without a family history, and defined by age of onset: infancy, childhood, adolescence, and adulthood [82,83]. Primary lymphedema can have a genetic basis, such as mutations of *VEGFR3* (Milroy disease) and *FOXC2* (lymphedema distichiasis). Infection and malignancy are responsible for most cases of secondary lymphedema [84]. The diagnosis is made by clinical history and physical examination. Lymphoscintigraphy is a useful adjunct; it can confirm the diagnosis and delineate the pathogenesis by defining anatomic and functional derangements [85]. Lymphedema is incurable. Treatment is focused on compression regimens, maintenance of a normal body mass index, hygiene, and protection of the limb from incidental trauma.

Ultrasonography can characterize superficial, well-localized LMs. MRI is useful to determine the extent and type of LM. LMs are hyperintense on T2-weighted and turbo short tau inversion recovery (STIR) images [86]. Cystic rims and septae are more apparent with contrast. The differential diagnosis of an LM in an infant includes teratoma, infantile fibrosarcoma, and infantile my-ofibromatosis. Magnetic resonance lymphangiography is a useful method for evaluating lymphatic channels. Conventional contrast lymphangiography has largely been abandoned because of its excessive morbidity and technical difficulties in small children.

LMs are associated with numerous intrinsic complications [77]. Superficial LMs may leak lymph and blood. Traumatic or spontaneous intralesional bleeding can cause an LM to expand, leading to pain, inflammation, and compression of adjacent organs. LMs can enlarge in response to viral or bacterial infection. Depending on the location of the LM, visual disturbance, airway compression, pain, dysphagia, and difficulty with ambulation can occur. Analgesia, rest, and time may be all that are needed. Localized swelling accompanied by erythema and/or systemic signs of infection requires prompt administration of antibiotics. Retroperitoneal and mesenteric LMs can present in frank septic shock.

Treatment of LMs is varied and includes observation, pharmacotherapy, sclerotherapy, and surgical excision. Treatment is tailored according to size, location, and extent. There is insufficient evidence to create treatment algorithms for management of LMs. The treatment plan is, therefore, based on acuity, patient and family preference, and experience of the team.

Many pharmacotherapies have been proposed for the treatment of vascular malformations [87–89]. Sirolimus (rapamycin) has emerged at the forefront. Mammalian target of rapamycin (mTOR) is a serine/threonine kinase regulated by phosphoinositide 3-kinase. mTOR acts as a master switch for numerous cellular processes, including cellular metabolism, cell motility, angiogenesis, and cell growth [90]. Patients with life-threatening vascular malformations treated with sirolimus have responded favorably. Ongoing research is under way to determine the efficacy of this medication.

Image-guided percutaneous sclerotherapy is the often-preferred primary treatment modality. Sclerotherapy causes direct endothelial damage with subsequent luminal obliteration and fibrosis [91]. Success depends in part on the efficacy of the sclerosant. Multiple agents have been used, including pure ethanol, sodium tetradecyl sulfate, doxycycline, OK-432, and bleomycin. In general, doxycycline is the sclerosant of choice for macrocystic LM based on its efficacy and safety profile [92,93]. Bleomycin is gaining more popularity for treatment of microcystic disease [77]. Sclerotherapy is performed in an interventional radiology suite because fluoroscopy is used during the procedure. Access into the LM is performed under real-time ultrasound visualization. The lymphatic fluid is then aspirated. The sclerosant, such as solubilized doxycycline, is usually reconstituted in water and then injected into the cystic cavity. Multiple punctures, aspirations, and injections are frequently necessary. Sclerotherapy should be performed by knowledgeable personnel familiar with the inherent risks and discomforts, such as need for general anesthesia; post-therapy swelling, especially near the airway or in contained anatomic compartments; and potential toxicities of the sclerosants. Edema and pain at the site of sclerotherapy are expected consequences. Sclerotherapy results are not instantaneous, requiring weeks for scarring and fibrosis. Multiple procedures spaced weeks apart may be necessary. Advantages of sclerotherapy include no incisional scars, decrease chance of nerve injury, minimal leakage of fluid from puncture sites, opportunity for outpatient procedures, and ability to repeat procedures. Disadvantages are need for anesthesia, multiple procedures, exposure to radiation, skin and soft tissue necrosis, blistering, swelling causing obstruction of vital structures (especially the airway), and inability to completely treat the LM.

The only potential for a definitive cure of an LM is surgical resection. Focal, well-localized LMs are more amenable to safe surgical resection. In general, microcystic LMs tend to more be infiltrative and more difficult to resect surgically [77]. Staged excisions are often required [8]. In each resection, a surgeon should aim to limit the resection to a defined anatomic region, perform as thorough a dissection as possible without injuring vital structures, minimize blood loss, and perform closed suction drainage of the resection cavity. Most LMs do not respect anatomic planes. This makes surgical excision difficult and leads to incomplete resection and recurrence [94]. Recurrence is thought to be due to growth and expansion of affected lymphatics in the remaining, seemingly normal-appearing tissue. After resection, typical cutaneous warty vesicles can develop seen in the scar; this can be managed with cauterization, laser coagulation, or scar excision. A multidisciplinary approach involving surgeons and interventional radiologists is needed for patients with LMs, keeping in mind the patient's treatment goals and expectations.

Venous malformation

VMs occur in a variety of forms: simple varicosities and ectasias, discrete masses, or complex collections of channels permeating any tissue or organ system. They are regularly incorrectly labeled *cavernous hemangioma*. This nomenclature is antiquated and is inappropriate. VMs are slow-flow lesions consisting of venous channels that can develop anywhere in the body. VMs are thought to be related to a developmental defect of the vasculature. VMs can be anomalous anatomic veins or venous anomalies that are separate from named venous branches. Superficial VMs often present as soft, bluish, easily compressible masses (Fig. 8). VMs grow proportionately with the child and do not involute. VMs can be encountered throughout the body. CMs, LMs, and more rarely AVMs may be found in combination with VMs.

Histologically, VMs are composed of attenuated thin-walled, dilated vascular channels. The vascular smooth muscle is attenuated, which may account for the progressive, gradual expansion of VMs. A majority (90%) of VMs occur sporadically. Somatic mutations in the tyrosine kinase receptor TIE2 have been discovered in approximately 50% of sporadic VMs [95,96]. Glomovenous malformations comprise 5% of VMs and are related to a mutation of the glomulin gene [97]. The lesions may be scattered occurring as multiple blue nodules or as confluent plaques with a cobblestone surface frequently affecting the trunk of extremities [98].

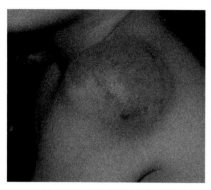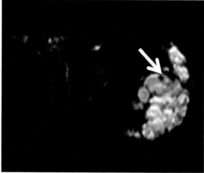

Fig. 8. VM. (*Left*) Six-year-old girl with VM of the right shoulder. (*Right*) MRI axial STIR images of the same VM. Pathognomonic phlebolith identified (*arrow*).

The most common symptom associated with VMs is pain. Patients frequently complain of pain and stiffness in the area of the VM [8]. The discomfort may be related to compression of adjacent structures like muscle, joints, and nerves. Venous stasis within VMs causes congestion. Phleboliths and small calcific thrombi and can also cause pain. VMs can be progressive, particularly during adolescence; pubertal hormones may contribute to expansion [99,100].

VMs can alter coagulation profiles, especially when extensive. A localized intravascular coagulopathy can occur due to blood stagnation in abnormal venous channels, leading to the production of thrombin and conversion of fibrinogen into fibrin. LIC is characterized by an elevated D-dimer level, normal to mildly diminished ($100,000–150,000/mm^3$) platelet count, and decreased fibrinogen level [101–103]. Patients with LIC are at risk of systemic thromboembolism. Consideration should be given to treatment with low-molecular-weight heparin during the perioperative period, pregnancy, bed rest, or travel to improve their hematologic status.

Complications of VMs are related to their location. Cervicofacial VMs can distort facial features. An extremity VM can result in leg length discrepancy or hypoplasia of the affected side due, in part, to disuse [98]. VMs in the synovial lining of the knee can cause episodic pain as a result of repeated bloody effusions. Hemarthrosis can be debilitating and can ultimately lead to degenerative arthritis [8]. Intraosseous VMs cause structural weakening of the bony diaphysis, predisposing to pathologic fracture. VMs of the GI tract can be solitary or multifocal and variably involve any or all layers of the bowel wall. A majority of GI VMs occur as transmural lesions of the left colon and rectum with variable local extension into pelvic structures [8,104,105]. GI VMs frequently present with lower GI bleeding. On physical examination, a bluish discoloration of the perineum can signal an underlying rectal VM. The presence of a rectal VM and associated ectatic mesenteric veins is a risk factor for developing portomesenteric venous thrombosis [106].

Blue-rubber bleb nevus syndrome (BRBNS) is a rare, sporadic disorder consisting of multifocal VMs in the skin, soft tissues, and GI tract. The cutaneous VMs of BRBNS are small—measuring 1 to 2 cm, are blue to purple in color, and range from several to hundreds [107]. The palmar and plantar surfaces are typically affected. The GI VMs of BRBNS are distributed throughout the gut, most commonly in the small bowel. Patients usually exhibit chronic GI bleeding, resulting in anemia and requiring lifelong iron replacement and repeated blood transfusions. Massive sudden hemorrhage is the exception. The intraintestinal VMs of BRBNS can also cause intussusception and volvulus [108].

Imaging modalities useful for the diagnosis of VMs include ultrasonography, MRI, and venography. Ultrasonography is typically the initial imaging modality of choice due to availability, cost, and lack of exposure to ionizing radiation. Monophasic low-velocity flow is observed using Doppler ultrasonography [98]. MRI documents the location, extent, and relationship to adjacent structures. MRI findings include focal or diffuse collections of high T2 signal, often containing identifiable spaces separated by septations. Fluid-fluid levels and phleboliths, seen as signal voids, may be present (see Fig. 8). Contrast enhancement of the vascular spaces of VMs distinguishes them from LMs.

Treatment of patients with VMs is individualized. A multidisciplinary approach is key. Pain, functional loss, bleeding, and appearance are a few indications for treatment. Therapeutic modalities include compression, anti-inflammatory medications, sclerotherapy, resection, and combined approaches. Graded elastic compression aids in reducing swelling and pain in VMs of the extremities. A garment can be worn while upright during the day and removed during recumbency. Garments should be tailored for the patient and replaced as children grow. Pain can be treated with anti-inflammatory medications. Aspirin is reported to improve pain and swelling [109]. It is best to limit narcotics.

Sclerotherapy is the mainstay of interventional treatment of most symptomatic VMs. Common sclerosants for VMs are dehydrated ethanol and sodium tetradecyl sulfate. Sclerotherapy of VMs is similar to that for LMs except that there may be large draining veins. Compression or tourniquets may be needed to limit venous drainage and prevent systemic delivery of the sclerosant. Sclerotherapy may be augmented by the use of coils and liquid embolic agents. These procedures should be performed by an experienced interventional specialist. Local and systemic complications of sclerotherapy include blistering, full-thickness cutaneous necrosis, nerve injury, sudden pulmonary hypertension, and hemolysis [110]. Cure with sclerotherapy is rare. VMs often recanalize and expand after treatment. Multiple sessions may be necessary. Compression garments, especially in the extremities, are required after sclerotherapy to enhance the effects post treatment. Results are usually stated in terms of patient satisfaction related to a decrease in pain, an improvement in appearance, or both.

Surgical excision of small, well-localized VMs is usually successful. Larger VMs may be treated with sclerotherapy initially to shrink the lesion prior to resection [110]. Staged subtotal resections can be performed. GI VMs of the bowel wall resulting in transfusion-dependent bleeding should be evaluated for surgical resection. Complete resection of multifocal VMs of BRBNS provides the only chance for possible cure. Bowel resection is rarely indicated. Rather, wedge excision and polypectomy by intussusception of successive lengths of intestine are preferred [107]. Colorectal VMs causing significant bleeding may be treated with colectomy, anorectal mucosectomy, and coloanal pull-through [111].

Arteriovenous malformation

AVMs are fast-flow malformations. The central core (nidus) is composed of abnormally connected arteries and veins (shunts) that bypass the high-resistance capillary bed. Most AVMs are sporadic. They can be associated with several syndromes, such as CM-AVM, caused by mutations in the *RASA1* gene, and CLOVES (key features of congenital lipomatous overgrowth, vascular malformations, epidermal nevi, and skeletal anomalies) syndrome (somatic mutation in *PIK3CA*) [112,113]. This discussion is limited to extracranial AVMs, which have a predilection for the head and neck followed by the extremities. AVMs are usually noted at birth due to the presence of a faint vascular stain. AVMs become evident during childhood and adolescence as a warm, pink cutaneous patch with an underlying palpable thrill or bruit (Fig. 9) [114]. As AVMs expand, they become more masslike and can be associated with ulceration of the overlying soft tissue, bleeding, pain, or heart failure.

Ultrasonography with color and spectral Doppler evaluation can reliably detect arteriovenous shunting. Radiographically, AVMs are characterized by the presence of dilated feeding arteries and draining veins. There is not a discrete parenchymal mass. MRI allows assessment of the adjacent soft tissue. The nidus may or may not be visible. Edema, increased fat, muscle enlargement, and bony changes are variably noted on imaging. Angiography can be used for diagnosis, but it should not be performed until intervention is scheduled [8].

Treatment of AVMs is challenging and reliant on an interdisciplinary approach. A majority of AVMs require treatment due to continued life-long expansion. The mainstays of treatment are angiographic embolization, surgical resection, or a combination of the 2. The main goal of AVM therapy is to control shunting and palliate symptoms. Evidence suggests that treatment of well-localized AVMs using excision with or without embolization is associated with better long-term control [114]. Regardless of stage or method of treatment, proximal feeding arteries must not ever be ligated or embolized. Ligation may temporarily improve heart failure, pain, or bleeding but precludes future embolizations. Furthermore, the nidus of the AVM recruits nearby arteries, resulting in continued growth and expansion [115].

Angiography should precede interventional therapy or surgical extirpation. Superselective arterial or retrograde venous embolization can ameliorate

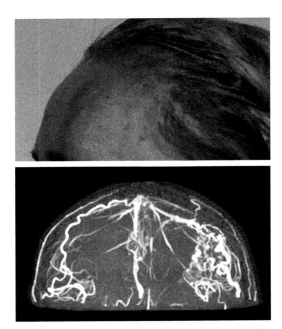

Fig. 9. AVM. (*Top*) Lateral view of an AVM of the left face and forehead in an adolescent girl. A pink stain is present above the left eye. (*Bottom*) Coronal magnetic resonance angiography tumble image of the same AVM demonstrating a tangle of vessels in the left scalp.

symptoms. Combined approaches for well-localized AVMs consist of embolization followed by surgical resection 2 to 3 days later. Preoperative embolization diminishes bleeding and may delineate the resection margin. The surgical goal is complete resection of the nidus and overlying soft tissue and skin to minimize the chance of recurrence. Complications of treatment include tissue necrosis, bleeding, and wound dehiscence. Early and continued follow-up with physical examination complemented by MRI, ultrasonography, and angiography may be necessary to evaluate for recurrence. Regrettably, many AVMs are extensive and permeate all tissue planes, rendering them unresectable. Embolization can be palliative. Amputation is a last resort for difficult to manage AVMs of the extremities [8,98,115].

COMBINED VASCULAR MALFORMATIONS
Combined vascular malformations are defined as lesions with 2 or more vascular anomalies. These more complex disorders are usually associated with hypertrophy and skeletal overgrowth. Klippel-Trénaunay syndrome (KTS) and CLOVES are both caused by somatic mutations in *PIK3CA* [113].

Klippel-Trenaunay syndrome
KTS is a well-known eponym for a complex overgrowth syndrome. Malformations include CMs, LMs, and VMs [8]. KTS usually affects the lower

extremity. Soft tissue overgrowth is mostly fatty and extrafascial. Skeletal hypertrophy tends to follow the soft tissue overgrowth. There is no fast-flow component. The CMs are often multiple, occurring predominantly on the lateral thigh and calf (Fig. 10). Lymphatic vesicles erupt through the CMs and frequently bleed or leak lymphatic fluid. Macroscystic, microcystic, or combined LM is often present. The LMs can cause recurrent pain and infection. The marginal venous system is the hallmark of VMs in KTS. The marginal venous system is a persistent embryologic network of veins that typically originates in the dorsal aspect of the foot and ascends in the lateral aspect of the calf and continues in the thigh as the sciatic vein. The system terminates in the deep iliac vein. Flow in the marginal venous system is often slow predisposing the patients to thromboembolism and thrombophlebitis. The deep venous system is often hypoplastic or absent.

Pelvic involvement is common. The lymphatic and venous components can involve the perineum, urethra, external genitalia, bladder, and rectum. Many patients remain asymptomatic; however, some present with recurrent infection with gut flora, hematuria, bladder outlet obstruction, hematochezia, and constipation.

Serial plain radiographs are used to evaluate and follow limb length discrepancies. MRI with contrast demonstrates extrafascial hypertrophic fatty tissue of the extremity, the marginal venous system, lymphatic anomalies of the limb, pelvis, and abdomen. The pelvic and perirectal fat is usually infiltrated with

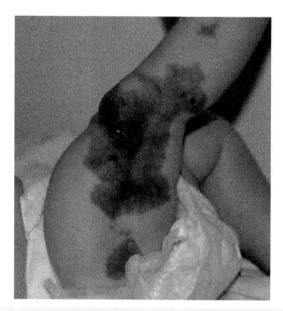

Fig. 10. KTS. Infant with classic laterally placed CM, lymphatic vesicles, and overgrowth of the leg.

LM. The sigmoid and anorectum are often thickened; the urinary bladder is elongated and displaced cranioventrally [116].

Treatment of KTS is usually conservative and managed collaboratively among the specialists. Compression garments minimize leg swelling, pain, and venous engorgement. Infection, cellulitis or lymphangitis is treated with antibiotics. Skin care and treatment of the lymphatic vesicles with sclerotherapy, carbon dioxide photovaporization, cauterization, or excision may reduce the risk of infection. Focal venous and LMs can be treated with sclerotherapy. Early identification and closure of the large phlebectatic veins diminishes the risk of thromboembolism. The marginal veins should be obliterated with excision or embolization or photocoagulated with endovenous laser in childhood prior to the veins becoming large and ectatic. Staged, contour resection of the extrafascial soft tissue overgrowth of the calf, thigh, and buttock can improve function and decrease infection [117]. Orthopedic follow-up is necessary for limb length discrepancy. Shoe lifts are used for mild differences in childhood. Epiphysiodesis of the longer limb can be performed for significant discrepancy in adolescence. Pelvic malformations causing transfusion dependent anemia can be treated with colectomy, anorectal mucosectomy, and coloanal pull-through [111].

Congenital lipomatous overgrowth, vascular malformations, epidermal nevi, and skeletal anomalies syndrome

CLOVES syndrome is a truncal lipomatous mass noted at birth [118,119]. The fatty growth extends from the trunk into adjacent areas, such as the mediastinum, retroperitoneum, thoracic cavity, and epidural space, which can compress the spinal cord, thecal sac, and nerve roots. CMs can be seen on the trunk. LMs and vesicles are frequently seen within and around the truncal lipomatous masses. VMs, in the form of central, limb, and thoracic phlebectasia, can result in pulmonary embolism [120]. Spinal and paraspinal AVMs have been observed. Acral deformities include large, wide feet and hands; macrodactyly; and a wide sandal gap. Scoliosis, neurologic, renal, and musculoskeletal malformations can also be present. The management of a patient with CLOVES is similar to one with KTS. Surgical debulking of large lipomatous masses and LMs can improve pain, appearance, and mobility. Ectatic veins should be closed when identified, particularly prior to procedures. AVMs can be embolized.

Parkes Weber syndrome (capillary malformation-arteriovenous malformation)

Parkes Weber syndrome is a capillary malformation-arteriovenous malformation (CM-AVM) caused by mutations in the *RASA1* gene [121]. The syndrome is evident at birth with symmetric enlargement of the involved limb, usually a lower extremity, associated with a confluent or patchy CM, hypervascularity of the affected limb, and osseous overgrowth, often resulting in limb length discrepancy. Stained areas are usually warm. The soft tissue overgrowth involves the muscle and bone, limiting the role for surgical debulking. On imaging, the affected extremity usually has fusiform subcutaneous, muscular, and bony overgrowth with diffuse microfistulae. Generalized arterial and venous dilation can be seen on angiography and venography. Correct diagnosis is essential because patients with CM-AVM can develop cardiac overload and cardiac failure. The cardiac overload is generally well tolerated. Infants and children are observed annually with monitoring for axial overgrowth, signs of cardiac failure, and cutaneous problems related to ischemia. Treatment is predicated on symptoms. Repetitive superselective embolization is the mainstay of therapy [8]. Rarely, significant reduction of cardiac failure may require limb amputation.

SUMMARY

A standardized classification system allows improvements in diagnostic accuracy. Multidisciplinary vascular anomaly centers combine medical, surgical, radiologic, and pathologic expertise. This collaborative approach tailors treatment and management of vascular anomalies for affected individuals.

References

[1] Mulliken JB, Glowacki J. Hemangiomas and vascular malformations in infants and children: a classification based on endothelial characteristics. Plast Reconstr Surg 1982;69(3):412–22.

[2] Available at: issva.org/classification. Accessed November 15, 2014.

[3] Greene AK. Current concepts of vascular anomalies. J Craniofac Surg 2012;23(1): 220–4.

[4] Greene AK, Kim S, Rogers GF, et al. Risk of vascular anomalies with Down syndrome. Pediatrics 2008;121(1):e135–40.

[5] Kanada KN, Merin MR, Munden A, et al. A prospective study of cutaneous findings in newborns in the United States: correlation with race, ethnicity, and gestational status using updated classification and nomenclature. J Pediatr 2012;161(2):240–5.

[6] Jinnin M, Medici D, Park L, et al. Suppressed NFAT-dependent VEGFR1 expression and constitutive VEGFR2 signaling in infantile hemangioma. Nat Med 2008;14(11): 1236–46.

[7] Boye E, Yu Y, Paranya G, et al. Clonality and altered behavior of endothelial cells from hemangiomas. J Clin Invest 2001;107(6):745–52.

[8] Mulliken JB, Fishman SJ, Burrows PE. Vascular anomalies. Curr Probl Surg 2000;37(8): 517–84.

[9] Drolet BA, Esterly NB, Frieden IJ. Hemangiomas in children. N Engl J Med 1999;341(3): 173–81.

[10] Chang LC, Haggstrom AN, Drolet BA, et al. Growth characteristics of infantile hemangiomas: implications for management. Pediatrics 2008;122(2):360–7.

[11] Haggstrom AN, Lammer EJ, Schneider RA, et al. Patterns of infantile hemangiomas: new clues to hemangioma pathogenesis and embryonic facial development. Pediatrics 2006;117(3):698–703.

[12] Liang MG, Frieden IJ. Infantile and congenital hemangiomas. Semin Pediatr Surg 2014;23(4):162–7.

[13] Mulliken JB, Young AE. Vascular birthmarks: hemangiomas and malformations. Philadelphia: Saunders; 1988.

[14] Tollefson MM, Frieden IJ. Early growth of infantile hemangiomas: what parents' photographs tell us. Pediatrics 2012;130(2):e314–20.

[15] Bowers RE, Graham EA, Tomlinson KM. The natural history of the strawberry nevus. Arch Dermatol 1960;82:667–80.

[16] Couto RA, Maclellan RA, Zurakowski D, et al. Infantile hemangioma: clinical assessment of the involuting phase and implications for management. Plast Reconstr Surg 2012;130(3): 619–24.

[17] Luu M, Frieden IJ. Haemangioma: clinical course, complications and management. Br J Dermatol 2013;169(1):20–30.

[18] Frieden IJ, Reese V, Cohen D. PHACE syndrome. The association of posterior fossa brain malformations, hemangiomas, arterial anomalies, coarctation of the aorta and cardiac defects, and eye abnormalities. Arch Dermatol 1996;132(3):307–11.

[19] Robertson RL, Chavali RV, Robson CD, et al. Neurologic complications of cerebral angiography in childhood moyamoya syndrome. Pediatr Radiol 1998;28(11):824–9.

[20] Pascual-Castroviejo I, Viano J, Moreno F, et al. Hemangiomas of the head, neck, and chest with associated vascular and brain anomalies: a complex neurocutaneous syndrome. AJNR Am J Neuroradiol 1996;17(3):461–71.

[21] Haggstrom AN, Garzon MC, Baselga E, et al. Risk for PHACE syndrome in infants with large facial hemangiomas. Pediatrics 2010;126(2):e418–26.

[22] Metry D, Heyer G, Hess C, et al. Consensus Statement on Diagnostic Criteria for PHACE Syndrome. Pediatrics 2009;124(5):1447–56.

[23] Stockman A, Boralevi F, Taïeb A, et al. SACRAL syndrome: spinal dysraphism, anogenital, cutaneous, renal and urologic anomalies, associated with an angioma of lumbosacral localization. Dermatology 2007;214(1):40–5.

[24] Girard C, Bigorre M, Guillot B, et al. PELVIS Syndrome. Arch Dermatol 2006;142(7): 884–8.

[25] Iacobas I, Burrows PE, Frieden IJ, et al. LUMBAR: association between cutaneous infantile hemangiomas of the lower body and regional congenital anomalies. J Pediatr 2010;157(5):795–801.e1–7.

[26] Drolet BA, Chamlin SL, Garzon MC, et al. Prospective study of spinal anomalies in children with infantile hemangiomas of the lumbosacral skin. J Pediatr 2010;157(5):789–94.

[27] Schumacher WE, Drolet BA, Maheshwari M, et al. Spinal dysraphism associated with the cutaneous lumbosacral infantile hemangioma: a neuroradiological review. Pediatr Radiol 2012;42(3):315–20.

[28] Paltiel HJ, Burrows PE, Kozakewich HP, et al. Soft-tissue vascular anomalies: utility of US for diagnosis. Radiology 2000;214(3):747–54.

[29] Meyer JS, Hoffer FA, Barnes PD, et al. Biological classification of soft-tissue vascular anomalies: MR correlation. AJR Am J Roentgenol 1991;157(3):559–64.

[30] North PE, Waner M, Mizeracki A, et al. GLUT1: a newly discovered immunohistochemical marker for juvenile hemangiomas. Hum Pathol 2000;31(1):11–22.

[31] Tanner JL, Dechert MP, Frieden IJ. Growing up with a facial hemangioma: parent and child coping and adaptation. Pediatrics 1998;101(3 Pt 1):446–52.

[32] Couto JA, Greene AK. Management of problematic infantile hemangioma using intralesional triamcinolone: efficacy and safety in 100 infants. J Plast Reconstr Aesthet Surg 2014;67(11):1469–74.

[33] Ruttum MS, Abrams GW, Harris GJ, et al. Bilateral retinal embolization associated with intralesional corticosteroid injection for capillary hemangioma of infancy. J Pediatr Ophthalmol Strabismus 1993;30(1):4–7.

[34] Sutula FC, Glover AT. Eyelid necrosis following intralesional corticosteroid injection for capillary hemangioma. Ophthalmic Surg 1987;18(2):103–5.

[35] Sans V, Dumas de la Roque E, Berge J, et al. Propranolol for severe infantile hemangiomas: follow-up report. Pediatrics 2009;124(3):e423–31.

[36] Leaute-Labreze C, Dumas de la Roque E, Hubiche T, et al. Propranolol for severe hemangiomas of infancy. N Engl J Med 2008;358(24):2649–51.

[37] Drolet BA, Trenor CC, Brandão LR, et al. Consensus-derived practice standards plan for complicated Kaposiform hemangioendothelioma. J Pediatr 2013;163(1):285–91.

[38] Holland KE, Frieden IJ, Frommelt PC, et al. Hypoglycemia in children taking propranolol for the treatment of infantile hemangioma. Arch Dermatol 2010;146(7):775–8.

[39] de Graaf M, Breur JM, Raphaël MF, et al. Adverse effects of propranolol when used in the treatment of hemangiomas: a case series of 28 infants. J Am Acad Dermatol 2011;65(2): 320–7.

[40] Kwon EK, Joachim S, Siegel DH, et al. Retrospective review of adverse effects from propranolol in infants. JAMA Dermatol 2013;149(4):484–5.

[41] Ahogo CK, Ezzedine K, Prey S, et al. Factors associated with the relapse of infantile haemangiomas in children treated with oral propranolol. Br J Dermatol 2013;169(6): 1252–6.

[42] Greene AK. Corticosteroid treatment for problematic infantile hemangioma: evidence does not support an increased risk for cerebral palsy. Pediatrics 2008;121(6): 1251–2.

[43] Boon LM, MacDonald DM, Mulliken JB. Complications of systemic corticosteroid therapy for problematic hemangioma. Plast Reconstr Surg 1999;104(6):1616–23.

[44] Bennett ML, Fleischer AB Jr, Chamlin SL, et al. Oral corticosteroid use is effective for cutaneous hemangiomas: an evidence-based evaluation. Arch Dermatol 2001;137(9): 1208–13.

[45] Dubois J, Hershon L, Carmant L, et al. Toxicity profile of interferon alfa-2b in children: a prospective evaluation. J Pediatr 1999;135(6):782–5.

[46] Barlow CF, Priebe CJ, Mulliken JB, et al. Spastic diplegia as a complication of interferon Alfa-2a treatment of hemangiomas of infancy. J Pediatr 1998;132(3 Pt 1):527–30.

[47] Nasseri E, Piram M, McCuaig CC, et al. Partially involuting congenital hemangiomas: a report of 8 cases and review of the literature. J Am Acad Dermatol 2014;70(1):75–9.

[48] North PE, Waner M, James CA, et al. Congenital nonprogressive hemangioma: a distinct clinicopathologic entity unlike infantile hemangioma. Arch Dermatol 2001;137(12): 1607–20.

[49] Berenguer B, Mulliken JB, Enjolras O, et al. Rapidly involuting congenital hemangioma: clinical and histopathologic features. Pediatr Dev Pathol 2003;6(6):495–510.

[50] Boon LM, Enjolras O, Mulliken JB. Congenital hemangioma: evidence of accelerated involution. J Pediatr 1996;128(3):329–35.

[51] Drolet BA, Frommelt PC, Chamlin SL, et al. Initiation and use of propranolol for infantile hemangioma: report of a consensus conference. Pediatrics 2013;131(1):128–40.

[52] Enjolras O, Mulliken JB, Boon LM, et al. Noninvoluting congenital hemangioma: a rare cutaneous vascular anomaly. Plast Reconstr Surg 2001;107(7):1647–54.

[53] Gorincour G, Kokta V, Rypens F, et al. Imaging characteristics of two subtypes of congenital hemangiomas: rapidly involuting congenital hemangiomas and non-involuting congenital hemangiomas. Pediatr Radiol 2005;35(12):1178–85.

[54] Marler JJ, Fishman SJ, Upton J, et al. Prenatal diagnosis of vascular anomalies. J Pediatr Surg 2002;37(3):318–26.

[55] Elia D, Garel C, Enjolras O, et al. Prenatal imaging findings in rapidly involuting congenital hemangioma of the skull. Ultrasound Obstet Gynecol 2008;31(5):572–5.

[56] Boon LM, Fishman SJ, Lund DP, et al. Congenital fibrosarcoma masquerading as congenital hemangioma: report of two cases. J Pediatr Surg 1995;30(9):1378–81.

[57] Christison-Lagay ER, Burrows PE, Alomari A, et al. Hepatic hemangiomas: subtype classification and development of a clinical practice algorithm and registry. J Pediatr Surg 2007;42(1):62–7 [discussion: 67–8].

[58] Kulungowski AM, Alomari AI, Chawla A, et al. Lessons from a liver hemangioma registry: subtype classification. J Pediatr Surg 2012;47(1):165–70.

[59] Morris J, Abbott J, Burrows P, et al. Antenatal diagnosis of fetal hepatic hemangioma treated with maternal corticosteroids. Obstet Gynecol 1999;94(5 Pt 2):813–5.

[60] Hsi Dickie B, Fishman SJ, Azizkhan RG. Hepatic vascular tumors. Semin Pediatr Surg 2014;23(4):168–72.

[61] Kassarjian A, Zurakowski D, Dubois J, et al. Infantile hepatic hemangiomas: clinical and imaging findings and their correlation with therapy. AJR Am J Roentgenol 2004;182(3): 785–95.

[62] Huang SA, Tu HM, Harney JW, et al. Severe hypothyroidism caused by type 3 iodothyronine deiodinase in infantile hemangiomas. N Engl J Med 2000;343(3):185–9.

[63] Mhanna A, Franklin WH, Mancini AJ. Hepatic infantile hemangiomas treated with oral propranolol–a case series. Pediatr Dermatol 2011;28(1):39–45.

[64] Haisley-Royster C, Enjolras O, Frieden IJ, et al. Kasabach-Merritt phenomenon: a retrospective study of treatment with vincristine. J Pediatr Hematol Oncol 2002;24(6):459–62.

[65] Gruman A, Liang MG, Mulliken JB, et al. Kaposiform hemangioendothelioma without Kasabach-Merritt phenomenon. J Am Acad Dermatol 2005;52(4):616–22.

[66] Chu CY, Hsiao CH, Chiu HC. Transformation between Kaposiform hemangioendothelioma and tufted angioma. Dermatology 2003;206(4):334–7.

[67] Lyons LL, North PE, Mac-Moune Lai F, et al. Kaposiform hemangioendothelioma: a study of 33 cases emphasizing its pathologic, immunophenotypic, and biologic uniqueness from juvenile hemangioma. Am J Surg Pathol 2004;28(5):559–68.

[68] Sarkar M, Mulliken JB, Kozakewich HP, et al. Thrombocytopenic coagulopathy (Kasabach-Merritt phenomenon) is associated with Kaposiform hemangioendothelioma and not with common infantile hemangioma. Plast Reconstr Surg 1997;100(6):1377–86.

[69] Christison-Lagay ER, Fishman SJ. Vascular anomalies. Surg Clin North Am 2006;86(2): 393–425, x.

[70] Smoller BR, Rosen S. Port-wine stains. A disease of altered neural modulation of blood vessels? Arch Dermatol 1986;122(2):177–9.

[71] Izikson L, Nelson JS, Anderson RR. Treatment of hypertrophic and resistant port wine stains with a 755 nm laser: a case series of 20 patients. Lasers Surg Med 2009;41(6):427–32.

[72] Lee MS, Liang MG, Mulliken JB. Diffuse capillary malformation with overgrowth: a clinical subtype of vascular anomalies with hypertrophy. J Am Acad Dermatol 2013;69(4): 589–94.

[73] Chapas AM, Eickhorst K, Geronemus RG. Efficacy of early treatment of facial port wine stains in newborns: a review of 49 cases. Lasers Surg Med 2007;39(7):563–8.

[74] de Serres LM, Sie KC, Richardson MA. Lymphatic malformations of the head and neck. A proposal for staging. Arch Otolaryngol Head Neck Surg 1995;121(5):577–82.

[75] Florez-Vargas A, Vargas SO, Debelenko LV, et al. Comparative analysis of D2-40 and LYVE-1 immunostaining in lymphatic malformations. Lymphology 2008;41(3):103–10.

[76] Bruder E, Perez-Atayde AR, Jundt G, et al. Vascular lesions of bone in children, adolescents, and young adults. A clinicopathologic reappraisal and application of the ISSVA classification. Virchows Arch 2009;454(2):161–79.

[77] Elluru RG, Balakrishnan K, Padua HM. Lymphatic malformations: diagnosis and management. Semin Pediatr Surg 2014;23(4):178–85.

[78] Edwards PD, Rahbar R, Ferraro NF, et al. Lymphatic malformation of the lingual base and oral floor. Plast Reconstr Surg 2005;115(7):1906–15.

[79] Rahbar R, Vogel A, Myers LB, et al. Fetal surgery in otolaryngology: a new era in the diagnosis and management of fetal airway obstruction because of advances in prenatal imaging. Arch Otolaryngol Head Neck Surg 2005;131(5):393–8.

[80] Greene AK, Slavin SA, Borud L. Treatment of lower extremity lymphedema with suction-assisted lipectomy. Plast Reconstr Surg 2006;118(5):118e–21e.

[81] Maclellan RA, Couto RA, Sullivan JE, et al. Management of primary and secondary lymphedema: analysis of 225 referrals to a center. Ann Plast Surg 2014. [Epub ahead of print].

[82] Greene AK, Schook CC. Primary lymphedema: definition of onset based on developmental age. Plast Reconstr Surg 2012;129(1):221e–2e.

[83] Schook CC, Mulliken JB, Fishman SJ, et al. Primary lymphedema: clinical features and management in 138 pediatric patients. Plast Reconstr Surg 2011;127(6):2419–31.

[84] Rockson SG. Diagnosis and management of lymphatic vascular disease. J Am Coll Cardiol 2008;52(10):799–806.

[85] Witte CL, Witte MH, Unger EC, et al. Advances in imaging of lymph flow disorders. Radiographics 2000;20(6):1697–719.

[86] Puig S, Casati B, Staudenherz A, et al. Vascular low-flow malformations in children: current concepts for classification, diagnosis and therapy. Eur J Radiol 2005;53(1):35–45.

[87] Burrows PE, Mulliken JB, Fishman SJ, et al. Pharmacological treatment of a diffuse arteriovenous malformation of the upper extremity in a child. J Craniofac Surg 2009;20(Suppl 1):597–602.

[88] Swetman GL, Berk DR, Vasanawala SS, et al. Sildenafil for severe lymphatic malformations. N Engl J Med 2012;366(4):384–6.

[89] Hammill AM, Wentzel M, Gupta A, et al. Sirolimus for the treatment of complicated vascular anomalies in children. Pediatr Blood Cancer 2011;57(6):1018–24.

[90] Vignot S, Faivre S, Aguirre D, et al. mTOR-targeted therapy of cancer with rapamycin derivatives. Ann Oncol 2005;16(4):525–37.

[91] Smithers CJ, Vogel AM, Kozakewich HP, et al. An injectable tissue-engineered embolus prevents luminal recanalization after vascular sclerotherapy. J Pediatr Surg 2005;40(6):920–5.

[92] Burrows PE, Mitri RK, Alomari A, et al. Percutaneous sclerotherapy of lymphatic malformations with doxycycline. Lymphat Res Biol 2008;6(3–4):209–16.

[93] Chaudry G, Burrows PE, Padua HM, et al. Sclerotherapy of abdominal lymphatic malformations with doxycycline. J Vasc Interv Radiol 2011;22(10):1431–5.

[94] Alqahtani A, Nguyen LT, Flageole H, et al. 25 years' experience with lymphangiomas in children. J Pediatr Surg 1999;34(7):1164–8.

[95] Limaye N, Wouters V, Uebelhoer M, et al. Somatic mutations in angiopoietin receptor gene TEK cause solitary and multiple sporadic venous malformations. Nat Genet 2009;41(1):118–24.

[96] Soblet J, Limaye N, Uebelhoer M, et al. Variable Somatic TIE2 Mutations in Half of Sporadic Venous Malformations. Mol Syndromol 2013;4(4):179–83.

[97] Brouillard P, Boon LM, Revencu N, et al. Genotypes and phenotypes of 162 families with a glomulin mutation. Mol Syndromol 2013;4(4):157–64.

[98] Marler JJ, Mulliken JB. Vascular anomalies. In: Mathes SJ, Hentz VR, editors. Plastic surgery, vol. 5, 2nd edition. Philadelphia: Elsevier; 2009. p. 19–68.

[99] Hassanein AH, Mulliken JB, Fishman SJ, et al. Venous malformation: risk of progression during childhood and adolescence. Ann Plast Surg 2012;68(2):198–201.

[100] Kulungowski AM, Hassanein AH, Nosé V, et al. Expression of androgen, estrogen, progesterone, and growth hormone receptors in vascular malformations. Plast Reconstr Surg 2012;129(6):919e–24e.

[101] Enjolras O, Ciabrini D, Mazoyer E, et al. Extensive pure venous malformations in the upper or lower limb: a review of 27 cases. J Am Acad Dermatol 1997;36(2 Pt 1):219–25.

[102] Dompmartin A, Acher A, Thibon P, et al. Association of localized intravascular coagulopathy with venous malformations. Arch Dermatol 2008;144(7):873–7.

[103] Mazoyer E, Enjolras O, Bisdorff A, et al. Coagulation disorders in patients with venous malformation of the limbs and trunk: a case series of 118 patients. Arch Dermatol 2008;144(7):861–7.

[104] de la Torre L, Carrasco D, Mora MA, et al. Vascular malformations of the colon in children. J Pediatr Surg 2002;37(12):1754–7.

[105] Fishman SJ, Fox VL. Visceral vascular anomalies. Gastrointest Endosc Clin N Am 2001;11(4):813–34, viii.

[106] Kulungowski AM, Fox VL, Burrows PE, et al. Portomesenteric venous thrombosis associated with rectal venous malformation. J Pediatr Surg 2010;45(6):1221–7.

[107] Fishman SJ, Smithers CJ, Folkman J, et al. Blue rubber bleb nevus syndrome: surgical eradication of gastrointestinal bleeding. Ann Surg 2005;241(3):523–8.

[108] Tyrrel RT, Baumgartner BR, Montemayor KA. Blue rubber bleb nevus syndrome: CT diagnosis of intussusception. AJR Am J Roentgenol 1990;154(1):105–6.

[109] Nguyen JT, Koerper MA, Hess CP, et al. Aspirin therapy in venous malformation: a retrospective cohort study of benefits, side effects, and patient experiences. Pediatr Dermatol 2014;31(5):556–60.

[110] Berenguer B, Burrows PE, Zurakowski D, et al. Sclerotherapy of craniofacial venous malformations: complications and results. Plast Reconstr Surg 1999;104(1):1–11 [discussion: 12–5].

[111] Fishman SJ, Shamberger RC, Fox VL, et al. Endorectal pull-through abates gastrointestinal hemorrhage from colorectal venous malformations. J Pediatr Surg 2000;35(6):982–4.

[112] Eerola I, Boon LM, Mulliken JB, et al. Capillary malformation-arteriovenous malformation, a new clinical and genetic disorder caused by RASA1 mutations. Am J Hum Genet 2003;73(6):1240–9.

[113] Kurek KC, Luks VL, Ayturk UM, et al. Somatic mosaic activating mutations in PIK3CA cause CLOVES syndrome. Am J Hum Genet 2012;90(6):1108–15.

[114] Liu AS, Mulliken JB, Zurakowski D, et al. Extracranial arteriovenous malformations: natural progression and recurrence after treatment. Plast Reconstr Surg 2010;125(4):1185–94.

[115] Smithers CJ, Fishman SJ. Vascular Anomalies. In: Ashcraft KW, Holcomb GW III, Murphy JP, editors. Pediatric surgery. 4th edition. Philadelphia: Elsevier Saunders; 2004. p. 1038–53.

[116] Uller W, Fishman SJ, Alomari AI. Overgrowth syndromes with complex vascular anomalies. Semin Pediatr Surg 2014;23(4):208–15.

[117] Kulungowski AM, Fishman SJ. Management of combined vascular malformations. Clin Plast Surg 2011;38(1):107–20.

[118] Alomari AI. Characterization of a distinct syndrome that associates complex truncal overgrowth, vascular, and acral anomalies: a descriptive study of 18 cases of CLOVES syndrome. Clin Dysmorphol 2009;18(1):1–7.

[119] Sapp JC, Turner JT, van de Kamp JM, et al. Newly delineated syndrome of congenital lipomatous overgrowth, vascular malformations, and epidermal nevi (CLOVE syndrome) in seven patients. Am J Med Genet A 2007;143A(24):2944–58.

[120] Alomari AI, Burrows PE, Lee EY, et al. CLOVES syndrome with thoracic and central phlebectasia: increased risk of pulmonary embolism. J Thorac Cardiovasc Surg 2010;140(2):459–63.

[121] Revencu N, Boon LM, Mulliken JB, et al. Parkes Weber syndrome, vein of Galen aneurysmal malformation, and other fast-flow vascular anomalies are caused by RASA1 mutations. Hum Mutat 2008;29(7):959–65.

Advances in Pediatrics 62 (2015) 257–282

ADVANCES IN PEDIATRICS

ELSEVIER
MOSBY

Hypo and Hyper
Common Pediatric Endocrine and Metabolic Emergencies

Jennifer M. Barker, MD[a], Lalit Bajaj, MD, MPH[b],*

[a]Section of Endocrinology, Children's Hospital Colorado, University of Colorado School of Medicine, 13123 East 16th Avenue, Aurora, CO 80045, USA; [b]Section of Emergency Medicine, Children's Hospital Colorado, University of Colorado School of Medicine, 13123 East 16th Avenue, Aurora, CO 80045, USA

Keywords
- Endocrine • Metabolic • Emergencies • Pediatrics

Key points
- The presentation of endocrine and metabolic emergencies represents one of the more challenging clinical scenarios faced by pediatricians and emergency providers.
- The clinical presentations of children with endocrine/metabolic disturbances are similar to those seen in children with other emergencies, especially in the newborn period and in infancy.
- Perhaps the most important point of this review is that the diagnosis of endocrine/metabolic disorders can only be made if appropriate critical and archival laboratory specimens are obtained *before* treatment (eg, intravenous glucose, calcium, or electrolytes) is begun.

INTRODUCTION
A wide variety of endocrine and metabolic emergencies may present to the pediatric emergency provider. These emergencies may be isolated occurrences, the initial manifestation of an endocrine/metabolic disorder (eg, diabetes mellitus), or an acute abnormality in a child with known endocrine/metabolic disease as a result of intercurrent illness, emotional stress, or noncompliance with medications. The pediatric emergency medicine provider is faced with a difficult task when evaluating a child with a suspected endocrine or metabolic disorder, especially a child with no known underlying condition, because the signs and symptoms of such disorders are varied and nonspecific. The lack

---

*Corresponding author. E-mail address: Lalit.Bajaj@childrenscolorado.org

0065-3101/15/$ – see front matter
http://dx.doi.org/10.1016/j.yapd.2015.04.008

of specific symptoms may lead to a delayed or missed diagnosis and can have serious consequences (eg, cerebral dysfunction leading to coma or death as seen in diabetic ketoacidosis, hypoglycemia, or adrenal insufficiency). Prompt diagnosis depends on the collection of critical and archival laboratory specimens before the administration of nonspecific therapy. Often the presentation of an endocrine or metabolic disorder is nonspecific altered mental status, which requires an extensive list of possible causes [1].

The clinical presentations of children with endocrine/metabolic disturbances are similar to those seen in children with other emergencies, especially in the newborn period and in infancy. A list of commonly found but nonspecific and nonsensitive signs and symptoms is shown in Box 1, and the signs and symptoms are described in each of the sections to follow. An altered level of consciousness and seizures are the most commonly seen signs and are characteristic of untreated diabetic ketoacidosis or other metabolic acidosis, hypoglycemia, and electrolyte abnormalities as well as of several nonendocrine/nonmetabolic conditions, such as sepsis, meningoencephalitis, poisonings, and trauma.

The altered level of consciousness may range from mild drowsiness to complete obtundation, and its degree may be classified by using the Glasgow coma scales in children (Box 2) and infants (Box 3) [2,3]. Changes in the pattern of respiration may be related to metabolic acidosis (rapid, deep Kussmaul respirations) or central nervous system (CNS) impairment (irregular, shallow

---

Box 1: Signs and symptoms of endocrine/metabolic emergencies

Central Nervous System Effects
   Lethargy, weakness
   Irritability, tremor
   Seizures
   Altered mental status, coma
   Hypotonia, hyperreflexia
   Spasticity
   Cheyne-Stokes respirations, apnea
General Metabolic Effects
   Kussmaul respirations
   Nausea, vomiting
   Poor feeding, weight loss, failure to thrive
Cardiovascular Effects
   Tachycardia
   Hypotension
   Shock

Box 2: Glasgow coma scale

Activity	Best response	Score
Eye opening	Spontaneous	4
	To verbal stimulation	3
	To painful stimulation	2
	None	1
Verbal	Oriented	5
	Confused	4
	Inappropriate words	3
	Nonspecific sounds	2
	None	1
Motor	Normal spontaneous	6
	Localizes pain	5
	Withdraws to pain	4
	Decorticate (flexion)	3
	Decerebrate (extension)	2
	None	1

Cheyne-Stokes respirations), and alterations in muscle tone (eg, hypotonia, hyperreflexia) may also be seen.

A history of poor feeding, vomiting, weight loss, or lethargy may be elicited in infants who are ultimately diagnosed with an endocrine/metabolic cause to their illness.

CRITICAL AND ARCHIVAL SPECIMENS

Perhaps the most important point of this review is that the diagnosis of endocrine/metabolic disorders can only be made if appropriate critical and archival

Box 3: Infant Glasgow coma scale

Activity	Best response	Score
Eye opening	Spontaneous	4
	To speech	3
	To painful stimulation	2
	None	1
Verbal	Coos, babbles, cries	5
	Irritable, cries	4
	Cries to pain	3
	Moans to pain	2
	None	1
Motor	Normal spontaneous	6
	Withdraws to touch	5
	Withdraws to pain	4
	Decorticate (flexion)	3
	Decerebrate (extension)	2
	None	1

laboratory specimens are obtained *before* treatment (eg, intravenous [IV] glucose, calcium, or electrolytes) is begun. Interpretation of laboratory data after the onset of treatment is misleading and may delay the identification of the child's specific disorder and its ongoing treatment. This point is particularly true of endocrine/metabolic disorders whose signs and symptoms are nonspecific [4,5].

Critical samples (blood and urine) are obtained soon after the child arrives in the emergency department or intensive care unit and IV access is obtained. Blood is sent for the laboratory determination of electrolytes, serum glucose, and other metabolites (eg, calcium) as part of a comprehensive metabolic profile, along with magnesium and phosphorus, venous pH and bicarbonate. Urine is sent for a routine urinalysis. These preliminary results enable the treating physician to establish or narrow the diagnostic possibilities of the child's disorder. They also allow for the calculation of the anion gap and serum osmolality, which may be helpful in the differential diagnosis, as is described in specific conditions later:

Anion gap: Na mmol/L − [Cl mmol/L + HCO$_3$ mmol/L], where Na is sodium, Cl is chlorine, and HCO_3 is bicarbonate.

Serum osmolality: 2 [serum Na mmol/L] + glucose mg/dL /18 + BUN/2.8, where BUN is blood urea nitrogen.

The relationship between serum and urine osmolality may also be initially estimated by using the calculated serum osmolality and urine specific gravity. Archival samples are obtained at the same time as the critical samples and are held in the laboratory for future measurements. Clues from the critical samples, therefore, allow the physician to use the archival samples for more specific diagnosis and treatment [4,5]. These archival samples may be sent for specific tests (eg, serum insulin, growth hormone, cortisol, and ketones in children with hypoglycemia) and are listed in the tables for each condition described later. The following review covers hypoglycemia, adrenal insufficiency, hyponatremia, hypernatremia, and hyperthyroidism. One of the most common endocrine emergencies, diabetic ketoacidosis, is not discussed in detail in this review as it is beyond the scope of this discussion and has been recently reviewed in the journal [6].

SPECIFIC CONDITIONS
Hypoglycemia
Definitions and causes
Symptoms in insulin-induced hypoglycemia have been recognized at plasma glucose concentrations of 60 mg/dL (3.3 mmol/L) and impairment of brain function at approximately 50 mg/dL (2.8 mmol/L) or 44 mg/dL (2.4 mmol/L) whole blood. In contrast to earlier studies, recent evidence suggests that whole blood glucose concentrations of less than 40 mg/dL (2.2 mmol/L) are rare in asymptomatic premature or term newborns who are fed immediately after birth [7]. As a safe approach, therefore, any patient with a whole blood glucose concentration of 50 mg/dL (2.8 mmol/L) or less should be monitored

closely; diagnostic and therapeutic procedures should be undertaken if the concentration is 40 mg/dL (2.2 mmol/L) or less. Hypoglycemia persisting past the first 48 hours of life is suggestive of an underlying disorder, and evaluation for the underlying cause of the hypoglycemia is recommended.

The causes of hypoglycemia vary with age (Box 4). Hyperinsulinism (transient and permanent) is the most common cause of intractable hypoglycemia from the newborn period to about 6 months of life, and inherited errors of fatty acid oxidation and organic/amino acid metabolism and hypopituitarism also make their appearance then. Infants born small for gestational age or premature may have transient hypoglycemia related to disorders of hepatic glucose production. These children have reduced glycogen stores and protein mass, along with immature enzymatic machinery for hepatic glucose production.

Ketotic hypoglycemia, a diagnosis of exclusion, is a cause of hypoglycemia presenting in older children and infants. It is hypothesized that the underlying pathophysiology is related to reduced muscle mass, which compromises the child's ability to mobilize amino acids as substrate for the gluconeogenesis. This condition is the most common cause of hypoglycemia in childhood and is eventually outgrown [8]. In adolescents, exogenous factors, such as insulin overdose in patients treated with insulin for type 1 or type 2 diabetes, ethanol ingestion, or intentional overdosing with oral hypoglycemic agents, become more prevalent causes of hypoglycemia. Rarely, an insulinoma can present with hypoglycemia.

Pathophysiology

Hypoglycemia results when there is an imbalance between total body glucose utilization and hepatic glucose production. The utilization rate of glucose is determined primarily by the brain, which, in contrast to most other body tissues, cannot acutely use ketones for its energy requirements. Because the brain is a larger proportion of total body weight in the newborn than in the adult, it is not surprising that glucose utilization rates based on body weight decrease with age (Box 5). Knowing these age-specific utilization rates helps to differentiate hypoglycemic disorders caused by increased utilization from those caused by decreased production because the rate of IV glucose administration necessary to maintain euglycemia in the latter should not exceed the normal utilization rate in a patient of corresponding age.

The utilization of glucose in most tissues is regulated by insulin and by the ability of the tissue to use ketones as an alternative energy source in the absence of glucose. Thus, disorders characterized by increased insulin secretion or by a relative inability to synthesize ketones (disorders of fatty acid oxidation) may lead to hypoglycemia caused by increased utilization. These disorders are usually associated with an absence of ketones in the blood or urine (ie, nonketotic hypoglycemias) [9]. When glucose utilization begins to exceed production, the counter-regulatory hormones (cortisol, growth hormone, epinephrine, and glucagon) are secreted to prevent hypoglycemia. These hormones, acting individually or in concert, stimulate glycogenolysis and gluconeogenesis to restore

Box 4: Causes of hypoglycemia by age

1. Up to 6 months
   a. Increased glucose utilization
      i. Hyperinsulinism
         1. Transient: SGA or asphyxiated neonates, infants of diabetic mothers, Beckwith-Wiedemann syndrome
         2. Persistent: focal islet cell hyperplasia versus diffuse, associated with mutations of the KATP channel genes (*ABCC8* and *KCNJ11*)
      ii. Defects in ketone production (fatty acid oxidation): carnitine deficiency, acyl-CoA dehydrogenase deficiencies (LCAD, MCAD, SCAD); inadequate fat stores (SGA and premature newborns)
      iii. Infections/Fevers
   b. Decreased hepatic glucose production
      i. Defects in glycogenolysis: enzyme deficiencies or inhibition of enzyme activities (glycogen storage diseases, galactosemia), inadequate glycogen stores (SGA and premature newborns), GH deficiency
      ii. Defects in gluconeogenesis: enzyme deficiencies or inhibition of enzyme activities (galactosemia, fructose intolerance, fructose-1, 6-bisphosphatase deficiency, alcohol or salicylate intoxication, hormonal deficiencies (GH, cortisol), inborn errors of organic or amino acid metabolism
      iii. Liver failure: many causes
2. Children (6 months to adolescence)
   a. Increased glucose utilization
      i. Drugs: insulin (Munchausen), oral hypoglycemic agents, other (illicit) drugs
      ii. Infections/fevers
      iii. Late-presenting disorders of fatty acid oxidation
   b. Decreased hepatic glucose production
      i. Ketotic hypoglycemia (decreased gluconeogenesis)
      ii. Infections/fever
      iii. Malnutrition, anorexia, bulimia
      iv. Alcohol or salicylate intoxication
      v. Reye syndrome
      vi. Late-presenting inborn errors in organic or amino acid metabolism
      vii. Liver failure

Abbreviations: GH, growth hormone; LCAD, long-chain acyl-CoA dehydrogenase; MCAD, medium-chain acyl-CoA dehydrogenase; SCAD, small-chain acyl-CoA dehydrogenase.

Box 5: Approximate glucose utilization rates versus age

Premature newborns	10 mg/kg/min
Term newborns	8 mg/kg/min
Young children	6–8 mg/kg/min
Older children/adolescents	4–6 mg/kg/min
Adults	2–4 mg/kg/min

and maintain normal serum glucose concentration. Deficiencies in the secretion of counter-regulatory hormones or in the enzymes or substrates involved in either of these 2 processes can result in hypoglycemia, usually accompanied by excessive breakdown of triglycerides and the production of ketones in the blood and urine.

History and physical examination
For the neonate with hypoglycemia, details of the pregnancy including maternal diabetes, preeclampsia, or other signs of fetal stress can point to transient causes of hypoglycemia. A family history of infant deaths may suggest an inherited metabolic disorder. On physical examination, infants of diabetic mothers and infants with hyperinsulinism are often large for gestational age. Hepatomegaly may be a clue to the presence of a glycogen storage disease or generalized liver disease; a small, premature newborn may be prone to develop hypoglycemia because of deficiencies in substrates (glycogen or muscle) or enzymes for hepatic glucose production. Hypoglycemia associated with decreased cortisol and/or growth hormone response can be seen in infants with congenital defects of the hypothalamic/pituitary region, including septo-optic dysplasia. Physical examination may reveal signs of pituitary hormone deficiencies (microphallus [normal phallic size is ≥ 2 cm in a term infant]), signs of optic nerve hypoplasia (nystagmus), or other midline defects.

In older children, a personal history of diabetes treated with insulin, drugs in the home that could cause hypoglycemia (eg, salicylates, insulin, or the oral hypoglycemic agents), or a history of alcohol abuse may be helpful in identifying the cause of hypoglycemia. Hepatomegaly raises the suspicious of glycogen storage diseases and/or generalized liver disease as the underlying cause of the hypoglycemia. Infection, especially sepsis, may also be found and may result in increased glucose utilization that cannot be compensated for, resulting in hypoglycemia.

The signs and symptoms of hypoglycemia may be related to its effects on the CNS or to the effects of increased secretion of epinephrine, one of the counter-regulatory hormones (see Box 1; Box 6) [7,10,11].

Laboratory evaluation
The information needed from the critical and archival samples is shown in Box 7. Although in an emergency setting, hypoglycemia can be screened for with the use of finger-stick reagent strips, hypoglycemia should be confirmed

Box 6: Effects of hypoglycemia beyond the newborn period

CNS effects

   Headache

   Irritability, confusion

   Fatigue

   Abnormal behavior, amnesia

   Altered mental status, coma

   Seizures

Adrenergic effects

   Sweating, cold extremities

   Tachycardia

   Anxiety, weakness

by a laboratory measure of the serum glucose in the critical blood sample. In addition, acid-base balance and liver function status may be obtained from the comprehensive metabolic profile obtained from this sample. The urinalysis helps to distinguish disorders of increased glucose utilization from disorders of glucose production by the absence or presence of ketones, respectively.

Box 7: Laboratory evaluation of hypoglycemia

Critical samples

   Bedside glucose, serum glucose

   Liver function tests

   Electrolytes

   Urinalysis (including ketones)

Archival samples

   Insulin

   Lactate

   Ketones

   Growth hormone

   Cortisol

   C peptide

   Carnitine profile

   Amino acids

   Toxins (salicylates, ethanol)

   Urine amino and organic acids, toxin screen

However, children whose hypoglycemia accompanies febrile illness may have increased utilization and decreased glucose production and show nonspecific ketonuria. Blood and urine that have been saved for future laboratory tests (archival samples) may be sent for other diagnostic measurements, as shown in Box 7. Of particular note should be the use of an archival blood sample for the measurement of serum C peptide in children with suspected hyperinsulinism (eg, nonketotic hypoglycemia in a child older than 6 months). The circulating C peptide results only from the conversion of proinsulin to insulin endogenously and is not found in commercial insulin preparations. Thus, a failure to find elevated serum C peptide levels in children with hypoglycemia caused by hyperinsulinemia suggests exogenous insulin overdose, either accidental or from child abuse. Medications that increase endogenous insulin production, such as sulfonylureas, will have an elevated C peptide. Additional testing to identify the underlying cause of the hypoglycemia may include glucagon stimulation testing (In hyperinsulinism, glucagon administration results in an increase in serum glucose because insulin suppresses glycogenolysis; in other forms of hypoglycemia, this suppression is not present and there is minimal increase in serum glucose at the time of glucagon administration.), assessment of the hypothalamic pituitary adrenal axis, growth hormone stimulation, cranial MRI, and genetic testing.

Treatment
Treatment of hypoglycemia is initially nonspecific because of the diverse causes in all age groups. The immediate goal is to restore normal circulating glucose concentrations with an IV glucose bolus (Box 8) to sustain CNS and renal metabolic needs. The IV glucose bolus is followed by ongoing IV glucose administration to maintain euglycemia and will vary depending on the cause

Box 8: Treatment of hypoglycemia

1. Nonspecific therapy (after critical and archival samples are obtained)
   a. IV glucose
      i. Emergent: 0.2 to 0.3 g/kg (10% dextrose 2–3 mL/kg)
      ii. Ongoing: 5 to 20+ mg/kg/min IV as required for maintenance of euglycemia
      iii. 5 mg/kg/min: D10 at 2 h maintenance fluid rate
      iv. 10 mg/kg/min: D10 at 1 and one-third maintenance rate
      v. 20 mg/kg/min: D20 at 1 and one-third maintenance rate
   b. Other nonspecific therapy: glucagon 0.5 to 1 mg/IM, or IV hydrocortisone 25 to 50 mg/m^2, or 2 to 3 mg/kg IV
2. Specific therapy for hyperinsulinism: diazoxide 10 to 15 mg/kg/d in 3 divided doses orally

Abbreviations: D10, 10% dextrose; D20, 20% dextrose; IM, intramuscular; SC, subcutaneous.

of the hypoglycemia. Disorders characterized by deficient hepatic glucose production may usually be corrected with IV glucose infusions approximating the normal utilization rate for the patients' age, usually less than 8 to 10 mg/kg/min (see Box 5), whereas much greater rates of IV glucose administration are required (>20 mg/kg/min) in states of increased glucose utilization (eg, hyperinsulinism).

If hypoglycemia persists, despite IV glucose administration, then other nonspecific parenteral agents (eg, glucagon or hydrocortisone) may be given at 4 to 6 hourly intervals as needed until more specific treatment can be instituted. If hyperinsulinism is strongly suspected (eg, in the large-for-gestational-age newborn or a child older than 6 months with nonketotic hypoglycemia), then oral diazoxide may be begun pending the return of results from the archival blood sample.

ADRENAL INSUFFICIENCY

Causes

The causes of adrenal insufficiency may be central (ie, related to abnormalities in the hypothalamus or pituitary gland) or primary to the adrenal glands themselves (Box 9). In addition, children receiving pharmacologic (oral or inhaled) steroids for the treatment of severe asthma, leukemia, organ transplantation, or autoimmune conditions and children who are taking physiologic replacement steroids for central or primary hypoadrenalism are all prone to adrenal insufficiency crises during acute, febrile illnesses, particularly when vomiting is present [12].

Pathophysiology

Control of aldosterone secretion has several steps. Hypovolemia and elevated serum potassium concentrations stimulate mineralocorticoid (aldosterone) release from the adrenal gland's zona glomerulosa under the stimulus of the renin-angiotensin II axis. Aldosterone then acts on the distal renal tubule to effect sodium and water retention and enhanced hydrogen ion and potassium excretion into the urine. Thus, aldosterone serves a critical function by maintaining normal levels of total body sodium and water and protecting the body from hyperkalemia, dehydration, and shock. A striking feature of mineralocorticoid deficiency at any age, especially in the dehydrated infant, is polyuria.

Corticotropin-releasing factor (CRF) is released from the hypothalamus during times of stress or hypoglycemia and stimulates the release of corticotropin (ACTH) from the pituitary gland. ACTH, in turn, stimulates the adrenal gland's zona fasciculata to secrete the glucocorticoid cortisol (hydrocortisone), which is one of the body's major defenses against hypoglycemia and shock and, thus, also has a critical function in the body. Adrenal insufficiency from any cause, therefore, results in a relative inability of the child to maintain electrolyte balance, plasma volume, blood pressure, and blood glucose during times of stress and may have a fatal outcome if glucocorticoid replacement is not administered in a timely manner.

Box 9: Causes of adrenal insufficiency

1. Central hypoadrenalism: abnormalities of the hypothalamus/pituitary gland
   a. Congenital
      i. Empty sella syndrome
      ii. Septa-optic dysplasia
      iii. Displaced pituitary/damage to hypothalamo-pituitary stalk
      iv. Tumors
         1. Craniopharyngioma
         2. Dysgerminoma
      v. Trauma/irradiation
      vi. Infection
      vii. Idiopathic
2. Primary hypoadrenalism
   a. CAHs: autosomal recessive enzyme deficiencies
      i. 21-hydroxylase: 95% of CAHs: salt-losing, virilizing
      ii. 11-hydroxylase: 4% of CAHs: salt-retaining, virilizing
      iii. 3-beta-ol dehydrogenase: ~1% of CAHs: salt-losing, undervirilizing
      iv. 17-hydroxylase/desmolase: ~1% of CAHs: salt-retaining, undervirilizing
      v. STAR: less than 1% of CAHs: salt-losing, undervirilizing
   b. Autoimmune: Addison disease, may coexist with insulin-dependent diabetes mellitus
   c. Rare conditions
      i. Adrenocortical hypoplasia congenita (congenital adrenal hypoplasia)
      ii. Allgrove syndrome: cortisol deficiency, alacrima, achalasia
      iii. Adrenal hemorrhage: trauma, meningococcemia
      iv. Other infections: histoplasmosis, tuberculosis
3. Central and primary
   a. Suppression from oral and/or steroids
   b. Transient suppression in infants of steroid-treated mothers

Abbreviations: CAHs, congenital adrenal hyperplasias; STAR, steroid acute regulatory protein.

Primary adrenal insufficiency in the newborn period is most commonly caused by one of the autosomally inherited congenital adrenal hyperplasias (CAHs). These have in common an inability to synthesize normal amounts of cortisol. The most common CAH is caused by a deficiency of 21-hydroxylase that also results in a relative inability to synthesize aldosterone (salt-losing tendency) and cortisol and in overproduction of androgens (virilization), whereas the less common CAHs may have either salt loss or salt retention and overvirilization or undervirilization associated with them, based on the specific enzyme deficiency (see Box 9). Transient adrenal insufficiency in the newborn may also be seen in infants born to steroid-treated mothers. Infants with septo-optic dysplasia may present with central adrenal insufficiency [13,14].

In childhood, the most common cause of adrenal insufficiency is seen in the steroid-dependent (oral or inhaled) child with asthma, an autoimmune disease, or hypopituitarism who fails to augment steroid dosage during times of stress (fever, trauma, surgery). Glucocorticoids administered for more than 10 to 14 days can suppress ACTH release for weeks and render the child susceptible to an adrenal insufficiency crisis. Primary adrenal insufficiency (both mineral-ocorticoid and glucocorticoid insufficiency) is rare in childhood but more common in adolescence and, when present, is most often caused by an autoimmune process (Addison disease). Addison disease may be associated with other auto-immune endocrinopathies, including type 1 diabetes and autoimmune thyroid disease (hypothyroidism or hyperthyroidism).

History and physical examination

Review of the medication history should include the use of steroids including a history of inhaled steroid use in children with asthma, particularly if the child is receiving relatively high dosages (>440 μg/d) of fluticasone (Flovent), since inhaled steroids may suppress ACTH and cortisol secretion as effectively as pharmacologic doses of oral steroids. Children with known autoimmune endo-crinopathies (type 1 diabetes or Hashimoto thyroiditis) may also be prone to develop autoimmune adrenal insufficiency (Addison disease), and those with known hypopituitarism are prone to adrenal insufficiency if compliance with replacement cortisol has been poor or if cortisol dosages have not been suffi-ciently increased during times of stress. Children with adrenal insufficiency may have a history of weakness, anorexia, vomiting, weight loss, salt craving, and hyperpigmentation (from the melanocyte-stimulating properties of the parent molecule of ACTH).

On physical examination, the child may have tachycardia and hypotension. Other clinical signs of shock may be present, including pallor; poor peripheral perfusion; cool, clammy skin; and disturbed consciousness or even coma. With dehydration there may be loss of normal skin turgor, sunken eyes, and dry mu-cous membranes. Hyperpigmentation of scars, flexion creases, gums, areolae, and nonexposed areas of skin reflects excessive secretion of the parent molecule of ACTH (proopiomelanocortin) and is suggestive of primary adrenal insuffi-ciency. Ambiguous genitalia in infant girls with virilizing CAH may be present; however, boys with virilizing CAH have no abnormalities on physical exami-nation, and the diagnosis is more likely to be missed, with the potential for heightened morbidity/mortality [13].

Laboratory tests

The comprehensive metabolic profile obtained as part of the critical blood sample (Box 10) may show the characteristic profile of adrenal insufficiency,

Box 10: Laboratory tests on evaluation of suspected adrenal insufficiency

Critical sample

    Electrolytes and glucose

    Plasma renin activity (on ice)

Archival sample

    Cortisol

    ACTH

    17-hydroxyprogesterone

    Free T_4 (if hypopituitarism is suspected)

Abbreviations: ACTH, corticotropin; CAH, congenital adrenal hyperplasia; T_4, thyroxine.

namely, hyponatremia with reduced bicarbonate and relatively increased chloride level (a normal anion gap metabolic acidosis) and a reduced glucose level. Approximately 50% of children presenting with primary adrenal insufficiency will have an elevated serum potassium level. If this pattern is found, blood should be drawn and put on ice for a determination of plasma renin activity. The archival blood sample may be sent for determination of serum cortisol and ACTH concentrations so that primary hypoadrenalism (decreased cortisol with elevated ACTH) may be differentiated from central causes (decreased cortisol without elevated ACTH). In infants suspected of having one of the CAHs, serum should be sent to measure 17-hydroxyprogesterone or (less commonly) a complete adrenal metabolic profile, so that the specific enzymatic block may be identified. Serum may be sent for determination of thyroid hormone status (free T_4) in children with known or suspected hypopituitarism.

Treatment

The first priority in the treatment of an adrenal insufficiency crisis is restoration of tissue perfusion. After an IV line is secured, a 20-mL/kg bolus of normal saline (0.9% sodium chloride [NaCl]) is given IV over a period of an hour or less, depending on the degree of hypotension or dehydration (Box 11). If hypoglycemia is present, a glucose bolus of 2 to 3 mL/kg of a 10% glucose solution may also be given to restore euglycemia. Stress doses of a glucocorticoid, specifically hydrocortisone, should then be given IV (25–50 mg/m^2 or 2–3 mg/kg). Hydrocortisone has a desirable mineralocorticoid effect as well as its glucocorticoid effect (20–35 mg hydrocortisone has the mineralocorticoid effect of 0.1 mg fludrocortisone), whereas methylprednisolone and dexamethasone have only a glucocorticoid effect and are not suitable therapies in this setting. Ongoing IV steroid therapy consists of hydrocortisone given as a total daily dose of 25 to 50 mg/m^2 or approximately 2 to 3 mg/kg in divided doses every 6 hours, if necessary [15].

Box 11: Treatment of adrenal insufficiency

Acute treatment

- IV fluid therapy: 20 mL/kg bolus of 5% dextrose/0.9% NaCl glucose: 200 to 300 mg/kg IV (2–3 mL/kg 10% glucose) as needed
- IV hydrocortisone: 25 to 50 mg/m^2 or 2 to 3 mg/kg: also has mineralocorti-coid effect[a]

Ongoing treatment

- IV fluid therapy: 2:2 × maintenance fluids as discussed previously, as needed
- Glucose: use 10% dextrose in IV fluids instead of 5% dextrose as needed
- hydrocortisone 25 to 50 mg/m^2/d or 2 to 3 mg/kg/d divided every 6 hours or continuous IV

[a] Methylprednisolone and dexamethasone are not satisfactory because they do not have the necessary mineralocorticoid activity in this setting.

Hyperkalemia of greater than 6 mEq/L can produce potentially fatal cardiac arrhythmias and requires aggressive therapy with sodium bicarbonate, 1 to 2 mEq/kg IV over 10 to 15 minutes; calcium gluconate, 50 to 100 mg/kg (maximum dose, 1 g) by slow (5–10 minutes) IV drip; or IV glucose, 500 mg/kg (2 mL/kg 25% glucose solution) plus insulin, 0.1 units/kg (monitor blood glucose). A potassium-binding resin, sodium polystyrene sulfonate (Kayexalate), 1 g/kg rectally or orally, may be given if tolerated.

HYPONATREMIA

Causes

The causes of hyponatremia (serum Na+ <135 mEq/L) are shown in Box 12. Disorders of sodium homeostasis are primarily the result of disturbances in water metabolism and their resultant changes in extracellular volume. Thus, hyponatremia results when the movement of free water into the extracellular space exceeds its loss. These disorders are usually characterized by extracellular hypo-osmolality. Several conditions, however, such as diabetic ketoacidosis or ethylene glycol poisoning, are not characterized by hypo-osmolality. These conditions result in an apparent hyponatremia caused by the accumulation of osmotically active substances (glucose and an organic alcohol, respectively) that move free water into the extracellular space and result in a dilution of other osmotically active entities, the most significant being sodium and chloride. Other conditions, such as hyperlipidemia, result in a pseudohyponatremia caused by a reduction in the plasma content of a given sample of blood [5].

Pathophysiology

As mentioned earlier, serum Na+ concentrations are primarily affected by changes in the extracellular fluid volume. Ordinarily, when an excess of free

Box 12: Causes of hypo-osmolar hyponatremia (serum Na+ <135 mEq/L)

Causes of hyponatremia

Hypovolemic

  Renal losses

    Diuretics, mineralocorticoid deficiency

    Renal tubular dysfunction

    Cerebral salt wasting

    Gastrointestinal losses: vomiting, diarrhea

    Skin losses: burns, cystic fibrosis

Normovolemic or hypervolemic

  SIADH or ADH overdose cortisol deficiency

  Nephrotic syndrome/cirrhosis

  Acute or chronic renal failure

  Water intoxication

Other states of apparent hyponatremia hyperosmolar (osmotic dilution)

  Hyperglycemia (DKA, nonketotic hyperglycemia)

  Organic alcohol intoxication (ethylene glycol, mannitol, ethanol)

  Factitious: hyperlipidemia

Abbreviations: ADH, antidiuretic hormone; SIADH, syndrome of inappropriate secretion of antidiuretic hormone.

water is present in the extracellular space, and hyponatremia (hypo-osmolality) develops, osmoreceptors in the hypothalamus respond by inhibiting the secretion of antidiuretic hormone (ADH). This secretopm results in the excretion of a dilute urine and a restoration of normal extracellular free water and Na+ concentration. A failure of this homeostatic mechanism (eg, syndrome of inappropriate secretion of ADH [SIADH]) may then lead to hyponatremia [16]. SIADH may be seen as a result of a CNS insult (tumor, meningitis, encephalitis, subarachnoid hemorrhage); respiratory disorders (pneumonia, asthma); with solid or hematologic malignancies; as a side effect of drugs (eg, vinca alkaloids, antiepileptic medications, such as carbamazepine or oxcarbazepine); or because of excessive use of an ADH analogue, desmopressin acetate (DDAVP), often used in the treatment of enuresis [17]. Conditions characterized by an inability to excrete a water load, such as ACTH/cortisol deficiency and the postoperative state, may also result in hyponatremia. Administration of hypotonic fluid in hospitalized patients has been associated with moderate hyponatremia [18,19].

Another mechanism involved in water and Na+ homeostasis is the renin/angiotensin/aldosterone pathway. This pathway is set in motion as a response to decreases in plasma volume and stimulates the renal tubular absorption of

Na+, resulting in obligatory water retention and a correction of the hypovolemia. Defects in this system, either renal tubular dysfunction or adrenal disorders (eg, Addison disease or one of the salt-wasting congenital adrenal hyperplasias), will also lead to hyponatremia. Other causes of renal salt loss (cerebral salt wasting) or gastrointestinal losses (hyponatremic dehydration) may also lead to hyponatremia and, rarely, panhypopituitarism with ACTH; secondary cortisol deficiency may compromise patients' ability to excrete free water normally and result in hyponatremia [16].

History and physical examination

A history of excessive free water intake (water intoxication) may be a manifestation of psychotic behavior or child abuse. Likewise, a search for excessive administration of hypotonic IV fluids postoperatively may be revealing in the hospitalized child. A history of known diuretic therapy, renal or adrenal disease, vomiting, or diarrhea may signify a potential for salt loss; known CNS trauma or infection may alert the physician to the possibility of SIADH, SIADH-like conditions, or cerebral salt wasting. This last condition is seen under the same circumstances as SIADH (ie, CNS insult) and may even be preceded by it but can be distinguished from SIADH by several criteria shown in Box 13.

Adolescents with Addison disease may have vomiting and complain of fatigue and loss of appetite. They may have darkening of the skin without tan lines and darkening of skin creases and along the gum line because of excessive secretion of CRF and ACTH.

The physical examination of children with hyponatremia should include an assessment of the state of their hydration or fluid balance because hyponatremia caused by salt loss is commonly associated with hypovolemia, whereas that caused by excess free water accumulation is not. The signs and symptoms seen in children with hyponatremia are proportional to the degree and the duration of this metabolic disturbance (Box 14). Acutely, the CNS effects are apparent; these worsen with the duration of the development of hyponatremia as well as its severity. In addition, gastrointestinal manifestations, such as nausea and

Box 13: Differential diagnosis of CSW and SIADH

	CSW	SIADH
Plasma volume	Decreased	Increased/norm
Clinical evidence of volume depletion	Present	Absent
Urine sodium concentration	Greatly increased	Increased
Urine flow rate	Greatly increased	Decreased
Net sodium loss	Greatly increased	Varies
Plasma renin activity	Decreased	Decreased/norm
Plasma ADH concentrations	Decreased	Increased
Plasma BNP concentration	Increased	Increased/norm

Abbreviations: BNP, brain natriuretic peptide; CSW, cerebral salt wasting.

vomiting, may be present; however, the latter may also be the cause of the disturbance. Generalized weakness may also be present. Of particular importance is the development of delayed CNS signs and symptoms during or after treatment, including a rarely seen and potentially fatal complication, central pontine myelinolysis, if care is not taken to correct the hyponatremia cautiously when the duration of the disturbance has exceeded 2 to 3 days (see Treatment). These delayed signs and symptoms are also shown in Box 6.

Laboratory evaluation

The critical blood sample should be sent for a comprehensive metabolic profile that will determine electrolyte, bicarbonate, glucose, BUN, and creatinine concentrations. Renal function can be estimated from these results. In addition, hyponatremia associated with mineralocorticoid deficiency is usually accompanied by hyperkalemia and a hyperchloremic (normal anion gap) metabolic acidosis. A calculated serum osmolality can also be obtained to document that the hyponatremia is associated with a hypo-osmolar state. It can also be compared with a measured osmolality, which should also be a part of the critical blood sample in the typical emergency department setting. Measured osmolalities that are more than 10 mOsm/kg greater than calculated are often associated with intoxications by osmotically active substances (eg, ethylene glycol).

Box 14: Signs and symptoms of hyponatremia or hypernatremia initially and during or after treatment

Initial signs and symptoms of hyponatremia
- (Note: These may also be seen during aggressive treatment of hypernatremia)
- CNS (reflects cerebral edema of varying degree): anorexia, lethargy, apathy
  - May progress to disorientation, agitation, delirium, seizures, Cheyne-Stokes respirations, hyporeflexia (hyponatremia) or hyperreflexia (hypernatremia), coma
  - Rarely: respiratory arrest and death caused by transtentorial herniation (hyponatremia)
- Neuromuscular: weakness
- Gastrointestinal: vomiting

Late-developing signs and symptoms: reflect CNS intracellular dehydration during treatment
- (Note: These may also be seen initially in hypernatremia)
- Mild: transient behavioral disturbances, movement disorders, seizures
- Severe: pseudobulbar palsy, quadriparesis, deepening coma
- Central or extrapontine myelinolysis, rare, may be fatal; occurs after 3 to 4 weeks

The archival blood sample may be sent for measurement of cortisol levels or a complete adrenal profile, serum ADH or brain natriuretic peptide concentrations, or both (see Boxes 12 and 13). The critical urine sample should be sent for a complete urinalysis, including specific gravity; the archival sample can be sent for urine sodium and creatinine concentrations, which may be helpful in the differential diagnosis by allowing the calculation of the fractional excretion of Na+.

Treatment

The treatment of hyponatremia, like the signs and symptoms, depends on both the degree (serum Na+ concentration) and duration of the disturbance (Box 15). As extracellular hyponatremia (hypo-osmolality) develops, the intracellular solute (organic osmolyte or idiogenic osmole) content of the brain slowly decreases to minimize fluid shifts into brain cells. The accumulation of idiogenic osmoles reduces the likelihood of severe cerebral edema but gradually (over 2–3 days) increases the potential for CNS dehydration if the hyponatremia is corrected rapidly. Thus, a more aggressive approach to treatment may be taken by using hypertonic (3%) saline in cases of hyponatremia developing over less than 1 to 2 days acutely (less than 1–2 days) (eg, with water intoxication, when serum Na+ concentrations are <105–110 mEq/L in a symptomatic patient, or both), because the risk of acute CNS decompensation in these patients is greater than the risk of late-developing complications, such as central or extrapontine myelinolysis. Serum Na+ concentrations should be monitored so that rapid changes in plasma osmolality (>1 mEq/L/h) do not occur [20].

The more common causes of hyponatremia usually develop over more than 2 days, and at that point patients are at greater risk of CNS pathology as a result of aggressive treatment. In these cases, treatment with fluid restriction and the use of isotonic rather than hypertonic saline is recommended, so that changes in serum sodium concentrations of less than 0.5 mEq/L/h (<12 mEq/L/d) are achieved. Rates of correction of hyponatremia may be adjusted based on the degree of symptoms exhibited by the patient, but changes in serum Na+ concentration should not exceed 1 mEq/L/h. The principle of changes in CNS intracellular solute concentrations that adjust to extracellular changes also applies to the correction of hypernatremia and is discussed later. Children with known or suspected adrenal insufficiency should also be given pharmacologic doses of IV hydrocortisone.

HYPERNATREMIA
Causes/Pathophysiology

As mentioned for hyponatremia, hypernatremia is also primarily a disorder of water metabolism. Loss of free water from the kidneys or gastrointestinal tract that exceeds the loss of Na+ will lead to hypernatremia. Conditions such as osmotic diuresis, diabetes insipidus (DI; central or nephrogenic), gastroenteritis, or excessive solute intake by mouth or IV may lead to hypernatremia (Box 16). In most persons with a normal thirst mechanism, hypernatremia rarely occurs,

Box 15: Treatment of hyponatremia

Acute hyponatremia (<2 days' duration) with serum Na+ less than 120 to 125 mEq/L

- Usually a hypervolemic hyponatremia due to water intoxication: polydipsia or excess hypotonic IV fluids postoperatively
  - ○ Hypertonic (3%) saline at 1 mL/kg/h IV: this will correct serum Na+ by 1 mEq/L/h
  - ○ Monitor serum Na+ and switch to fluid restriction rates of isotonic (0.9%) saline when serum Na+ greater than 125 mEq/L
  - ○ If initial serum Na+ greater than 120 to 125 mEq/L, use fluid restriction in hypervolemic states (see Box 4) or
  - ○ Isotonic saline in less common hypovolemic states (eg, adrenal insufficiency or hyponatremic dehydration)
- Note: If adrenal insufficiency is suspected (eg, in patients with known Addison disease or congenital adrenal hyperplasia) or if hyperkalemia, hypoglycemia, and metabolic acidosis coexist with hyponatremia, use pharmacologic glucocorticoid as IV hydrocortisone sodium succinate (Solu-Cortef), 25 to 50 mg/m^2 (2 to 3 mEq/kg)

Chronic hyponatremia (>2 days' duration) with serum Na+ less than 120–125 mEq/L and symptomatic patient (may be a hypovolemic or hypervolemic hyponatremia)

- Hypertonic (3%) saline at 0.5 mL/kg/h IV: this will correct serum Na+ by 0.5 mEq/L/h
- Monitor serum Na+ and switch to isotonic (0.9%) saline when serum Na+ greater than 125 mEq/L
- Rate of fluid administration should be tailored to patients' diagnosis: that is, fluid restriction in SIADH, cortisol deficiency, acute or chronic renal disease, or fluid overload, or fluid replacement in hypovolemic states, such as adrenal insufficiency, renal tubular dysfunction, CSW, or losses from the skin (burns) or GI tract

Special circumstances

- SIADH: If fluid restriction is not effective in increasing serum Na+ sufficiently, a loop diuretic (eg, furosemide [Lasix] 1 mg/kg IV) may be given. Total urine Na+ excretion should be measured for 3 to 4 hours after the diuretic and the Na+ replaced with 3% saline.
- CSW: Vigorous fluid and salt replacement should be provided, based on measured urine volume and calculated Na+ excretion every 1-4 hours. Replacement of Na+ loss often requires use of 3% saline.

Abbreviations: CSW, cerebral salt wasting; GI, gastrointestinal; SIADH, syndrome of inappropriate secretion of antidiuretic hormone.

Box 16: Causes of hypernatremia (serum Na+ >145 mEq/L) and their urine sodium concentrations

Cause	Urine sodium concentration
Hypovolemic (water loss > sodium loss)	
Renal losses: osmotic diuresis	Increased
Gastrointestinal losses: diarrhea	Decreased
Diabetes insipidus: central or nephrogenic	Decreased
Hypervolemic	
Mineralocorticoid excess: Cushing syndrome, exogenous steroids	Increased
Excess solute intake: IV or PO	Increased

even in DI. Thus, those children at risk are those with impaired thirst (eg, burn patients) or those with inanition accompanying moderately severe gastroenteritis. In children with excessive mineralocorticoid secretion or action (Cushing syndrome, exogenous steroids), the hypernatremia is modest, usually less than 150 mEq/L, because of sodium's osmotic activity that draws water into the extracellular space. Therefore, hypertension and hypokalemia are seen.

History and physical examination
A history of known DI or gastroenteritis may be elicited, as can a history of steroid intake or one of the salt-retaining forms of CAHs [4]. The examination should include an estimate of the state of hydration (hypovolemic or hypervolemic). The signs and symptoms associated with hypernatremia are those of the resultant intracellular CNS dehydration because the brain gradually loses intracellular water (and gains intracellular solute) to achieve a new equilibrium with the extracellular space.

Laboratory evaluation
As with hyponatremia, a comprehensive metabolic profile should be part of the critical blood sample so that renal function can be assessed. In addition, a calculated serum osmolality can be obtained and compared with the critical urine sample's specific gravity or osmolality. In children with DI, there is a characteristic dissociation between the two, so that the urine specific gravity (osmolality) is inappropriately low (<800 mOsm/kg) when the serum osmolality is greater than 300 mOsm/kg. The finding of hypernatremia and hypokalemia suggests excess mineralocorticoid secretion (Cushing syndrome) or effect (exogenous steroids).

Further studies (archival) may include measurement of plasma renin activity (PRA; suppressed in states of excess mineralocorticoid), ADH, and adrenal function. Urine Na+ excretion can also be calculated if Na+ and creatinine are measured. In children with suspected DI, a trial of aqueous vasopressin (Pitressin) (0.1 U/kg, <5 U) given subcutaneously may distinguish central DI (ADH deficiency) from nephrogenic DI secondary to renal tubular dysfunction or, rarely, caused by an X-linked recessive condition. In central DI, an increased concentration of the urine and a decreased urine output are seen within 30 minutes, whereas in nephrogenic DI, the kidneys are incapable of responding to the test dose.

Treatment

The approach to treatment should take into account the duration of the development of the hypernatremic state. As with hyponatremia or other changes in extracellular osmolality, the CNS can adjust by changing its content of organic osmolytes (idiogenic osmoles). When hyperosmolality develops, the brain slowly accumulates these osmolytes to reach equilibrium with the extracellular space. Rapid correction of hypernatremia, therefore, may result in movement of water into the brain, resulting in cerebral edema and its deleterious effects. In general, it is best to correct serum Na+ concentration by less than 0.5 mEq/L/h in chronic (duration >2 days) hypernatremia [21].

In hypovolemic patients, correction may be made by using isotonic (0.9%) saline, switching to 0.45% saline after volume deficits have been replaced, usually over 36 hours or more (Box 17). In central DI, DDAVP is the drug of choice, whereas in nephrogenic DI, a trial of hydrochlorothiazide is often useful. In hypervolemic states, such as Cushing syndrome, diuretic therapy may be helpful; reduction in dosage may be needed (if possible) in children on pharmacologic doses of steroids.

HYPERTHYROIDISM

Causes

Hyperthyroidism in children may be caused by stimulating antibodies directed at the thyroid gland (Graves disease or Hashimoto thyroiditis), by

---

Box 17: Treatment of hypernatremia

Hypovolemic states
- Isotonic (0.9%) saline IV to provide maintenance and to correct fluid deficits over 36 to 48 hours
- Switch to 0.45% saline to provide for maintenance and ongoing fluid losses
- Treat known central DI with DDAVP, 5 to 30 µg/d intranasally; give in divided doses twice a day
- Treat nephrogenic DI with hydrochlorothiazide, 2 to 3 mg/kg/d PO; give in divided doses every 12 hours

Hypervolemic states
- Adjust IV fluid/sodium content as necessary
- Adjust exogenous steroid dose, if possible, based on patients' primary condition
- Diagnose/treat Cushing syndrome with endocrine consult
- Diuretics and water replacement

excessive thyroid hormone intake in a hypothyroid child, by autonomous hypersecretion of thyroid hormone (eg, in McCune-Albright syndrome), by massive release of stored thyroid hormones after treatment with I131 in the treatment of Graves disease, by production of thyroid hormone by a functioning nodule, or by autoimmune destruction of the thyroid gland releasing preformed thyroid hormone [22–24]. Transplacental passage of thyroid-stimulating immunoglobulins from pregnant women with Graves disease to their newborns may also occur. This condition may present with signs of hyperthyroidism in the newborn period and may persist for the first 6 to 8 weeks of life.

Pathophysiology

The major emergency problems associated with hyperthyroidism are related to the positive inotropic effects of thyroid hormones (thyroxine [T_4] and triiodothyronine [T_3]) on the heart, leading to tachycardia, systolic hypertension, and secondary high-output congestive heart failure. It is thought that these are mediated by an upregulation of β-adrenergic receptors by thyroid hormones.

History and physical examination

Children with hyperthyroidism may present in the emergency setting with neurologic and/or cardiovascular symptoms. A history will reveal nervousness, agitation, inability to concentrate, insomnia, delirium, or overtly psychotic behavior. Major cardiovascular complaints include palpitations and dyspnea. Other complaints include heat intolerance, diarrhea, headaches, amenorrhea or dysmenorrhea, hair and skin changes (hair thinning and smooth, dry, warm skin), and weight loss or failure to thrive in the infant. In the child with previously diagnosed hyperthyroidism, noncompliance with antithyroid medications may lead to a rapid reemergence of symptoms.

Neurologic findings include agitation, tremor, and hyperactive reflexes. Cardiopulmonary examination can reveal tachycardia, a systolic flow murmur or the murmur of aortic or mitral valve insufficiency, widened pulse pressure with systolic hypertension, cardiomegaly, and tachypnea. With severe high-output failure, edema, rales, and hepatomegaly are noticeable.

Dehydration warrants fluid therapy in addition to other modalities (see later discussion). Severe hyperthermia may be present and, with severe cardiovascular abnormalities, has been termed *thyroid storm*, a rare presentation of hyperthyroidism in children. Almost all patients have a goiter, or rarely, a toxic nodule; a flow murmur may be audible over the gland. Lid lag and exophthalmos may be present. In patients without a goiter, excessive thyroid hormone intake should be considered. Goiters may also not be visible or palpable in newborns with transplacentally acquired Graves disease, and a history of maternal Graves disease should be elicited in all infants younger than 2 months who are seen with the signs or symptoms described earlier. Similar presentations may be seen in infants of cocaine- or methadone-addicted mothers.

Laboratory evaluation

Children with the signs and symptoms described earlier may have hysteria, psychiatric disturbances, drug abuse, or pheochromocytoma; however, a routine thyroid profile plus a serum T_3 concentration should easily differentiate hyperthyroidism from these other conditions. In the child with hyperthyroidism, abnormalities in circulating thyroid hormones may readily be demonstrated as considerable elevations in serum T_4 (often >18 µg/dL), free T_4 (>3 ng/dL), and T_3 (>250 ng/dL). In addition, serum thyroid-stimulating hormone concentrations are suppressed (<0.03 mU/L). If hyperthyroidism is confirmed by the results of these laboratory tests, archival serum may be sent for measurement of antithyroid antibodies (antithyroglobulin and antithyroid peroxidase) and for thyroid-stimulating immunoglobulin. Children with McCune-Albright syndrome, a rare disorder of constitutively active polypeptide hormone receptors, may present with hyperthyroidism; but precocious puberty is the most frequent finding and may be assessed on physical examination [5].

Treatment

Nonspecific acute treatment

In the child with severe systolic hypertension and tachycardia with or without congestive heart failure, β-adrenergic blocking agents should be administered in the emergency department (Box 18). β-Blockers antagonize the increase in the catecholaminelike positive inotropic effects of elevated thyroid hormones. Propranolol, the β-blocker most widely used, can be given IV over 10 minutes in doses of 0.1 to 0.15 mg/kg, maximum dose of 1 mg/dose in infants and 3 mg/dose in children and adolescents. Oral propranolol is given in doses of 0.5 to 1 mg/kg/d divided every 6 to 8 hours. Its IV use requires electrocardiogram monitoring for the development of bradycardia or arrhythmias. In more severe cases, stress-level IV doses of a glucocorticoid (eg, methylprednisolone) may be administered because it inhibits the conversion of T_4 to its more active metabolite, T_3. Hyperthermia should be treated with a cooling blanket, acetaminophen, or both but not with aspirin because it uncouples oxidative phosphorylation, which may accentuate the hyperthermia.

Specific acute treatment

Once propranolol (and steroids as necessary) is given, thiourea therapy can be initiated even before laboratory results are available if hyperthyroidism is highly likely clinically (see Box 18). The thiourea drugs, propylthiouracil (PTU) and methimazole (Tapazole), interfere with the synthesis of thyroid hormone; PTU also inhibits the conversion of T_4 to T_3. Given the risk for hepatotoxicity with PTU, it is no longer recommended for the treatment of hyperthyroidism in pediatrics. The initial dose of methimazole is 0.8 to 1.2 mg/kg orally followed at 8-hour intervals by 0.6 to 0.8 mg/kg for the first day. If the child is unable to swallow, the drugs can be given via a nasogastric tube. Iodides block the production of thyroid hormones more rapidly than do the thiourea drugs and may be used in addition to these drugs acutely. A saturated solution of potassium iodide or of Lugol solution, 2 to 10 drops based on

---

Box 18: Treatment of hyperthyroidism

Nonspecific acute treatment

1. Propranolol: 0.015 mg/kg IV given over 10 minutes, may be repeated × 3 as necessary ECG monitoring required
2. If cardiovascular signs are severe: IV methylprednisolone (Solu-Medrol): 10 to 15 mg/m^2 or ≈1 mg/kg initially, then 0.25 mg/kg IV q6 hours
3. Cooling blanket as necessary

Specific acute treatment

1. SSKI or Lugol solution 2 to 10 drops (based on body weight) every 6 hours

Long-term treatment

1. Until cardiovascular status is normal
   a. Propranolol initial of 0.5–1 mg/kg/d titrate to a maximum of 4 mg/kg/d PO divided into 3 doses or
   b. Atenolol 25 to 50 mg PO at bedtime

Abbreviations: ECG, electrocardiogram; PTU, propylthiouracil; SSKI, saturated solution of potassium iodide.

---

the weight of the patient, can be given orally 3 times a day, starting several hours after the first dose of methimazole, for the first 1 to 2 days of treatment. General support, as mentioned, may include cooling by hypothermic blanket, administration of acetaminophen, and infusion of IV fluids as needed to correct dehydration.

Long-term treatment
Methimazole is given at a dosage of 0.5 to 0.7 mg/kg/d divided into 2 doses (see Box 18). Symptoms of hyperthyroidism usually improve within 1 to 2 weeks, but laboratory studies may take 4 to 6 weeks to become normal. Propranolol, 1 to 2 mg/kg/d divided into 3 doses, or atenolol, 25 to 50 mg at bedtime, can be used in the first weeks of treatment until the child's cardiovascular status is normal. The thiourea drugs can produce significant side effects, such as allergic reactions, oral mucosal ulcerations, thrombocytopenia, and leukopenia. With acute infections, children taking a thiourea drug should have a complete blood cell count with differential and a platelet count to rule out significant hematologic abnormalities that could compromise their clinical status.

SUMMARY

The presentation of endocrine and metabolic emergencies represents one of the more challenging clinical scenarios faced by pediatricians and emergency providers. In this review, the authors attempt to describe some of the more common entities that a provider may see and provide a guide for the recognition and management of these difficult-to-assess and often very ill children.

References

[1] MacNeill EC, Vashist S. Approach to syncope and altered mental status. Pediatr Clin North Am 2013;60(5):1083–106.

[2] Teasdale G, Maas A, Lecky F, et al. The Glasgow coma scale at 40 years: standing the test of time. Lancet Neurol 2014;13(8):844–54.

[3] Wing R, James C. Pediatric head injury and concussion. Emerg Med Clin North Am 2013;31(3):653–75.

[4] Kappy MS, Bajaj L. Recognition and treatment of endocrine/metabolic emergencies in children: part I. Adv Pediatr 2002;49:245–72.

[5] Kappy MS, Bajaj L. Recognition and treatment of endocrine/metabolic emergencies in children: part II. Adv Pediatr 2003;50:181–214.

[6] Rewers A. Current controversies in treatment and prevention of diabetic ketoacidosis. Adv Pediatr 2010;57(1):247–67.

[7] Rozance PJ. Update on neonatal hypoglycemia. Curr Opin Endocrinol Diabetes Obes 2014;21(1):45–50.

[8] Daly LP, Osterhoudt KC, Weinzimer SA. Presenting features of idiopathic ketotic hypoglycemia. J Emerg Med 2003;25(1):39–43.

[9] Magoulas PL, El-Hattab AW. Systemic primary carnitine deficiency: an overview of clinical manifestations, diagnosis, and management. Orphanet J Rare Dis 2012;7:68.

[10] Claudius I, Fluharty C, Boles R. The emergency department approach to newborn and childhood metabolic crisis. Emerg Med Clin North Am 2005;23(3):843–83, x.

[11] Park E, Pearson NM, Pillow MT, et al. Neonatal endocrine emergencies: a primer for the emergency physician. Emerg Med Clin North Am 2014;32(2):421–35.

[12] Charmandari E, Nicolaides NC, Chrousos GP. Adrenal insufficiency. Lancet 2014;383(9935):2152–67.

[13] Finkielstain GP, Kim MS, Sinaii N, et al. Clinical characteristics of a cohort of 244 patients with congenital adrenal hyperplasia. J Clin Endocrinol Metab 2012;97(12):4429–38.

[14] Merke DP, Poppas DP. Management of adolescents with congenital adrenal hyperplasia. Lancet Diabetes Endocrinol 2013;1(4):341–52.

[15] Grossman A, Johannsson G, Quinkler M, et al. Therapy of endocrine disease: perspectives on the management of adrenal insufficiency: clinical insights from across Europe. Eur J Endocrinol 2013;169(6):R165–75.

[16] Oh JY, Shin JI. Syndrome of inappropriate antidiuretic hormone secretion and cerebral/renal salt wasting syndrome: similarities and differences. Front Pediatr 2014;2:146.

[17] Lucchini B, Simonetti GD, Ceschi A, et al. Severe signs of hyponatremia secondary to desmopressin treatment for enuresis: a systematic review. J Pediatr Urol 2013;9(6 Pt B):1049–53.

[18] Foster BA, Tom D, Hill V. Hypotonic versus isotonic fluids in hospitalized children: a systematic review and meta-analysis. J Pediatr 2014;165(1):163–9.e2.

[19] McNab S, Ware RS, Neville KA, et al. Isotonic versus hypotonic solutions for maintenance intravenous fluid administration in children. Cochrane Database Syst Rev 2014;(12):CD009457.

[20] Moritz ML, Ayus JC. Management of hyponatremia in various clinical situations. Curr Treat Options Neurol 2014;16(9):310.

[21] Bockenhauer D, Zieg J. Electrolyte disorders. Clin Perinatol 2014;41(3):575–90.

[22] Hays HL, Jolliff HA, Casavant MJ. Thyrotoxicosis after a massive levothyroxine ingestion in a 3-year-old patient. Pediatr Emerg Care 2013;29(11):1217–9.

[23] Majlesi N, Greller HA, McGuigan MA, et al. Thyroid storm after pediatric levothyroxine ingestion. Pediatrics 2010;126(2):e470–3.

[24] Rohrs HJ 3rd, Silverstein JH, Weinstein DA, et al. Thyroid storm following radioactive iodine (RAI) therapy for pediatric graves disease. Am J Case Rep 2014;15:212–5.

Advances in Pediatrics 62 (2015) 283–293

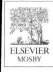

ADVANCES IN PEDIATRICS

Pediatric Headaches

Robin Slover, MD*, Sheryl Kent, PhD

University of Colorado, Children's Hospital of Colorado, 13123 East 16th Avenue, B615, Aurora, CO 80045, USA

Keywords
- Migraine • Headache • Aura

Key points
- Pediatric headaches are common, and many may never require intervention by a health care provider.
- However, migraines can become more difficult to treat, especially if they become chronic daily headaches.
- Pediatric headache is a subjective and unique experience that requires attention to both psychological and physiologic components in diagnosis and treatment.

INTRODUCTION

Headaches are one of the most common types of pediatric pain. The frequency of headaches increases with age, ranging from 20% [1] in children younger than 5 years to 75% in children aged 15 years [2]. The frequency of migraines is less, averaging from 3.9% to 7%. Three other reports suggest that 4% to 20% of adolescent boys and 10% to 27% of adolescent girls will develop migraines [3]. Although the International Headache Society has adjusted its definition of migraine headaches over the year, the basic distinction between migraine headaches and tension headaches persists.

MIGRAINE DEFINITION

A migraine headache without aura is defined as multiple attacks (at least 4 or 5) of headaches with a temporal throbbing sensation, usually unilateral but sometimes bilateral. These headaches (especially in younger patients) are accompanied by nausea, vomiting, photophobia, and phonophobia and are made worse by movements. These attacks can occur at anytime (even waking the patient) and last from 1 hour (in younger patients) to 48 to 72 hours. Sleep can help

*Corresponding author. E-mail address: Robin.Slover@childrenscolorado.org

0065-3101/15/$ – see front matter
http://dx.doi.org/10.1016/j.yapd.2015.04.006

ameliorate symptoms. Younger patients may have motion sickness, vomiting, and abdominal pain before developing head pain. Only about 15% of children have auras with their migraines. Auras are defined as unilateral reversible symptoms in visual, sensory, speech or language, motor, brainstem, or retinal areas that spread gradually over 5 minutes and last 5 to 60 minutes followed by a migraine headache. Patients can have 2 or more symptoms occurring in succession [4].

PATHOPHYSIOLOGY

Migraines seem to be due to a combination of inherited genetic susceptibility (60%–70%) and environmental factors. Insights into the responsible mechanisms and the interrelationship with neuronal components such as astrocytes have come from studies of familiar hemiplegic migraine, in which several responsible genes have been identified: CACNA1A, ATP1A2, and SCN1A [5–7]. Abnormalities in calcium metabolism are thought to be involved in some migraines.

There are 2 current explanations for migraine pain: the vasogenic theory and the neurovascular theory. The vasogenic theory is based on the observation that migraines have painful, distended, pulsing extracranial vessels during attacks. Stimulation of intracranial vessels has been shown to cause an ipsilateral migraine [8]. In addition, vasodilatory substances such as nitrates can cause headaches, whereas vasoconstrictive compounds such as ergotamines and caffeine can abort migraines. It is important that migraineurs have uniform exposure to caffeine (preferably none). Even though caffeine is vasoconstrictive, frequent exposure can trigger migraines because of rebound vasodilation.

In the neurovascular theory, the aura (if present) is due to an altered cerebral susceptibility to migraine attacks. Vascular changes observed are the result rather than the cause of the attack. Aura changes are seen as focal neurologic effects. The expanding neurologic effects covering many different areas of the brain are attributed to a spreading cortical depression [9]. Spreading cortical depression results from hyperpolarization followed by suppression and blood flow decreases [10]. Fluid changes in the cells also occur in the wake of the spreading cortical depression, increasing the pain.

Recently, PET imaging performed at the start of several migraines (without aura) has shown increased blood flow in an area in the ipsilateral brainstem, leading to speculation that this could be a migraine generator [11]. In these patients, areas usually associated with aura have shown decreased blood flow (visual cortex and auditory regions). Neocortex activation leads to release of nociceptive substances into the interstitial space. Released substances activate pain nerves and trigeminovascular fibers that surround pial vessels. As more nociceptive compounds accumulate, the trigeminal nerves are activated, along with C fibers. Fibers travel from the activated trigeminal ganglion to other areas of the brain involved in the headache responsible for the patients' perception of pain.

PRESENTATION

Migraines can be divided into 4 stages: prodrome, aura (if present), headache and termination or postdrome [12]. The prodrome is evident up to 24 hours before any headache and may be the earliest sign of dysfunction in the brain. Prodrome may be expressed by irritability, change in sleep patterns, change in appetite, or temporary personality change. An aura occurs within an hour of the start of the headache. Migraineurs who have auras do not have them with every headache. Common auras include visual changes in scotomata, decreasing visual fields, blurred vision, smell, or speech changes. Depolarization of perivascular and meningeal C fibers from the spreading cortical depression is thought to contribute to the gradual intensification and prolongation of a headache as well as to decreased blood flow.

Migraines are intense, painful (10 out of 10), throbbing headaches that can be unilateral, but become bilateral as they increase in intensity. Occipital and temporal pain locations are common. In younger patients, migraines can be bilateral and located in the frontal temporal area. Younger patients also have periodic variants such as abdominal migraines, cyclic vomiting, and vertigo. The timing and pattern of the periodic variant is the same as that of a migraine and responds to similar interventions. Head pain usually develops as the child ages, but the child can continue to have abdominal pain and vomiting with headaches. Sleep and dark quiet rooms are sought by patients until the episode has passed. Headaches are thought to be due to the continued peripheral and central sensitization of the trigeminal nerves. Sphenopalatine blocks, which directly target the trigeminal nerves, can be effective in decreasing headache intensity if performed early enough.

TREATMENT

Once set in motion, C fibers release neuropeptides (substance P, calcitonin gene related protein) which have neuroinflammatory effects within the meninges, causing increased plasma leakage, vasodilation, and mast cell activation. Once this system is activated, less stimulation is needed to keep it activated. Sleep and abortive medication (Table 1) can be helpful in breaking the cycle.

Table 1
Migraine abortives

Name of drug	Dose	Timing
Ibuprofen	10 mg/kg	q 4–6 h
Acetaminophen	10–12.5 mg/kg	q 4–6 h
Naproxen	5.7 mg/kg	q 8–12 h
Sumatriptan oral	25–100 mg	May repeat once
Sumatriptan nasal	5–10 mg <12 y	—
	20 mg >12 y	
Rizatriptan	5–10 mg older adolescents	May repeat once every 2 h
Almotriptan	6.25–12.5 mg	May repeat once every 2 h

The sooner the abortive medication is given, the more effective it will be because the area of neural inflammation and central sensitization required to be calmed will be smaller. Given the widespread changes throughout the brain, it is not surprising that migraineurs do not feel like themselves for a period of time after the main headache and may still have pain, although to a smaller degree. This area has not been studied well in pediatrics.

Most families with migraines recognize children who have migraines and may not even see a care provider unless migraines are severe. There are some known environmental triggers for migraines that should be considered and modified. For example, a regular sleep schedule, good stress management (cognitive behavioral techniques may be helpful), attending school, avoiding monosodium glutamate, minimizing caffeine, and regular exercise are very helpful for reducing migraines. Increased migraine frequency has also been associated with obesity, sleep apnea, asthma and allergies, epilepsy, and psychological emotional disorders. In addition to environmental and psychosocial factors, avoiding overmedication treatment of headaches is also important. No more than 2 headaches per week should be treated with medication. An MRI or computed tomography should be done during the child's course of treatment [13], particularly because sinusitis is a common cause of similar headaches. Imaging only needs to be done once, unless there is a very severe change in the presentation of the headaches. Youth presenting with motor weakness, numbness, temporary vision loss, or severe speech difficulties definitely need imaging, probably an MRI/magnetic resonance angiography/magnetic resonance venography to rule out venous sludging as well as other pathologic conditions. Papilledema should be checked for as part of the neurologic evaluation.

Migraines can be primary or secondary. Secondary migraines include headaches associated with depression, lupus, arteriovenous malformation, cancer, human immunodeficiency virus infection, drugs associated with cystic fibrosis, and pseudotumor cerebri [14]. These headaches are treated by dealing with the underlying issues.

An interdisciplinary team evaluation is important for primary migraines. Psychological correlates such as depression and anxiety should be evaluated and appropriately treated. A physical therapy program is also helpful. After a full medical history and evaluation rules out other medical causes, patients should be encouraged to keep a headache diary for a month to look for triggers and patterns. If the headaches are fewer than 1 per week, abortive medication can be used. If individuals have 2 or more headaches per week, then a preventive as well as an abortive medication can be used. Some of the preventive medications are natural such as vitamin B_2, magnesium, and coenzyme Q10 (Table 2). Topiramate is very effective in decreasing headaches. Pediatric efficacy can be seen in a meta-analysis of topiramate and trazodone [15]. Administration of 50 mg topiramate at night can be helpful for headache reduction. Regardless of the dose, weight should be monitored because topiramate frequently causes weight loss. Nonsteroidal antiinflammatory drugs

Table 2
Migraine preventives

Name of drug	Dose	Side effects
Topiramate	1–2 mg/kg/d (the authors use 50 mg) headache	Sedation Appetite suppression Kidney stones
Amitriptyline	0.1–1 mg/kg/d	Sedation Weight gain Get ECG Dry mouth Constriction abnormalities
Nortriptyline	0.1–1 mg/kg/d	Sedation Dry mouth Mood changes, including suicidality
Lamotrigine	50 mg for two weeks before increasing if desired up to 1-2 mg per kg	Sedation Use in patients older than 12 y
Cyproheptadine	0.25–1.5 mg/kg/d	Sedation Dry mouth
Co Q10	100–300 mg	Minimal Check blood level
Vitamin B_2	200–400 mg	Yellow-orange urine
Magnesium	100–150 mg	Check blood level Diarrhea
Propranolol	2–4 mg/kg/d	Hypotension
Atenolol	0.5–1 mg/kg/d	Hypotension
Valproic acid	20–40 mg/d	Sedation Weight gain Mood changes Hepatotoxicity, bone marrow changes
Gabapentin	10–40 mg/d tid dose	Sedation Mood changes Weight gain

Abbreviations: Co Q10, coenzyme Q10; ECG, electrocardiogram.

(NSAIDs) are often the most effective abortive medication for younger patients with migraine.

TENSION HEADACHE
Tension headaches occur in approximately 10% to 15% of youth [16] and are usually less painful than migraines. These headaches have a pressing or band-like quality rather than throbbing, as well as a different location compared with migraines. Tension headaches are shorter in duration, bilateral, usually posterior in location, and do not meet criteria for migraines; they are typically worst in the afternoon or evening. There may be a muscular component to them, especially in the neck and trapezius. Pericranial tenderness may be present. Tension headaches can co-occur with migraine headaches and lead to

chronic daily headaches. Tension headaches are usually treated with NSAIDs.

OPIATES

Opiates should be used sparingly in treating any headache. Prolonged opiate use can lead to development of chronic headaches as well as addiction and dependence. Opiates can be used to treat underlying anxiety and not the headache itself. If abortive medications have not worked, a visit to the emergency room for a migraine cocktail, often consisting of metoclopramide, ketorolac, and an antinausea agent, can be effective. This cocktail should be used judiciously. Ergotamine infusions and Depakote infusions are also available in the emergency room. A patient's first exposure to these agents should be in a monitored setting.

CHRONIC DAILY HEADACHE

The term chronic daily headache does not define any particular type of headache such as migraine or tension headache but rather a continuum of central sensitization, neuronal inflammation, and myalgia that is constant. The pain may vary somewhat, but is usually high in intensity. Causes of chronic daily headache or transformed migraines include overuse of analgesic medications, depression, and poorly treated migraines or tension headaches (often with poor compliance to the outlined treatment plan) so that persistent neuronal inflammation and desensitization of C fibers, with concomitant anxiety and depression, because of unrelieved pain, dominate the picture. In the authors' interdisciplinary clinic, discontinuing the overuse of analgesics has successfully treated some patients. Lidocaine patches or Lidoderm gel along the neck, trapezius, and occipital prominence can also be helpful in the reduction of pain. If medications have not been effectively used before, adding topiramate or amitriptyline can be helpful. Lamotrigine can be another helpful medication. Trigger point injections into areas of severe muscle spasms of neck, trapezius, para scapular and posterior strap muscles, as well as the occipital nerves, periauricular nerves, and supraorbital nerves have been helpful for the patients treated by the authors. Many of these patients are particularly tender over the C3 area and mastoid processes. A combined treatment approach of injections under sedation, physical therapy program, appropriate medications, and psychological interventions is often helpful. Most patients usually need injections only once. However, if physical therapy is not being actively used, then these injections are of less value. If local anesthesia and steroid injections do not help, or help only briefly, then chemodenervation with onabotulinum toxin type A is considered.

ONABOTULINUM TOXIN

The use of onabotulinum toxin type A in adolescents younger than 18 years is an off-label use, but it has been effective for patients with chronic daily headaches. Chan and colleagues [17] studied 12 adolescents aged 14 to 18 years, of whom 6 received botulinum toxin. All reported improvement of 33% to 75%. Two had complete relief between injections. Bernhard and colleagues [18] treated 10 patients aged 10 to 17 years, of whom 7 showed improvement. The authors have treated 55 adolescents with transformed migraines, aged 14 to 18 years, with 200 units of botulinum toxin type A, in a standard "migraine and follow-the-pain" pattern; 50 of these patients showed improvement in terms of headache frequency and duration. Double-blind randomized studies of onabotulinum toxin in adolescents should be carried out. Chemodenervation seems to be useful in patients who are resistant to other therapies. A combination of topiramate and onabotulinum toxin type A is more effective than individual use of either of these drugs [19].

CLUSTER HEADACHE

Cluster headaches are rare in children, but distinctive. Adolescents with cluster headaches have multiple severe headaches (up to 8 per day) in a period of several weeks or months, followed by relatively long headache-free intervals. These headaches tend to occur on a regular schedule, even waking patients from a sound sleep; they are more common in spring and fall. Usually the pain is frontal in location and does not have a throbbing quality. Patients cannot lie still; they walk, bang their head with their fists, or rock back and forth. The headache is always unilateral. It is more common in males, and there is a hereditary component. Breathing oxygen through a nonrebreather mask is effective for about 3 of 4 patients [20]. Subcutaneous sumatriptan is equally effective. Sumatriptan nasal sprays are sometimes effective. Lithium has also been used.

ADDITIONAL INTERVENTIONS

Other interventions are effective for treating pediatric headaches in addition to medications and injections. Multiple systematic reviews demonstrate that psychological treatments can effectively reduce pain frequency and intensity in youth with headache [21–23] and lead to an approximately 3-fold greater likelihood of clinically significant improvement in headache compared with control conditions [24]. These same interventions can be effective for many comorbidities of headache in children and adolescents, such as impaired social interaction, school absences, and anxiety and depression [25]. Importantly, these psychological treatments focus on self-management skills, and data suggests that treatment gains are sustained after termination of treatment, leading to stable decrease in headache intensity. Most research on psychological treatment of pediatric headaches has focused on effectiveness of cognitive behavioral interventions, relaxation techniques, and biofeedback. In many cases, these treatment strategies have been shown to be as effective as pharmacologic treatment in pediatric migraine treatment [22,26].

COGNITIVE BEHAVIORAL THERAPY

Cognitive behavioral therapy (CBT) is the most commonly researched and empirically supported psychological treatment for the management of pediatric pain, including headache. CBT is a brief, goal-oriented psychotherapy based on the concept that thoughts, feelings, and behaviors are interrelated and changeable. Individuals learn cognitive strategies to identify and restructure illogical or maladaptive thoughts related to pain (especially the concept that pain cannot be controlled), as well as behavioral strategies to relieve physiologic discomforts and relearn healthy functioning. Goals of CBT include gaining a sense of control over pain, reducing fear of pain, enhancing function, increasing feelings of hopefulness and resourcefulness, and improving mood. Individuals focus on application, generalization, and maintenance of learned coping skills to pain-producing situations. Many reviews [24,27] have demonstrated that CBT can reduce intensity of headache in adolescents. A recent randomized controlled trial [28] expanded upon these results by demonstrating reduced frequency of headache as well as decrease in headache-related disability in adolescents receiving CBT. Acceptance and commitment therapy (ACT) is a psychotherapy that is often considered a new wave of CBT. ACT is based on the premise that acceptance (and not avoidance) of pain results in decrease in pain and pain-related disability. ACT uses mindfulness and values clarification to identify and reduce pain-avoidance-based behavior [29], and there is a growing body of empirical literature to indicate that ACT may be helpful for pediatric chronic pain and headaches [30].

RELAXATION TECHNIQUES

Relaxation skills increase a sense of control over physiologic processes and increase both physical and psychological well-being to counteract pain states. Relaxation slows the heart rate and breathing rate, reduces the need for oxygen, increases blood flow to muscles, and decreases muscle tension [31]. Relaxation-based therapies have been empirically shown to decrease headache in youth [32]. Research demonstrates that progressive muscle relaxation (tensing and relaxing each muscle group in order to learn the difference between discomfort and relaxation) effectively reduces pediatric headache [33,34], often in conjunction with diaphragmatic breathing (to maximize the amount of oxygen that goes into the bloodstream and interrupt the fight-or-flight response). Guided imagery (mental imagery to take a visual journey to a nonpainful environment) has also demonstrated reduction in pediatric headache [27]. Hypnosis is defined as a state of heightened awareness and focused attention in conjunction with suspension of peripheral awareness (to lessen pain signals). This technique has also been shown to effectively manage headaches in children [35].

BIOFEEDBACK

Biofeedback measures and provides auditory and/or visual feedback to patients about an individual's physiologic activity (indicators of autonomic arousal, such as heart rate and skin temperature). The goal is to increase awareness of and voluntary control over physiologic processes that are activated by pain or stress [36] so that patients can intentionally change the targeted physiologic function to a desired direction. For pediatric pain control, biofeedback is often taught in conjunction with relaxation strategies (called biofeedback-assisted relaxation therapy) and has been shown to reduce headache [37]. According to recent meta-analyses, there are strong evidence levels for the effectiveness of biofeedback in the treatment of pediatric migraine or tensiontype headaches [23,38,39]. In particular, research demonstrates excellent evidence for the effectiveness of thermal biofeedback (produces changes in peripheral and cranial blood flow) in treating pediatric migraine headaches [40], and electromyographic biofeedback (monitoring the electrical activity of the skeletal muscles and helps to increase self-control of muscle tension) in treating pediatric tension-type headaches in which there is more of a myofascial component [41]. In general, children with headache benefit from biofeedback more than adults [42], and data suggest that biofeedback also improves children's ability to cope, attend school, and sleep better, leading to reduction in headache-related disability [23].

ACUPUNCTURE

Acupuncture involves the insertion of thin needles into the skin to help stimulate and rebalance the flow of natural energy (Qi) along energy pathways (meridians). Western practitioners often view acupuncture points as places to stimulate nerves, muscles, and connective tissue in order to boost the activity of body's natural pain killers and increase blood flow. Growing research in adults has supported the efficacy of acupuncture for headaches [43,44]. Literature on acupuncture in children with headaches is growing but limited, and further studies are needed with rigorous research standards. However, 2 randomized controlled trials of acupuncture of children with chronic headaches have demonstrated a reduction in severity and frequency of headaches [45].

SUMMARY

Pediatric headaches are common, and many may never require intervention by a health care provider. However, migraines can become more difficult to treat, especially if they become chronic daily headaches. Pediatric headache is a subjective and unique experience that requires attention to both psychological and physiologic components in diagnosis and treatment. A biopsychosocial, multidisciplinary approach, including both medication management and psychological treatment, is considered essential for effective management [46,47].

References
[1] Silanpoo M, Piekkala P. Prevalence of headache at preschool age in an unselected child population. Cephalagia 1991;11:239–42.
[2] Bille B. Migraine in school age children. Acta Paediatr 1962;51:16–151.
[3] Carlsson S. Prevalence of headache in school children: relation to family and school factors. Acta Paediatr 1996;85:692–6.
[4] Carol-Artal FJ. Tackling chronic migraine: current perspectives. J Pain Res 2014;7:185–94.

[5] Ophoff RA, Terwindt GM, Vergouwe MN, et al. Familial hemiplegic migraine and episodic ataxia type-2 are caused by mutations in the Ca ++ channel gene CACNL1A4. Cell 1996;87:544–52.

[6] De Fusco M, Marconi R, Silvistri L, et al. Haploinsufficiency of ATP1A2 encoding the Na+/K+ pump alpha2 subunit associated with familial hemiplegic migraine type 2. Nat Genet 2003;33(2):192–6.

[7] Dichgans M, Freilinger T, Eckstein G, et al. Mutation in neuronal voltage-gated sodium channel SCN1A in familial hemiplegic migraine. Lancet 2005;366(9483):371–7.

[8] Gasparini CF, Heidi G, Griffiths LR. Studies on the pathophysiology and genetic basis of migraine. Curr Genomics 2013;14(5):300–15.

[9] Cui Y, Kataoka Y, Watanabe Y. Role of cortical spreading depression in the pathophysiology of migraine. Neurosci Bull 2014;30(5):812–22.

[10] Ferrari MD, Klever RR, Terwindt GM, et al. Migraine pathophysiology: lessons from mouse models and human genetics. Lancet Neurol 2015;14(1):65–80.

[11] Weiller C, May A, Limmroth V. Brain stem activation in spontaneous human migraine attacks. Nat Med 1995;1:658–60.

[12] Cutrer FM, O'Donnell A. Pathophysiology of headaches. In: Warfield C, Bajwa ZW, editors. Principles and practice of pain medicine. 2nd edition. New York: McGraw-Hill; 2004. p. 204–8.

[13] Hockeday JM, Barlow CF. Headache in children. In: Olesen J, Tfelt-hansen P, Welch KM, editors. The headaches. Philadelphia: Raven Press; 1993. p. 705–808.

[14] Antilla P. Tension-type headache in childhood and adolescence. Lancet Neurol 2002;5(6): 268–74.

[15] El-Chammas K, Keyes J, Thompson N, et al. Pharmacologic treatment of pediatric headaches: a meta-analysis. JAMA 2013;167(3):250–8.

[16] Matthew PG, Garza L. Headache. Semin Neurol 2011;31(1):5–17.

[17] Chan VW, McCabe EJ, MacGregor DL. Botox treatment for migraine and chronic daily headache in adolescents. J Neurosci Nurs 2009;41(5):235–43.

[18] Bernhard MK, Bertsche A, Syrbe S, et al. Botulinum toxin injections for chronic migraine in adolescents – an early therapeutic option in the transition from neuropaediatrics to neurology. Fortschr Neurol Psychiatr 2014;82(1):39–42.

[19] Matthew NT, Jaffri SF. A double-blind comparison of onabotulinum toxin A (BOTOX) and topiramate (TOPMAX) for the prophylactic treatment of chronic migraine: a pilot study. Headache 2009;49(10):1466–78.

[20] Blume HK. Pediatric headache: a review. Pediatr Rev 2012;33(12):562–76.

[21] Eccleston C, Morley S, Williams A, et al. Systematic review of randomized controlled trials of psychological therapy for chronic pain in children and adolescents, with a subset meta-analysis of pain relief. Pain 2002;99:157–65.

[22] Palermo TM, Eccleston C, Lewandowski AS, et al. Randomized controlled trials of psychological therapies for management of chronic pain in children and adolescents: an updated meta-analytic review. Pain 2010;148(3):387–97.

[23] Trautmann E, Lackschewitz H, Kroner-Herwig B. Psychological treatment of recurrent headache in children and adolescents-a meta-analysis. Cephalalgia 2006;26: 1411–26.

[24] Grazzi L, D'Amico D, Usai S, et al. Disability of young patients suffering from primary headaches. Neurol Sci 2004;25:111–2.

[25] Damen L, Bruijn J, Koes B, et al. Prophylactic treatment of migraine in children. Part 1. A systematic review of non-pharmacological trials. Cephalalgia 2006;26(4):373–83.

[26] Holden E, Deichmann M, Levy J. Empirically supported treatments in pediatric psychology: recurrent pediatric headache. J Pediatr Psychol 1999;24(2):91–109.

[27] Powers SW, Kashikar-Zuck SM, Allen JR, et al. Cognitive behavioral therapy plus amitriptyline for chronic migraine in children and adolescents: a randomized clinical trial. JAMA 2013;310(24):2622–30.

[28] Hayes S, Smith S. Get out of your mind and into your life: the new acceptance and commitment therapy. Oakland (CA): New Barbinger Publications, Inc; 2005.

[29] Wicksell R, Melin L, Lekander M, et al. Evaluating the effectiveness of exposure and acceptance strategies to improve functioning and quality of life in longstanding pediatric pain-a randomized controlled trial. Pain 2009;141(3):248–57.

[30] McCaffery R, Beebe A. Pain, clinical manual for nursing practice. London: Mosby; 1994.

[31] Larsson B, Carlsson J, Fitchel A, et al. Relaxation treatment of adolescent headache sufferers: results from a school based replication study. Headache 2005;45(6):692–704.

[32] Engel J, Rapoff M, Pressman A. Long-term follow-up of relaxation training for pediatric headache disorders. Headache 1992;32:152–6.

[33] Varkey E, Cider A, Carlsson J, et al. Exercise as migraine prophylaxis: a randomized study using relaxation and topiramate as controls. Cephalalgia 2011;31(14):1428–38.

[34] Kohen D, Zajac R. Self-hypnosis training for headaches in children and adolescents. J Pediatr 2007;150:635–9.

[35] Olson RP, Schwartz MS. A historical perspective on the field of biofeedback and applied physiology. In: Schwartz MS, Andrasik F, editors. Biofeedback: a practitioner's guide. 2nd Edition. New York: Guilford Press; 2003. p. 3–19.

[36] Yucha C, Gilbert C. Evidence Based Practice in Biofeedback and Neurofeedback. Colorado Springs (CO): Association for Applied Psychophysiology and Biofeedback; 2004.

[37] Evans S, Zeltzer K. Complementary and alternative approaches for chronic pain. In: Walco GA, Goldschneider KR, editors. Pediatric pain management in primary care: a practical guide. Totowa (NJ): The Humana Press; 2008. p. 153–60.

[38] Blume H, Brockman L, Breuner C. Biofeedback therapy for pediatric headache: factors associated with response. Headache 2012;52(9):1377–86.

[39] Hermann C, Blanchard E, Flor H. Biofeedback treatment for pediatric migraine: prediction of treatment outcome. J Consult Clin Psychol 1997;65(4):611–6.

[40] Scharff L, Marcus D, Masek B. A controlled study of minimal-contact thermal biofeedback treatment in children with migraine. J Pediatr Psychol 2002;27(2):109–19.

[41] Hermann C, Blanchard H. Biofeedback in the treatment of headache and other childhood pain. Appl Psychophysiol Biofeedback 2002;27(2):143–62.

[42] Sarafino EP, Goehring P. Age comparisons in acquiring biofeedback control and success in reducing headache pain. Ann Behav Med 2000;22(1):10–6.

[43] Linde K, Allais G, Brinkhaus B, et al. Acupuncture for tension-type headache. Cochrane Database Syst Rev 2009;(1):CD007587.

[44] Melchart D, Linde K, Fisher P, et al. Acupuncture for recurrent headaches: a systematic review of randomized controlled trials. Cephalalgia 1999;19:89–94.

[45] Pintov S, Lahat E, Alstein M, et al. Acupuncture and the opioid system: implications in management of migraine. Pediatr Neurol 1997;17(2):129–33.

[46] Powers S, Gilman D, Hershey A. Suggestions for a biopsychosocial approach to treating children and adolescents who present with headache. Headache 2006;46(S3):S149–50.

[47] Seshia S, Phillips D, von Baeyer C. Childhood chronic daily headache: a biopsychosocial perspective. Dev Med Child Neurol 2008;50(7):541–5.

Moving?

Make sure your subscription moves with you!

To notify us of your new address, find your **Clinics Account Number** (located on your mailing label above your name), and contact customer service at:

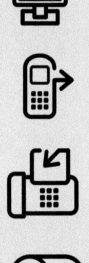

Email: journalscustomerservice-usa@elsevier.com

800-654-2452 (subscribers in the U.S. & Canada)
314-447-8871 (subscribers outside of the U.S. & Canada)

Fax number: 314-447-8029

Elsevier Health Sciences Division
Subscription Customer Service
3251 Riverport Lane
Maryland Heights, MO 63043

*To ensure uninterrupted delivery of your subscription, please notify us at least 4 weeks in advance of move.

ELSEVIER